Anatomy Live

The production of this book was made possible by the support of Het Oranjehotel and the Netherlands Society for Scientific Research (NWO)

Final editing: Fleur Bokhoven and Laura Karreman
Cover: Sacha van den Haak and Floris Schrama
Lay-out: V3-Services, Baarn

ISBN   978 90 5356 516 2
NUR   670

Anatomy Live:

Performance and the Operating Theatre

Edited by Maaike Bleeker

AMSTERDAM UNIVERSITY PRESS

Contents

Acknowledgements

The beginning of my fascination with the anatomical theatre dates back almost ten years when I attended Mike Tyler's performance *Holoman; Digital Cadaver* and a lecture by José van Dijck. I am very happy that both are represented in this book. Four years later, the School for New Dance Development (SNDO, Amsterdam) invited me to teach a theory class about the body. This was the first time I used the title *The Anatomical Theatre Revisited* to frame my explorations into the relationship between the history of anatomy and current issues in theory, philosophy and the performing arts. I would like to thank the SNDO for giving me this opportunity, and my students for their challenging questions and remarks. In 2005, I continued this course at the University of Amsterdam as part of the MA program in Theatre Studies as well as in a PhD seminar. In 2006, they were followed by the international conference *The Anatomical Theatre Revisited* (www.anatomicaltheatrerevisited.com), a joint project by the Department of Theatre Studies of the University of Amsterdam, the Amsterdam School for Cultural Analysis, Waag Society, the School for New Dance Development, the MA program Dance Unlimited and Marijke Hoogenboom's research group Art Practice and Development, the last three all part of the Amsterdam School of the Arts. This book is the outcome of that conference. It contains the plenary lectures presented at *The Anatomical Theatre Revisited* as well as a selection of the other papers, and one text (by Gianna Bouchard) that was not presented at the conference but fortunately could be included in this volume. Added to this is a series of performance documentations informing the reader about performative explorations of the theatre of anatomy.

The Anatomical Theatre Revisited conference and this book were supported by the Netherlands Society for Scientific Research (NWO). Both are part of my NWO-funded Veni research project (provisionally) titled *See Me, Feel Me, Think Me: The Body of Semiotics*.

José van Dijck's 'Digital Cadavers and Virtual Dissection' is part of her book *The Transparent Body. A Cultural Analysis of Medical Imaging* (Washington, Washington University Press, 2005) and is reprinted with kind permission of Washington University Press. I would also like to thank the University of Michigan Press for permission to reprint Francis Barker's 'Men with Glass Bodies' (from his *The Tremulous Private Body: Essays on Subjection*, Ann Arbor, University of Michigan Press, 1995), Toer van Schayk for his permission to reproduce two of his drawings for René Vincent's book *Klassieke Ballettechniek. De techniek en de terminologie van het akademische ballet* (Zutphen, Uitgeverij De Walburg Pers, 1982), Vivienne van Leeuwen for granting us the right to include two of Ger van Leeuwen's photographs, and all the other artists and photographers whose work features on the pages of this book.

I would like to thank the editorial board of the Amsterdam University Press for their trust in this project and Jeroen Sondervan and Christine Waslander for all their help and support.

Last but not least, I want to thank two people who have been indispensable to both the conference and this book: Fleur Bokhoven and Laura Karreman. Their double signature Fleur & Laura was the trademark of the conference. Their care and attention are behind every single word of this book. Without them I would never have been able to complete this manuscript in time, and it would definitely not have been such a pleasure. Therefore, I dedicate this book to them.

Prologue
Men with Glass Bodies

Francis Barker

Dr Nicolaes Tulp, surgeon and representative of the civil authority, anatomist and frequent office holder in the bourgeois government of Amsterdam. But also a general practitioner who, like Freud, left behind his casehistories, the *Observationes*, where the body is made text, and in which one of the patients is constrained to spend a winter in bed suffering from the insight that his bones were made of wax and would buckle if he stood up. The sick man was a painter to whom Tulp refers in a way that suggests it was Rembrandt, the most prolific producer of self-portraits ever, who was obsessed by the story of Samson and Delilah – that narrative of symbolic castration of treachery of women – and whose first important canvas depicted Tulp's magisterial dissection of the executed criminal Aris Kindt. At which event Descartes was probably present; anatomist himself, philosopher and legislator for modern subjectivity, who, mediating by the stove, considering strangely whether his body exists, uses the wax at hand to prove that corporeal objects have no consistency or essentiality but extension in space. And Caspar Barlaeus was almost certainly there at the dissection too, a leading intellectual and noted neurotic, who wrote poetry in praise of Tulp's dissection of Kindt, and dared not sit down for fear that his buttocks, which were made of glass, would shatter.

While in England, their brothers: Hamlet calling on his flesh to melt; Marvell, Member of Parliament, who let aggressivity write in his poem. And Milton and Pepys: each committed in their different ways to inexorable textuality; riven by equivocal desire. A revolutionary poet and censor, who also wrote a Samson, and a secret diarist narrating himself and his world in private. Both eventually blind...

But these are anecdotes and in some respects improbable, or at least not susceptible of proof. Surely not worth serious historical attention. And yet is there not something at once risible and haunting about a poet of the bourgeois class who thought that his body was made of glass (for Descartes, of course, strictly a madness); or salutary in an image of the public dissection of a man who had

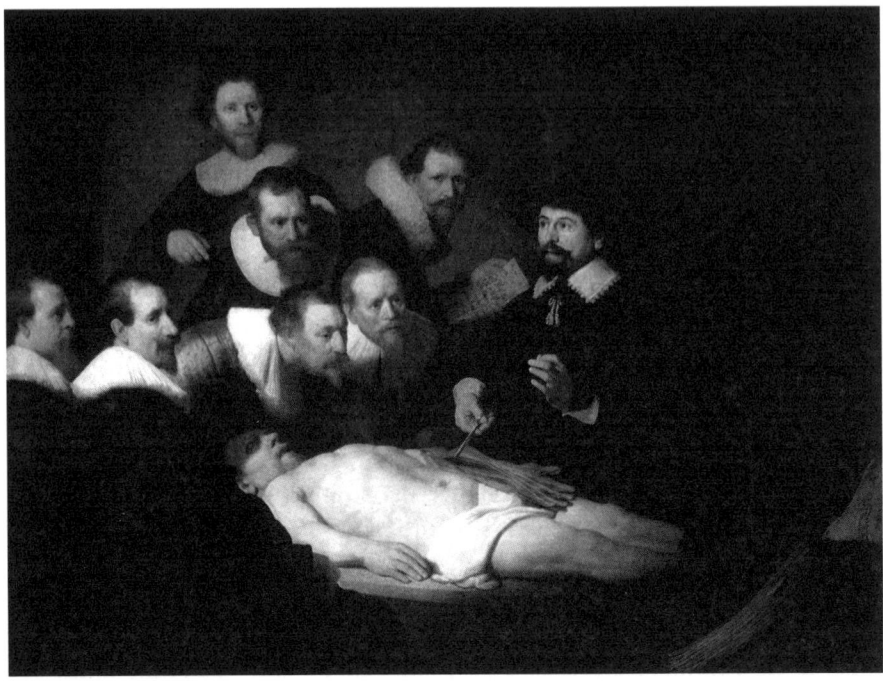

Rembrandt van Rijn, *The Anatomy Lesson of Dr Nicolaes Tulp*, 1632.

no respect for the law? Or revealing in men driven blind by writing? When we consider these conditions in the representatives of an historical order, is there not some reflection to be made on the rationality and freedom in the elaboration of which the period is said to have made important advances?

Then do these fragments not begin to figure the outline of an historical fable, even a structure: at the foundations of our own epoch a conjunction of themes and powers which is still ours to live, and, if enough time remains, undo, today?

(From: Francis Barker, *The Tremulous Private Body: Essays on Subjection*. Ann Arbor, University of Michigan Press, 1995, pp. 103-104.)

Introduction

Maaike Bleeker

In his classic 1947 ethnography of New Caledonia, *Do Kamo: Person and Myth in a Melanesian World*, Maurice Leenhardt reports on a conversation between himself and an elderly indigenous philosopher regarding the impact of European civilization on the cosmocentric world of the Canaques. Leenhardt suggested that the Europeans had introduced the notion of 'spirit' to indigenous thought. His interlocutor did not agree and remarked that on the contrary, they have 'always acted in accord with the spirit.' What the Europeans brought to the Canaques was the notion of body (Csordas in Weiss & Haber, 1999, p. 143). Of course, the Canaques had already been bodies; they existed as bodily beings before and after their 'discovery' by Europeans. However, the character of this existence is what was altered by 'discovery', and it is that alteration that is at stake in the difference of opinion to which Leenhardt's text testifies.

When discussing Leenhardt's observations, Thomas Csordas remarks that, for Leenhardt, the Canaque philosopher's remark is a startling pronouncement. It overturns a stereotypical presumption that the body is allied with nature, and that spirit belongs to the civilized. Quoting Leenhardt, Csordas interprets the philosopher's remark as follows:

> [The body] had no existence of its own, nor specific name to distinguish it. It was only support. But henceforth the circumscription of the physical being is completed, making possible its objectification. The idea of a human body becomes explicit. The discovery leads forthwith to a discrimination between body and the mythic world. (Weiss & Haber, 1999, p. 143)

The Canaques became body through European intervention. It is only with the arrival of European civilization that 'the human body becomes explicit', which involved the objectification of the body. For Csordas, this implies that the very possibility of individuation, or the creation of the individual that we understand as the core of the ideological structure of Western culture, has as its condition of possibility a particular mode of inhabiting the world as a bodily being. This brings Csordas to an elaboration of a methodological distinction between the body as a biological, material entity and embodiment as an indeterminate methodological field 'defined by perceptual experience and by mode of presence and engagement in the world' (Csordas in Weiss & Haber, 1999, p. 145).

But isn't this distinction precisely what is questioned by the Canaque philosopher? It presupposes that 'bringing the body to the Canaques' involved making them aware of something they already were but of which, prior to the arrival of European civilization, they were not aware. This seems to confirm Leenhardt's idea that what the Europeans brought was 'spirit', or the spiritual capacity to conceive of themselves and the world (including their bodies) in new ways. The Canaque philosopher, however, argues that the Europeans brought 'body', not spirit. In equating body with matter and nature, and opposing body (defined as involving perceptual experience and engagement in the world) to embodiment, what is overlooked is the cultural character of the material and biological body; how this biological body 'matters' according to culturally specific parameters. And how the concept of the body as matter distinguished from spirit is an invention of European civilization, an invention they brought to the Canaques.[1]

In his seminal *The Body Emblazoned: Dissection and the Human Body in Renaissance Culture* (1995), Jonathan Sawday argues that it is the invention of the anatomical body, understood as the material basis of our existence, that provokes, as a psychical consequence of this body, the coming into being of modern subjectivity. The anatomization of the body in early modernity was part and parcel of the development of Cartesian subjectivity as the powerful spirit or 'ghost' in the machine. Sawday describes how this was accompanied, in fact made possible, by the deployment of a new language with which to describe the body's interior. Nowadays, this language is primarily associated with the post-Cartesian formulation of the body as a machine. But, Sawday observes:

> [t]o the natural philosophers of the earlier seventeenth century, it was not a mechanistic structure that they first encountered as they embarked upon the project of unraveling the body's recesses. Rather, they found themselves wandering within a geographical entity. The body was territory, an (yet) undiscovered country, a location which demanded from its explorers skills which seemed analogous to those displayed by the heroic voyagers across the terrestrial globe. (Sawday, 1995, p. 23)

During this first phase of the development of the modern understanding of the body, anatomists, like Columbian explorers, 'dotted their names, like place names on a map, over the terrain which they encountered.' Sawday explains:

> In their voyages, they expressed the intersection of the body and the world at every point, claiming for the body an affinity with the complex design of the universe. This congruence equated scientific endeavour with the triumphant discoveries of the explorers, cartographers, navigators and early colonialists. And in the production of a new map of the body, a new figure was also to be glimpsed – the scientist as the heroic voyager and intrepid discoverer. The body was a remote and strange terrain into which the discoverer voyaged. (Sawday, 1995, pp. 23-24)

When the body was opened, it was alien territory into which the scientist journeyed. This sense of the body as alien to the sensibility that inhabited it, provided the material for the construction of the natural philosopher as the heroic explorer, the civilizing force within the boundaries of the natural body. His task was to voyage within the body to reveal its secrets. Once discovered, the body-landscape could be harnessed to the service of its owner. This process, according to Sawday, was part of a larger process of 'dominion over nature' and was truly colonial, in that it reproduced the stages of discovery and exploitation simultaneously taking place within the context of the European encounter with the New World.

> Like property, the body's bounds needed to be fixed, its dimensions properly measured, its resources charted. Its 'new' owner – which would eventually become the thinking process of the Cartesian *cogito* – had to know what it was that was owned before use could be made of it. (Sawday, 1995, p. 26)

Sawday thus explains how the process of colonization within the body's interior paved the way for the Cartesian machine body. He also shows that this involved much more than discovering and giving names to what was already there. In this process of colonization, the body and the world are actually produced as the savage, and the natural other of the mind, and of civilization. They are thus what precedes and is merely discovered. This invention is further perfected in the Cartesian image of the body as a machine operating according to the laws of mechanics. As a machine, the body became objectified and fully divided from the Cartesian subject. The result is paradoxical, to say the least. The division between the 'I' that thinks and the 'it' or body in which 'we' reside, turns the relationship between them into a question.

Sawday illuminates the intimate connection between the body of anatomy, the philosophical discourse of Western modernity, and a subject which, as Francis Barker (1995) puts it, 'is skeptical of its body and guilty of its sexuality; which is committed to writing and to the domination of the object world; but one which is forever constrained to its own self-alienation and is conscious, in the end, of so very little' (Barker, 1995, p. vi). Like Barker, Sawday locates the emergence of this constellation, this 'historical fable' (Barker), in the anatomy theatres of the early Renaissance.

In the early modern period, a 'science' of the body had not yet emerged. Instead what was to become science – a seemingly discrete way of ordering the observation of the natural world – was at this stage no more than one method amongst many by which human knowledge was organized. Dissection, Sawday argues, played a crucial role in reorganizing the cultural 'map' of knowledge, and to understand its role involves acknowledging the two-sided nature of dissection. On the one hand, dissection is 'an insistence on the partition of something (or someone) which (or who) hitherto possessed their own unique organic integrity' (Sawday, 1995, p. 3). This aspect of dissection can be seen reflected in the ways in which the 'scientific revolution' of the Renaissance encouraged seemingly endless partitioning of the world and all that it contained. The pattern of all these different forms of division was derived from the human body. Therefore, Sawday argues, the body must lie at the very centre of our inquiry into what might be called the other side of this process of partitioning, which is how the world, including the body, is constructed, or given a concrete presence through dissection (Sawday, 1995, p. 3). The divisionary procedures of dissection are the other side of the unified sense of selfhood typical of the construction of modern individuality.

The popularity of anatomy, according to Sawday, cannot be understood solely from raising the ban on the formerly forbidden practice of dissection, nor simply as a result of the superior quality of the knowledge thus produced. Rather, the anatomical body is part and parcel of the development of modern individualism, and of the modern scientific world view. Dissection turns the body into a mute corporeal object, separated from and opposed to the Cartesian disembodied I/eye as the site of subjectivity, thought and knowledge. Additionally, the 'culture of dissection' (Sawday) marks the beginnings of what Michel Foucault has analyzed as the 'surveillance' of the body within regimes of judgment and punishment, as well as an early crystallization of the modern Western sense of interiority. The public dissections in the historical anatomy theatre mark the emergence of this constellation of ideas and practices underlying what became the dominant conception of the body, including prevailing notions of how the body can be known, and what it means to know. This inaugural moment was highly theatrical in character, and occurred in a theatrical space.

During the centuries that followed, this theatrical character disappeared from view, as theatre and theory drifted apart. New developments onstage, in contemporary theory as well as in philosophy, suggest the productivity of bringing theatre and theory back into the same room in order to explore alternative conceptions emerging at the intersection of artistic practices and philosophical, theoretical and scientific ideas. Many artists use (or have used) performance, theatricality, staging, or re-enactment as means to challenge conceptions of the body as a mere object. They argue for a new understanding of the body as an agent actively involved in world-making and in the production of thought and knowledge. Sometimes, their work presents an explicit critique of the history of the anatomical body. In other cases the implications of their work can be read as an implicit commentary on the constellation of ideas and practices concerning bodies, thought and knowledge, neatly summarized in Sawday's notion of the 'culture of dissection'. This volume contains documentation on such artistic projects by Mike Tyler, Sasha Waltz, Ivana Müller, Glen Tetley, Marijs Boulogne, Eric Joris/CREW, Emil Hrvatin, Stefan Kunzmann, Isabelle Jenniches, and Renée Copraij. These performance documentations are presented alongside a series of theoretical reflections addressing the relationships between anatomy, theatre and the culture of dissection from a theoretical point of view.

In the historical anatomy theatre, the body is not only demonstrated but also performed. Anatomy involves cutting into bodies, studying their interiors, and making visualizations of what is inside. Yes, but anatomy does more. Anatomy performs constative acts that produce knowledge by means of a public demonstration of 'how it is' with the body. This demonstration is what Mieke Bal (1996) has termed a 'gesture of exposing' that involves the authority of a person who knows (epistemic authority), who points to bodies and seemingly says 'Look, that is how it is'. These constative acts are constructed according to a logic that finds its theatrical expression in the *mise en scène* of the historical anatomy theatre, as well as in the composition of the painted anatomy lessons by Rembrandt van Rijn, among others.

Analogous to speech acts, these constative acts of producing the body 'as it is' can be analyzed in terms of three different positions, or persons, involved. The first person speaking is the anatomist, demonstrating the body to an audience. The audience takes the position of the second person, the one addressed. The body demonstrated to this audience is the third person, the one who is talked about, but not speaking him- or herself. This third person is dead, a mute object there to prove the authority of the anatomist.

As Bal points out, the success or failure of expository activity is not a measure of what one person 'wants to say' but of what a community and its subjects think, feel or experience to be the consequences of the exposition (Bal, 1996, p. 8). In order to understand the implications of the ways in which bodies matter in and through the cultural performances that produce them, it is necessary to consider how the body is discursively installed as ontological. José van Dijck ('Digital Cadavers and Virtual Dissection') demonstrates how, at this point, the explicit theatrical character of the historical anatomy theatre allows for a perspective on late twentieth-century visualizations of the anatomical body in the *Visible Human Project*. Van Dijck elucidates how current practices of compiling and disseminating digital body data reflect and construct persistent cultural norms involving age, gender, spectacle, identity, transparency and crime and punishment, cultural norms that can be traced back to the public dissections in the Renaissance anatomy theatres.

Ian Maxwell ("'Who Were You?': The Visible and the Visceral') further elaborates one particular aspect of the relationship between the public dissections in the historical anatomy theatres and contemporary practices, namely the complex intertwining of science, education and entertainment. Following Jane Goodall (2002), he argues that the performances in the historical anatomy theatre were a forum in which scientific debates of the day were played out both in the imaginations and visceral responses of popular audiences. With respect to these historical performances, Maxwell observes a tension between ideas about visibility (through which human bodies yield knowledge in an aestheticized, putatively democratized display) and an idea about alternative, perhaps coexisting, if challenging, knowledge derived from more tangible, performative, and embodied graspings of those same bodies. This brings him to a critical evaluation of the relationship between public dissections in the historical anatomy theatre and Gunther von Hagens's present-day re-enactments of such demonstrations in his television series *Anatomy for Beginners*.

Von Hagens explicitly inscribes his project in the history of the Renaissance anatomy theatres. Not only does his performance in *Anatomy for Beginners* recall the public anatomy lessons of the Renaissance, in 2002 Von Hagens staged the first public autopsy in 170 years. The autopsy was performed in a former brewery in London, under a copy of Rembrandt's *The Anatomy Lesson of Dr Nicolaes Tulp*. In Von Hagens's exhibition *Body Worlds*, plastinated human bodies are staged next to enlarged images from Renaissance anatomical atlases. Several of the figures are in poses that correspond to the bodies depicted in these images. In a promotional video accompanying his exhibition, Von Hagens argues that the historical anatomists of the late Middle Ages and early Renaissance knew the power of aesthetics to reach and teach their audiences. Not only did they perform their work in the often elaborately decorated setting of anatomy theatres, they also worked with artists to produce representations of their anatomy lessons as well as images and atlases in which the anatomical understanding of the human body was demonstrated. In the course of time, however, the connection between art and science got lost as representations of the human body in anatomy and medicine became more and more 'objective'. As a result, Von Hagens argues, people are no longer able to relate these images to their personal experience. With *Body Worlds*, Von Hagens promotes a return to the early stages of anatomy, and an undoing of this alienation through 'Anatomy that is Alive.'

Von Hagens certainly knows how to reach his audience. His exhibitions draw huge crowds of visitors all over the world. His work also raises many questions, for example concerning the ethical implications of using human body material. Other issues include the normative character of what his exhibition presents as 'the human body' and the ways in which his method of preserving and staging the body obscures differences and erases prominent features of embodied presence like fat, skin, fluids and hair. The result is a sterile athletic body of unspecified race and without traces of personal history except from injuries and medical procedures like artificial knees, moments that testify to the marvels of medical technology, capable of competition with Creation.

In the promotional video and in related texts, Von Hagens argues that he is not universalizing, but rather that his way of showing human figures makes visible the individuality of each person beneath the skin.[2] No body is similar. Yet, his project erases the connection with the histories that might have made (and once did make) these differences meaningful. Von Hagens's project stages difference as variations on a universal standard, thus confirming the status of the body of anatomy as a universal and an ahistorical given. Made to look like the historical images exhibited next to them, these plastinated bodies serve as proof of the knowledge and understanding handed down to us by historical tradition, a tradition in which it is the dead body that is used to teach us about living ones. So much for anatomy that is alive.

Karen Ingham ('The Anatomy Lesson of Professor Moxham') also points to the ways in which the historical anatomy theatre, far from being a relic of the past, is flourishing under new surgical and digital façades. She too argues for the importance of renewed collaboration between artists and scientists. Unlike Von Hagens, however, she demonstrates how such collaboration may actually serve to revitalize the allegorical potential of what she terms anatomo-art. The architecture and metaphysics of the anatomy theatre influenced and continue to influence the way the anatomo-clinical body is located within hierarchies of power and surveillance. These hierarchies are the subject of artworks which turn the anatomy lesson into lessons that provoke, stimulate and question the very notion of what it is to be human. Such critical gestures undermine the claim to truth by the constative gesture of which the historical anatomy theatre presents a spatial metaphor, precisely by exposing the construction of this gesture.

This complicated relationship between the theatre of anatomy and the truth claim performed by it is also the subject of Gianna Bouchard's '"Be not faithless but believing": Illusion and Doubt in the Anatomy Theatre.' The corpse dissected within the theatre of anatomy, she argues, is fundamentally a pedagogical prop, utilized by medical science to educate and elucidate through elaboration and proof. In the anatomy theatre, this proof is provided by means of acts of persuasion and demonstration that are staged to deliver truth but are nevertheless embedded within structures of illusion. Bouchard engages with the construction of such acts of persuasion through a reading of, on the one hand, Caravaggio's painting *The Incredulity of Saint Thomas* (1603) and, on the other, Romeo Castellucci's version of Shakespeare's *Julius Caesar* (2001). In both, bodies are definable as props in the sense that they may be read as theatrical objects with material presence in the moment of performance or display. In both, the body is acted upon and interrogated in a way that subverts and destabilizes the realism of anatomical science as a non-illusionary field of knowledge, instead animating more doubt.

Anja Klöck ('Of Dissection and Technologies of Culture in Actor Training Programs – an Example from 1960s West Germany') also engages with the relation between theatrical staging, the truth claim performed within and by this staging, and Renaissance practices of producing truthful representations of the human body. She demonstrates how residual fractures of the 'culture of dissection' have played out on the bodies of actors and actresses since then. Focusing especially on actor training programs in 1960s Germany, she shows how the actor's body becomes the site wherein the border between the externally perceivable social order and the internally concealed and possibly unordered aspects of being is explored and negotiated.

The relationship between truth, spectatorship, and the theatre is also the subject of Pannill Camp's 'Ocular Anatomy, Chiasm and Theatre Architecture as a Material Phenomenology in Early Modern Europe'. Whereas Bouchard and Klöck focus on the ways in which bodies are staged in order to deliver proof of the truth, Camp draws attention to the theatrical architecture constitutive of such proof. He observes remarkable structural similarities between the structure of modes of thought typical of Husserlian phenomenology and certain spatial attributes of theatre architecture in the Renaissance and Modern eras. He traces the relationship between this phenomenological mode of thought and a series of early modern theatre buildings that manifest clear isomorphic resonances with the human eye. Within this logic, the stage appears as a continuity that divides. This technology enables us to encounter the present, but in such a way as to separate it from ourselves.

With his analysis, Camp directs attention to the other bodies involved in the production of (anatomical) knowledge and demonstrates how the need to account for the role of these bodies in observing and recognizing phenomenological truths resulted in the incorporation of a theatrical model in which seeing is equated with knowing. My own contribution ('Martin, Massumi, and The Matrix') also engages with this relationship between the architecture of the theatre and modes of thinking, approaching this relationship from the question of movement. The theatrical architecture of Husserlian phenomenology involves a bracketing of movement, reducing transformation and change to successions of static moments. The practice of bracketing stages a stable relationship between an objective world and a stable point of view, a position from which the world can be defined by means of pinning isolated phenomena down on the grid of culturally constructed significations. This is what Massumi terms the problem of positionality. Positionality involves a denial of movement/sensation as constitutive of the way in which the world appears to us as an object of cognitive perception. These perceptual-cognitive practices are the subject of my text, and I approach them through, on the one hand, John Martin's *Introduction to the Dance* (1939) and on the other Neo's introduction to Kung Fu in *The Matrix*, both examples read through Massumi's distinction between mirror vision and movement vision.

Susan Foster in her '"Where Are You Now?": Locating the Body in Contemporary Performance' further historicizes the relationship between the static architecture of theatre and ways of knowing the world. She points out that the reorganization of the cultural map of knowledge in the early modern period not only involves profound transformations in how the world is known but also manifests itself in decisive changes in the practice of mapping. These changes coincide with a new kinaesthetic awareness of one's positionality in the world. Whereas earlier techniques had required either the reader or the map to move continually, new cartographic techniques, such as Mercator's implementation of a horizontal and a vertical grid to contain and locate the world's land masses, privileged the single and stationary subject. Foster compares the ways that bodies discerned their locatedness in the world prior to the establishment of the anatomical subject with current trends in mapping and orienting by means of the Global Positioning System and the mobile phone. She traces the implications of these developments for contemporary performance practices through a reading of Rimini Protokoll's *Call Cutta* (2004).

Sally Jane Norman ('Anatomies of Live Art') continues this exploration of the relationship between turn-of-the-century information and communication technologies, new conceptions of the body, and corresponding theatre architectures. She observes that our constant invention of machines and interactive processes to multiply and extend bodily relations to the world can be read in parallel transformations of theatre architectures that turn the theatre into a place for staging the peculiar cut-ups or splicings of space, time, persona, and more or less embodied presence afforded by networks. Technologies linking previously isolated moments and places alter our sense of presence and embodiment essential to the live art of the theatre and allow for hybrid relations between human and electromechanical and informational resources. The theatre offers ideal ground for exploring fringe zones between the natural and the artificial, between living and inanimate phenomena, and between humans and other autonomous evolving creatures.

Architectures that have marked theatre history since the Renaissance reflect the anatomy of the body politic that they convene and contain. This body politic and its ethical implications are the subject of the three remaining contributions to this volume. In 'Restaging the Monstrous', Bojana Kunst points out how the 'culture of dissection' has been instrumental in turning the monstrous – as that which does not fit within scientific, social or political categories – into a kind of quasi-object, a perversion of the natural order of things, as well as a perversion of authority. From having been an object of scientific attention, the monstrous (pretending to be something it is not and with its excessive presence disturbing the given order of things) now becomes a player on the political stage. Kunst traces the consequences of this change in the status of the monstrous, and connects those consequences to the present situation. Today, the divisions between life and death, human and non-human, are created by expelling the human out of the human body, leaving that inert life to the mercy of the contemporary flaws of political and corporative ownership. The question is how, within this situation, theatre might contribute to disclosing the generative potentiality of the monstrous while still avoiding becoming an empty spectacle.

Michal Kobialka ('Delirium of the Flesh: "All the Dead Voices" in the Space of the Now') argues this potential of the theatre is to be found in the ways in which it can create a space (literally and metaphorically) in which categories and concepts are wrested from the use-value and invoke what Lyotard calls 'the unrepresentable in presentation itself'. Kobialka cites how the Renaissance 'culture of dissection' divided the bodies (or their parts) into those that mattered or did not matter, turning those that did matter into complete and rational objects delimited by particular political and social coding, corporeal investigations and ideological structures. This process is taken further in the work of many theorists and philosophers, reducing the body to the ways in which it is inscribed by social meaning, and assigned psychical or indexical significance. Making bodies visible or readable is to gloss over that moment when something happens which cannot be fully folded into the known. What happens when the very materiality, the fidgety 'liveness' of the flesh, or the lack thereof, disrupts this coding? Such moments perturb the order of things in the space of the now.

Rachel Fensham, in 'Operating Theatres: Body-bits and a Post-apartheid Aesthetics', observes a close connection between the history of modern states (and their body politics) and a specular regime based on dissection. She suggests that political theatre in this globalized and postcolonial phase of modernity has to be one of body parts, not seen as intensely physical totalities, but rather as bits that provide evidence of our current non-human history. The unintelligibility of these organs without bodies (Žižek) needs a theatre that sutures the bits together again. She finds such theatre in a staging of Monteverdi's 1640 opera *Il Ritorno d'Ulisse* by the Handspring Puppet Company, in association with visual artist William Kentridge. This puppet-opera is set in a scale replica of Vesalius's anatomy theatre, complete with mortuary table and raked seating. In this theatre, Ulysses's journey is represented as a kind of postoperative delirium endured by the modern, white subject.

Organs without bodies, the delirium of the flesh perturbing the order of things in the space of the now, Ulysses returning to Vesalius's anatomy theatre, hybrid relations between human and electromechanical and informational resources, anatomo-art and new kinaesthetic awareness: do these fragments begin to conjure the outline of a new conjunction of themes and powers, a transformation of the historical fable at the foundation of our epoch, a transformation that may be ours to live?

Notes

1   See for a further elaboration of this example my 'Of Passing and Other Cures: Arjan Ederveen's Born in the Wrong Body and the Cultural Construction of Essentialism'. In: Murat Aydemir (ed.), *Indiscretions: At the Intersection of Postcolonial and Queer Theory*. Amsterdam, 2008.
2   See for example the promotional video *Anatomy Art. Fascination Beneath the Surface. A Tour Through the Exhibition*, and Gunther von Hagens and Angelina Whalley, *Prof. Gunther von Hagens' Anatomy Art: Fascination Beneath The Surface. Catalogue on the Exhibition*. Heidelberg, 2000.

References

Anatomy Art. Fascination Beneath the Surface. A Tour Through the Exhibition. Institute for Plastination, Heidelberg, 1999.

Bal, M., *Double Exposures. The Subject of Cultural Analysis*. New York and London, 1996.

Barker, F., *The Tremulous Private Body: Essays on Subjection*. Ann Arbor, 1995.

Goodall, J. R., *Performance and Evolution in the Age of Darwin: Out of the Natural Order*. London and New York, 2002.

Hagens, G. von and A. Whalley, *Prof. Gunther von Hagens' Anatomy Art: Fascination Beneath The Surface. Catalogue on the Exhibition*. Heidelberg, 2000.

Sawday, J., *The Body Emblazoned: Dissection and the Human Body in Renaissance Culture*. New York and London, 1995.

Weiss, G. and H. F. Haber, *Perspectives on Embodiment. The Intersections of Nature and Culture*. New York and London, 1999.

Performance Documentation 1:
Holoman; Digital Cadaver

Mike Tyler's *Holoman; Digital Cadaver* began as a collection of songs about a fictional character named J.P. Holoman whose life and death parallel that of real-life murderer J.P. Jernigan. Jernigan received the death penalty in Texas in 1993, but not before donating his body to science. After undergoing MRI scanning and computer tomography (CT), Jernigan's frozen body was sliced into thousands of paper-thin sections and photographed. When digitally reassembled, he became the 'universal human meat': his digitalization resulted in a bloodless, dissectible cadaver for anatomy students and, perhaps, the first immortal man.

In *Holoman; Digital Cadaver*, the digital images of Jernigan's interior are confronted with the living body of actor Frank Sheppard. Sheppard 'embodies' the convicted criminal whose body was used to produce the digital images. Tyler's lyrics suggest that Jernigan's mind has also survived the ordeal. It speaks to us as disembodied psyche, trapped within the computer, reduced to digital information to be accessed by anyone anytime.

(Mike Tyler to audience)
    Remember when human dissections were outlawed by the Church?
    If the authorities showed up during the operation, the corpse could be
    lowered through a trap door at a moment's notice, gone no more,
    and in his place a goose or a boar.

    Many sleeves were rolled,
    much skin was peeled and bones were sawed,
    stomachs turned.
    Others gaped in awe at the dark innards turned to face the light
    (like a shovel's blade in the dark earth turns up the wondrous hidden
    roots).

A man cut from the gallows and still in his boots would be the
universal human meat. And it was quickly shown that the hearts
of wicked men were not smaller than their own: those who would
pride themselves healers and defy God's will that all life should
return to dust.

(to Holoman)   Lie still!
    Now the rigid stiff in the CAT scanner turns
    Rigor mortis network burns
    The new digital cadaver is frozen and sliced...
    It's time for the Anatomical Theater to begin!

(Holoman, voice on tape)
    Consciousness is a subtler form of material
    and death is the sister of sleep (I know I met her).
    (...)
    Death is the skinny sister of sleep
    and this dreamer knows he's dreaming (in her bed).

    When a hologram is broken
    each piece becomes a smaller version of the original,
    each fragment contains the whole, it seems.

    I was carried away on a data stream, put back together,
    pixel by polygon,
    yes many times gone.

(Holoman, live)
    Holoman, Hollow-man
    Digified stiff on the fly.
    I ask you why was I picked for the hard disk?
    To be crunched like a silicon snack chip:
    A convenient cadaver for the queasy.
    Click on the mouse (you can cut me that easy).
    You're talking to the number 1, the culprit. O.K. I am guilty.
    Yeah, my first crime was being born dirt.

    When the magnets spun round my corpse I left the body
    or awoke (?)
    from the needle poke
    beam me up Scotty no joke

I'm a phantom.
No rest for the restless, just patterns vibrating.

I am a traveler.
No computer will ever be my home!
Every organism was just a machine to me.
Now I've become a spook
comin with the program,
a fluke.
Got eternal life in the jesusbytes.
So behold. The last cowboy!
Whipping a ghost horse with the reins.
Para-magnetic suntan, isotope whiskey in my veins.
I'm the last cowboy.

(Mike Tyler to Holoman)
Think it over Mr. Holoman ... You wanna be another John Doe?

(Holoman)
Computerized Tomography?

(Mike Tyler to Holoman)
It's like skin mapping. Think of yerself as a landscape and we're like archeologists crawled down to your mouth to look for bones.

(Holoman)
MRI?

(Mike Tyler to Holoman)
Ahhh, Magic Ressurrection Instrument... No, just kidding, MRI stands for: Magnetic Resonance Imaging. It's a way of turning you inside out.
Eternal life just sign here.

(Holoman)
I'm patented?

(Mile Tyler to Holoman)
You're more than that. Why you gotta trademark: 'the Visible Man'
TM
All rights reserved.

(Father's voice)

'Hey you selfish swine, do something kind for humankind, something good this time'

(Mike Tyler to Holoman)

You'll be applied to scores of educational, diagnostic, mathematical, industrial and artistic uses!

(Holoman)

Watta you mean by 'artistic uses'?

(Mike Tyler to Holoman)

(pleading) It's about science, man! Hard science!

(Mother's voice)

'Good can come out of bad sometimes, even you, Joseph'

(Holoman)

Is that you, ma?

(Mike Tyler to Holoman)

Think about it... Joe Paul Holoman, professional data set, like that?
Has got a ring to it, doesn't it?
O.K. Yeah. Yer what's known as public domain.

(Holoman)

Public Domain?

(Mike Tyler as Holoman)

That means everyone can use you free of charge.

(aside to audience)

We'll hyperlink the hell outta ya.
The J.P. Holoman interactive freestyle kick boxing buddy state of the art crash test dummies
(oh, I mean, passenger injury model)
Virtual porn stud Joe Paul! Guys with dick mounted displays 'll be wishing they were you, getting into those little cyber-honies!

(Holoman)

I don't know…

(Mike Tyler to Holoman)

Where are you going anyway… to some murderers' plot rotten with death? You know where you're gonna go? Everywhere.

(Holoman)

I'll be top man on D-Row!

I'm Holoman, I'm Hollowman,
my volume been rendered, I'm off-centered.
My flesh been erased, but I'm standing.
Got my face in the database
and as another day breaks somewhere, somebodies getting into my megabytes.

(Holoman to Mike Tyler)

Do you remember those visible guys in the encyclopedia?
Those overlapped, clear plastic guys where you could look at their guts and skeletons and brains and stuff?

I'm Holoman, I was trapped in a hologram beam.
My soul crashed (on the principle of uncertainty).
Got a job working as a mechanic after I was thrown out of the service.
Give you some advice: It's for suckers.

(Mike Tyler)

The ghost who's your host! Master of this ceremony: Mr MC Ghost!

(Holoman)

I'm the ghost who's yer host,
MC Ghost. Master of this ceremony.
Naked love coming at you from a dead heart on this ellipse, this creaky wood.
I stand here alive as any man

I'm a candle, white wax filled with light,
stiff, waxy and white … look at me!

Only the dead know this, but shadows also cast shadows!
That's me. I'm a shadow's shadow thrown on the wall of some kinda 25-dimensional cave. I suck light like lesser monsters suck blood.

(Mike Tyler to Holoman)
  Got any close relatives?

(Holoman)
  Relativity is my next of kin!
  Can't imagine where Holoman's been.

Between 1994 and 2004, **Mike Tyler** had an artist's practice that encompassed works of installation, sculpture, garden/cemetery design, photography and video, with the occasional foray into songwriting, performance and theatrical productions, of which *Holoman; Digital Cadaver* is an example. He participated in solo and group exhibitions at the Stedelijk Museum, Amsterdam; Kunsthalle, Bern; Instituto Tomie Ohtake, Sao Paulo; Location One, NYC; and the 49th Venice Bienalle, among others, and taught at the Design Institute, Eindhoven; Piet Zwart Institute, Rotterdam; and Goldsmith's College in London. He now lives in California and is working on his first feature film production, *The Moving*.

Performance Data

With Frank Sheppard as Holoman
Mike Tyler (concept, director, lyrics, drums, voice)
Isabelle Jenniches (animations, video)
Meindert Meindertsma (guitars)
Peter Kuitwaard (percussion)
Frank van der Ven (choreography)
First version: Festival a/d Werf, Utrecht, May 1997; second version: De Balie, Amsterdam, May 1998.

More on *Holoman; Digital Cadaver*: http://www.9nerds.com/isabelle/HOLO-MAN/index.html and Maaike Bleeker, 'Death, Digitalization and Dys-appearance. Staging the Body of Science'. In: *Performance Research* 4 (2) Summer 1999, pp. 1-7.

Digital Cadavers and Virtual Dissection

José van Dijck

Anatomical dissection is considered an essential ingredient of medical training. By looking at and cutting into dead bodies, future doctors learn to distinguish between healthy and diseased tissue in living bodies, while also gaining an understanding of the three-dimensional shape of organs, veins, and bones. Anatomical dissection literally means to separate the body into pieces; this systematic disassembling of the physical body is justified because it results in an entirely new body – a body of knowledge.[1] More generally, the confrontation with human cadavers functions as an important initiation rite for medical students: not until they have familiarized themselves with the face of death can they embark on a long educational journey that ends with a solemn dedication to life – the Hippocratic oath. Anatomy, from the outset, has been surrounded by sacral and secular symbolism; to this very day, the medical specialty has a morbid public image, associated as it is with the smell of decay and the aura of death.

Cadaver dissection does not provide the only occasion for students to become acquainted with human organic architecture. Anatomical illustrations help them conceptualize the form and structure of various organs before they actually touch them. Without these two-dimensional representations, a thorough understanding of the body's physiology would be inconceivable. Ever since the fifteenth century, knowledge derived from close observation of cut-up cadavers has been recorded in drawings and anatomical atlases.[2] To convey their empirical findings, anatomists depended on the precision and craft of their illustrators. Accordingly, anatomical illustration is commonly viewed as mediated knowledge. Even the most sophisticated anatomical drawings, like those by Leonardo da Vinci and Andreas Vesalius, were considered a derived form of knowledge – idealized representations of real bodies.

From the early days of anatomy, then, anatomical training has relied on a combination of learning to dissect bodies and learning to read anatomical illustrations. But this basis has become too limited, argue the initiators of the *Visible*

Human Project (VHP), who in the 1990s developed a new instruction tool that will purportedly revolutionize anatomy (Ackerman, 1999, pp. 667-70). Funded by the American Congress and the National Science Foundation, the Center for Human Simulation (CHS) at the University of Colorado, Boulder, created the first digital database of a complete human cadaver.[3] The production of a complete virtual body involves a range of complicated, state-of-the-art techniques. First, the body needs to be digitized by means of magnetic resonance imaging and computed tomography. Then the cadaver is immersed in a special fluid and deep frozen to minus seventy degrees Celsius. Next, lab workers use a precision planing device, a cryogenic macrotome, to shave off millimetre-thin slices of the body. After each slice, the cross-sected profile is photographed digitally and scanned into a computer. The resulting data set constitutes the basis for an unlimited series of three-dimensional simulations. In 1995, the digital body of the Visible Male became available for public use, followed one year later by the even more detailed data set of the Visible Female. Both data sets are accessible through the National Library of Medicine's Internet site.[4]

The VHP has presented the digitized Visible Human as a revolution in anatomy. According to its director Michael Ackerman, the creation of digital cadavers signals a radical break with traditional anatomical education.[5] However, I will argue that virtual dissection and digital cadavers constitute a distinct continuation of age-old anatomical practices. The VHP is firmly rooted in historical conceptions of the body and its representation, of crime and punishment, and of physiology and art. Rather than suggesting a break with educational traditions, the VHP reflects a renaissance of public anatomy lessons. In order to develop this argument, we have to return to early sixteenth-century Europe, where the first public anatomy lessons took place and where, slightly later on, in cities like Padua, Bologna, Amsterdam and London, special anatomical theatres were built to accommodate the large crowds these lessons attracted. In those days, public dissections not only served educational purposes, but they were also linked up with the criminal justice system, and they taught moral lessons. In this way, the early anatomical theatre incorporated three institutional settings: it clearly functioned as a school or educational site, it was firmly embedded in a legal context, and it formed a locus for entertainment or public spectacle. A close consideration of these three settings will bare the VHP's cultural roots; it will reveal how this digital American project, that in many ways seems so characteristic of our postmodern day and age, directly hooks up with European Renaissance tradition.

The Anatomical Theatre as a School

The first and foremost goal of the *Visible Human Project* is educational: it should help medical students to become better doctors. Digital anatomy, VHP director Michael Ackerman posits, has considerable advantages over both conventional dissection and anatomical illustration (Ackerman, 1999, p. 668). The Visible Human, he claims, offers a standard model for twenty-first-century anatomy, enabling students to obtain valuable clinical training without the need for pre-pared cadavers. Real cadavers are expensive, perishable, and commonly tainted by diseases. Moreover, cutting into dead bodies remains an uncomfortable ex-perience for students, many of whom are bothered by feelings of uneasiness when confronted with corpses. Anatomical illustrations, for their part, reduce anatomical structures to two-dimensional flat surfaces and are therefore insuf-ficient as teaching tools. The Visible Human purportedly emulates paper repre-sentations because digitization allows viewers a three-dimensional perspective on body parts and organs. Before qualifying these claims, I need to elaborate on the role of anatomical dissection in the history of medical education.

Cadaver dissection as part of the medical curriculum dates back to the fif-teenth century, but Katherine Park firmly rejects the myth that cutting into dead bodies rarely happened before that time (Park, 1994). In Italy, for in-stance, dissections are recorded as early as 1286. Autopsies formed a regular part of medical practice in order to detect unknown causes of death, and post-mortems are known to have taken place in the early fourteenth century at the University of Bologna's medical school. Dissection was sometimes warranted by suspicions of sainthood: a recently deceased person's body was cut open in the hope of finding physical signs and symbols of sacredness.[6] The educational value of postmortems and autopsies, as Park contends, was still rather limited. University professors taught their students the principles of human anatomy by dissecting cadavers, yet: 'Their goal was not to add to the existing body of knowledge concerning human anatomy and physiology but to help students and doctors understand and remember the texts in which that knowledge was enclosed' (Park, 1994, p. 14). As we can tell from fourteenth-century depic-tions of anatomical lessons, the transmission of knowledge was hierarchically structured.[7] Galen's theory of the body – accepted since the fourth century as the only valid theory of physiology – had the highest authority, and it was explicated ex cathedra by a professor or lector. A so-called 'ostensor' pointed a stick at the organs in the laid-open body on the table. The actual dissection was left to relatively unimportant menials, so-called 'dissectors' or 'butchers', who were considerably lower in status than the lector or ostensor, because the demonstration of dissected body parts played a minor, purely ornamental role.

In the early sixteenth century, anatomical dissection changed from a private educational practice into a public lesson. The Flemish anatomist Andreas Vesalius was one of the first to dissect cadavers in public; more importantly, he upset the assumed hierarchy between anatomical theory and manual anatomical skill.[8] He dismissed the dominant system of classification and relied, instead, on empirical evidence to disprove Galen's theocentric theory.[9] Vesalius's view and practice not only meant an unscrupulous sacrilege of Galen, but also implied an outright condemnation of Galen's followers and their uncritical acceptance of his theories – that is, without empirically verifying them. Vesalius simultaneously performed the acts of dissection and explication, undermining the authority of the text by prioritizing the tactile dimensions of the body (Carlino, 1999, pp. 206-207). By the time the British anatomist William Harvey established his famous school, around 1650, it was common practice for anatomists to handle instruction and dissection in tandem.[10] Hands-on contact with the cadaver was the exclusive privilege of the anatomist. During public dissection students were not allowed to touch any body parts; only afterwards, behind closed doors and in small sessions, were they given the opportunity to train their manual skills. The anatomist's personality and oratory talent largely determined the educational value of public lessons, but it is safe to say that they were of little instructional use to anyone except, perhaps, the anatomist himself.

The anatomist, rather than the cadaver, constituted the focal point of a public dissection in the theatre. It was his task to lead the public from observation of a single dead body to abstract theories about living bodies. Some anatomists proved to be excellent performers and were capable of convincingly translating their concrete tactile and visual perceptions into imaginative, oratory narrative. But without expert explanation there was little to learn for students and the general public. Although the dissecting professor literally visualized physiology by demonstrating body parts and viscera to the crowds, only those who sat up front, close to the dissection table, could actually observe his operations. Those further at the back had to rely on the anatomist's verbal explications, which were comprehensible only to the already initiated. For the ordinary spectator, who was generally illiterate, the anatomist's elucidation in Latin did not add anything to the visual demonstration (Sawday, 1995, p. 64).

The *Visible Human Project* is conceived as a simulation of anatomical dissection or, more precisely, as its emulation in a virtual environment. Three-dimensional reconstructions of real cadavers enable medical students to connect theoretical and empirical knowledge. Like a surgeon who examines radiological information on the screen, students could perform virtual dissections on dead bodies to get a better sense of anatomical structure. At a later stage, the University of Colorado's CHS will create a virtual surgical unit, complete with radiological and anaesthesiological simulators.[11] This simulation unit will resemble virtual cockpits designed for Starfighter pilots. Both virtual environments offer hands-on experience without having to endanger real people's lives. The term 'hands-on' suggests that virtual dissection is seen as a perfect replacement for the tactile experience obtained by regular dissection; manipulating digital pictures with a computer mouse is seen as the equivalent of handling a dissector's knife.

The cultural history of anatomical dissection, however, invites us to put into proper perspective the overtly ambitious claims advanced by the VHP. In the early sixteenth century, Vesalius challenged the dominant Galenic paradigm by putting practice before text, but at the end of the twentieth century, tactile experience is on the verge of being replaced by the visual. The three elements of text, image, and body may completely coalesce in a digital cadaver, yet in the hierarchy of the senses, the visual has clearly vindicated the dimensions of both reading and touching. The VHP presents itself as a visual reference book – a standard body for the twenty-first century. However, it is rather presumptuous to equate actual cadavers to digital reconstructions, and to treat virtual dissections as equally valid as their real-life counterparts. Nevertheless, this does not mean that working with the VHP's data sets constitutes a lesser or less valuable preparatory tool for future doctors. On the contrary, getting acquainted with human anatomy through digital cross-sections perfectly fits everyday practice in contemporary medicine, which already relies heavily on looking at scanned cross-sections of patients' bodies. The particular significance of the Visible Human for medical education, then, may be less in the digitization of human cadavers than in the digitization of medicine as a whole.

The superiority of anatomical instruction through three-dimensional representations over actual dissection is hard to substantiate. Digital cross-sections of the Visible Male mean as much to a layperson as the anatomist's explications in Latin meant to the spectator in the Renaissance anatomy theatre. For one thing, the data set itself is nothing but a series of bits and bytes, and it takes competent medical software specialists as well as large computer storage space in order to translate and recompile those data into usable fly-throughs. Moreover, the interpretation of cross-sections requires substantial viewing experience; the less-than-a-millimetre slices mean little or nothing if the viewer cannot relate these slices to actual three-dimensional organs. Just as decoding ultrasound images or X rays requires training, one needs an experienced eye to translate MRI and CT scans into anatomical structures. Since virtual anatomy instruction takes place through the visual rather than the tactile, 'eyes-on experience' seems a better term for virtual anatomy than the actual 'hands-on experience' it advertises.

Besides the bold promise that the Visible Human will replace conventional dissection in medical training, its proponents also claim that digitized cadavers emulate classical anatomical illustrations. Because anatomists were rarely gifted illustrators, atlases commonly resulted from close collaboration between an artist and an anatomist.[12] For a faithful and accurate depiction of anatomical knowledge, lectors depended on the precision of their illustrators, yet artistic interference detracted attention from physiology to art, and from the scientist to the artist. In the eyes of many – the initiators of the VHP among them – this has two major drawbacks: it has led to idealized, abstracted, and often 'distorted' representations of the human body, and most importantly, it always involved the projection of three-dimensional structures onto a flat surface.

By contrast, the digital data sets offer three-dimensional images that can be rotated so that the projected body parts may be seen from any plane or perspective. On the computer screen, students can manipulate the images with their mouse, and pre-modelled fly-throughs enable a smooth look inside or between organs.[13] A digital cadaver, the VHP claims, is no longer a *representation*, tainted by the subjective interpretation of an artist, but a *simulation* – a digital reconstruction of a real body. Or, as the VHP suggests, its digital simulations constitute 'unmediated inscriptions' of cadavers that are neither distorted by the pencil of the illustrator nor by the knife of the dissector.

Asserting that digital inscription is beyond representation, however, seems exaggerated, if not unwarranted.[14] Introductions of new visualizing techniques, starting with X rays in 1895, have in fact always been accompanied by enthusiastic claims of increased transparency. But in each case this has proven to be illusory. Even a combination of all available perspectives will never produce an undistorted, transparent body. Invariably, our view of the body is informed by the modality of its visualizing instruments. The Visible Human is not beyond representation because digital imagery imitates body shapes better than conventional anatomical illustration; rather, its illusion of verisimilitude is primarily due to the fact that digital images are now a common visual currency in medical practice.

The Anatomical Theatre as a Criminal Court

Most people who donate their body after death regard their gift as a contribution to science. Signing a codicil is generally considered a noble act, one that enables medical students to practise dissection, which in turn will help them save lives later on. The provenance of cadavers, in Western teaching hospitals, is regulated by strict protocols and is rarely a subject of discussion; as a rule, the cadaver's anonymity is guaranteed, so students can concentrate exclusively on the scientific dimension of the dead body. By the same token, scientific articles referring to the Visible Human omit any information regarding the creation of these databases. However, the provenance of these digital bodies – the actual bodies on which they are based – forms a crucial subtext for understanding the historical and cultural roots of the *Visible Human Project*.

Until the late fifteenth century, anatomists generally used unclaimed cadavers for dissection; this usually involved individuals without relatives or friends to take care of their burial. The supply of unclaimed cadavers kept pace with the number of bodies needed for dissection each year. This changed around 1500, when public dissections began to attract larger crowds, and the demand for fresh cadavers increased accordingly (Park, 1994, pp. 14-15). To keep up with demand, anatomists started to recruit cadavers of convicted and executed criminals, in addition to the bodies of individuals who had died of some kind of disease and whose body was donated or left unclaimed (Lassek, 1958). But for judicial, moral, and scientific reasons, anatomists preferred bodies of executed criminals. In the early sixteenth century, public dissection became directly connected to the criminal justice system, as the courts wielded it as a form of extra punishment on top of the death penalty. By the seventeenth century, public dissection was common practice in most European countries (Lassek, 1958, p. 32). In Britain, it was explicitly incorporated in the famous Murder Act of 1752, which was designed to teach shameless bandits a moral lesson. Death by hanging or execution was considered too mild a deterrent, but public dissection appeared a daunting instrument that signified double punishment. Besides public humiliation, it implied that the executed criminal was denied a decent burial – a final resting place for the soul. The notion of double punishment was based on the assumption that, after the criminal's execution, his or her soul would be floating around the body for several more days. Public dissection meant that the criminal's soul suffered its second indignity after the execution, witnessed by a large crowd. This combined public execution and dissection constituted, as Jonathan Sawday aptly put it, 'two acts in a single drama' (Sawday, 1995, p. 63).

From a disciplinary point of view, the anatomist's job functioned as an extension – sometimes even literally – of the executioner's job: they were both in charge of executing the sentence imposed by the judge.[15] Although anatomists explicitly distanced themselves from ordinary executioners, they had a similar professional interest in capital punishment. It may not be a coincidence that the establishment of anatomical theatres often led to an increase in the number of death row convictions (Richardson, 1987, pp. 30-51). Public dissections, like executions, also worked as a moral deterrent; it gave spectators the sense that those who had harmed society were forced to give something in return. Murderers in particular were sentenced to death plus dissection. This punishment in the service of medical science had considerable moral and symbolic value. Moreover, by paying his dues to society, the convicted criminal's chances of ending up in purgatory or even in heaven increased considerably.[16]

The moral and scientific implications of a criminal's dissection were inextricably intertwined. For scientific purposes, Renaissance anatomists preferred corpses of executed criminals. This preference suggests two interesting paradoxes. First, cadavers had to be both identified and anonymous. They had to be identified as criminals in order to function as a moral deterrent, yet they had to be anonymous to serve as a scientific object. In most of Europe it was common practice to safeguard the anonymity of corpses for dissection; the British Murder Act even legally stipulated it. Contrary to public execution, which usually took place in the convicted criminal's hometown, cadavers used for public dissection were brought in from nearby towns.[17] Out of respect for the criminal's family – to spare them the added shame – the cadaver's identity was not disclosed. Identification of the body would also have distracted from the scientific nature of the anatomy lesson, since the audience would see a dead criminal instead of a scientific object on the dissection table. The anatomist solved this dilemma by listing, at the beginning of the dissection, the crimes for which this body had been sentenced to death, so the moral lesson was made explicit without the identity of the criminal being exposed. Yet there was another reason for withholding the criminal's name: it increased the body's representativeness rather than emphasizing its uniqueness. After all, dissection was not meant to expose the interior of a particular corpse, but to extract general knowledge about the human body.

Anatomist's preference for corpses of criminals yielded another interesting paradox: while obviously dead, the cadaver had to be representative of the living body. In contrast to 'found' or donated bodies, which were commonly disease-ridden, the bodies of executed criminals were usually in good shape. It is known that anatomists told judges they were specifically interested in bodies of average length, age, and size.[18] In order to be representative, the bodies used at dissection had to fit the audience's sense of what constituted a normal healthy body. But the criminal's moral repugnancy was at least as important as his or her mint physical condition. Although his crimes had to be utterly heinous in order to set a moral standard, his body had to be untainted, either by disease or by the execution of the death sentence.[19] As a rule, the judge granted the anatomist's request to have the criminal hanged rather than executed, because the gallows left fewer physical marks and hardly disfigured the body.

Female bodies were especially in demand, but they were scarcer as there were fewer women convicted. Male criminals mostly received capital punishment for murder, female convicts for infanticide or theft. In general, female criminals were sentenced to the dissection table for smaller offences than their male counterparts, perhaps because their bodies were more in demand. Female corpses offered an opportunity to demonstrate the reproductive system, and the younger their bodies, the better. In a society where the veiled female body is associated with chastity and honour, whereas the naked female body is linked to seduction and shame, female cadavers obviously provided an attractive spectacle for a mostly male audience (Park, 1994, p. 13). In the gendered social order of the Renaissance, it should come as no surprise that female cadavers were held up against different standards of punishment and moral judgment to male cadavers.[20]

The cultural and historical ties between the medical and the judicial system, as discussed above, elucidate our understanding of contemporary virtual anatomy. The VHP confronts us with similar paradoxes concerning the body's representativeness and anonymity. To start with the latter: the identity of the Visible Male remained anything but a secret. When the CHS put the man's digital data on the Internet, it refused to disclose his identity; the only fact they revealed was that the Visible Male was modelled after the body of a 39-year-old Texan prisoner who had been sentenced to death. Yet, since the CHS had released the date of the prisoner's conviction, it was fair game for journalists to trace his identity: the 'real' Visible Male turned out to be Joseph Paul Jernigan, who had been sentenced to death for murder and robbery on August 26, 1993. While still on death row, he had agreed to donate his body to science, and specifically to the *Visible Human Project*. In exchange for his collaboration, his sentence to the electric chair was changed into death by lethal injection. Just like Renaissance judges who sentenced criminals to the gallows to please anatomists, the milder sentence for the Texan prisoner was primarily motivated by a desire to serve the interests of science rather than those of the convict: lethal injection causes minimal effects on the otherwise perfect body. In line with sixteenth-century European conventions, the body was not dissected in his hometown in Texas, but was transported to Colorado, where the cryogenic macrotome saw cut it into 1,872 thin slices.

For the scientific status of the VHP, the identity of the man whose material body constituted the basis of the digital data set was absolutely irrelevant, if not harmful. Therefore, the initiators of the VHP were reluctant to release the Visible Male's identity. However, the ease with which journalists tracked down Jernigan's personal record renders this intention questionable. The media instantly turned Jernigan into a posthumous celebrity. Without the Visible Man's criminal past, the Project would most likely have received half as much media attention.[21] When we look more closely at the VHP's media coverage, it is remarkable to notice how Renaissance morality resonated in 1995 newspaper clippings.[22] Jernigan's dissection into slices was described as 'extra punishment' on top of his death sentence. Some newspapers commented that, by donating his body to this educational-scientific project, Jernigan at least paid his dues to society. Other commentators appeared outraged that this murderer was granted eternal life on the Internet – virtual reanimation as a reward for his hideous crime.[23] In whatever capacity, the mythology of the convicted criminal has become an integral part of the Visible Male data set; Jernigan's digital representation is a constant reminder of American capital punishment, of the body disciplined through crime and punishment, forever exposed to the scopic regime of science.

The second paradox concerns Jernigan's alleged representativeness for the average living body, while the virtual cadaver undeniably exhibits some very distinct idiosyncratic features. According to the initiators, it proved rather difficult to find a suitable body for the Visible Male, and it took them more than two years to find a body that could serve as a 'standard for anatomy', that is, a body of average size, length, weight, and height, with no visible physical imperfections. Joseph Jernigan was chosen from five other potential candidates because of his mint condition: a healthy 39-year-old, 170-pound male who had lifted weights in prison on a daily basis. Yet his body, as it turns out, was not exactly perfect: besides a missing appendix, one testicle was removed to prevent a benign tumour from growing, while Jernigan was still in prison. Apparently, these abnormalities did not qualify this body as unrepresentative. On the other hand, some outward features, like a tattoo on his arm, signal the criminal's 'authenticity,' as they are clearly visible on the screen.

In the data set of the Visible Female, we may perceive similar paradoxes concerning anonymity and representativeness.[24] Her model was not recruited from the circles of criminals; the material basis for the Visible Female originated from a Maryland woman who had signed a codicil to donate her body to science after death. Unlike Joseph Jernigan, she had not specifically intended her body to be used for the VHP, but her husband decided after her death that this was a noble and important cause. Through the CHS, her husband confirmed her apparent excellent condition by stating that his wife had never been sick a single day until she was struck by a heart attack. The female cadaver underwent the same treatment as Jernigan's body, the only difference being that she was cut into slices of one-third of a millimetre, resulting in an even more refined database.[25]

In contrast to Jernigan's case, we know nothing about the Visible Female's identity but her age and status; the CHS revealed that the cadavermodel for the Visible Female came from a '59-year-old housewife from Maryland who had died of a heart-attack'. In the media attention that followed, the Visible Female was primarily evaluated on the basis of these gender-specific features.[26] The label 'housewife' suggested the normalcy of the woman, one whose body is unaffected by intellectual or otherwise 'untypical' female activities. Yet the woman's representativeness is clearly undermined by her age: since she is post-menopausal, her body cannot serve to illustrate the female reproductive functions, and the directors of the VHP have agreed they should make up for this deficiency by searching for a younger sample. Apparently, there are different standards for determining the normalcy of virtual males and females. Despite his missing testicle, Jernigan is still presented as a 'standard', while the Visible Female is looked upon as imperfect, because she is no longer fertile. Even though menopause is not the pathological equivalent of a missing testicle, the Visible Female is not considered representative of the average female body. Significantly, the gender-specific cultural criteria that we use to differentiate between living men and women are unilaterally projected onto these virtual cadavers.

The major paradoxes prevalent in Renaissance anatomy resonate in the VHP. Like the Renaissance anatomical theatre, the VHP is bound up with the criminal court system. Whereas formerly in Europe criminals were sentenced to death and dissection, today in the United States criminals are sentenced to death and asked if they mind being cross-sectioned. By confronting the audience of public anatomy lessons with the body's criminal past, moral content was added to the practice of anatomical dissection. Similarly, in contemporary virtual anatomy, contextual information on the Visible Male's and Visible Female's identities turned out to be a major factor in popularizing the project and disseminating its data sets.

The Anatomical Theatre as a Public Spectacle

In addition to having ties to the educational and justice systems, anatomical dissection also counts as an early form of mass entertainment – of public spectacle. Although this dimension virtually disappeared from anatomical practice after the late eighteenth century, it is surprising to find how the VHP has contributed to its return. In the sixteenth century, Vesalius's dissections – giving rise to an empirical turn in anatomy – also induced a shift from private to public instruction. Most likely due to the change in emphasis from textual to personal authority, the public appeal of the anatomy lesson increased from a handful of students to large crowds of spectators. In this new popular setting, the anatomist attracted spectators from all social strata. To accommodate large crowds, theatres built particularly for this purpose mushroomed in Europe during the seventeenth century, especially in towns and cities with universities that had medical faculties, such as Bologna, Padua, London, Leiden, and Amsterdam.[27]Architecturally, anatomical theatres were designed after typical Renaissance stages – round stages and gradually ascending seats – enabling the audience to literally gaze into the cadaver from a high angle.

Illustrations and drawings from Vesalius's famous anatomy atlas *De humani corporis fabrica* show how large and varied crowds surrounded the anatomist and the cadaver.[28] Attributes like skeletons and Vanitas symbols decorated the open space, underscoring the moralistic intentions of the public anatomy lesson. It was not uncommon for a banquet, a concert, or other performances to adorn dissections, contributing to an event that lasted up to several days. It usually took place during the cold season, February being the most popular month; obviously, the low temperatures helped conserve the cadaver for several days,

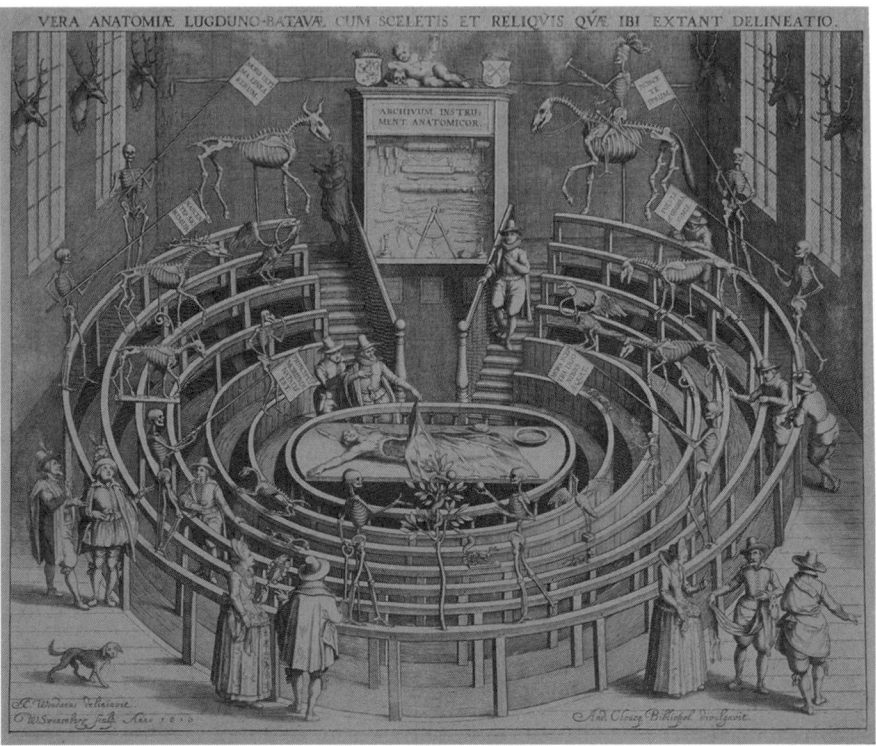

The anatomical theatre in Leiden. Drawing by J.C. Woudanus, 1610.

while some historians have also associated the spectacle of dissection with the annual carnival.[29] Tickets for anatomical festivals did not come cheap and were much in demand; we know from historical tracts that rituals and ceremonies added lustre to anatomical lessons.[30]

The public anatomy spectacle was highly influenced by the conventions of the Renaissance morality play. In seventeenth-century dramas, like those by Shakespeare in Britain and Vondel in Holland, catharsis or purification of the soul was a central element of the play. Anatomy lessons, much like the Elizabethan tragedies that ended with the death of all characters, had a decidedly morbid plot, moving from a fresh and preferably perfectly intact corpse to what was basically not more than a gnawed-off skeleton. Illustrious skeletons on the walls of the anatomical theatre foreshadowed the cadaver's inevitable fate. The anatomist, in his public lesson, articulated the relation between the dead body on the table and the living body of the spectator. Catharsis was only immanent if crime and punishment were theatrically packaged in a moral performance.

Anatomical theatres played a major role in the dissemination of science to a large lay audience. The popularity of anatomical theatres in the Renaissance should be regarded in the context of the rise of *Kunst-* and *Wunderkammer* and botanical gardens, which also exposed large crowds to the marvels of nature and science. However, in their public dissections, anatomists did not so much intend to share their knowledge with a general audience, as to impress them and command respect and awe. As anatomical theatres flourished, they turned into cultural centres, where scientists and artists worked side by side, inspiring one another. Many famous painters and writers, most notably Rembrandt, attended public dissections and recorded the anatomical spectacle in their art works. Scientists and artists used the same 'raw material', only for different purposes. Although few artists really understood the Latin oracle in front of the cadaver, they were fascinated by the combination of scientific aura, moral transformation, and morbid entertainment.

The same cocktail of science, morality, and morbidity can be retraced in the *Visible Human Project*. This expensive virtual anatomy project was evidently

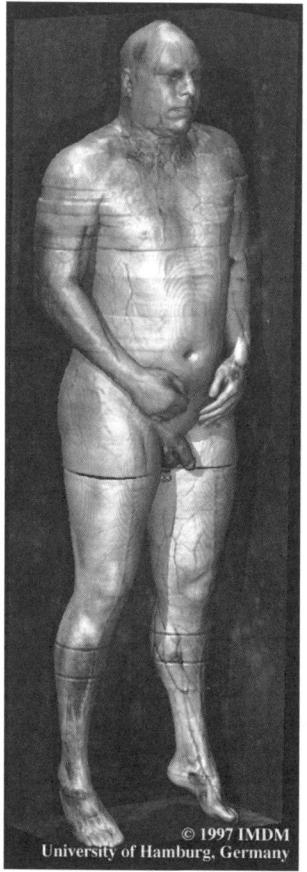 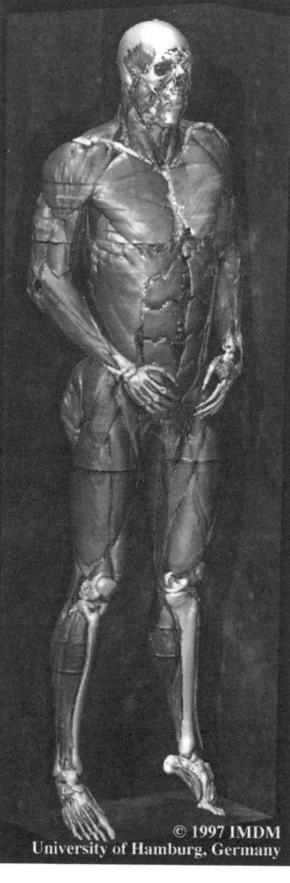

VOXEL-MAN computer-based anatomy model. Torso with and without skin. Institute for Medical Informatics, University of Hamburg, Germany. Courtesy of Karl Heinz Höhne. www.uke.uni-hamburg.de/voxel-man

designed for educational purposes, but through the release of its results on the Internet, the data have become public property, and they have – perhaps inadvertently – been used already by a variety of professionals for very different purposes.[31] And, just like in the Renaissance, artists have deployed the Visible Human data sets to create their own versions of corporeal imaging with artistic and entertainment goals in mind.

When we take a closer look at one of these popularized products, it is easy to find historical echoes of the anatomical theatre's function as a public spectacle. The CD-ROM and its companion book *Body Voyage* vaguely pretends to disseminate anatomical knowledge to a lay audience, but its educational value proves very low indeed.[32] Except for a few general medical facts and figures, this CD-ROM contains no serious information on either physiology or anatomy. The user has to understand and interpret colourful cross-sections without any further explanation. For laypersons with little prior knowledge of physiology, the educational value of this product is close to zero. The high entertainment value of *Body Voyage* is undoubtedly due to its spectacular presentation and dramatic plotting: the recompiled data set of the Visible Male is presented as the lugubrious 'inside experience' of a dead criminal's body. The only explanations we get from scrolling through the disk are juicy details about Jernigan's background and criminal past. We learn how he was sentenced to death after robbing and killing a 75-year-old man, and that he never showed any remorse for his cold-blooded crime. Minutely, the CD-ROM describes the details of Jernigan's execution, including his last words and information on his last meal (a cheeseburger). The actual dissection device, the cryogenic macrotome, is shown on a quick time video display. Just like the anatomical theatre, *Body Voyage* capitalizes on the spectacle of dissection: the spectator can virtually dissect Jernigan's cadaver layer by layer, and thus execute the dissection 'hands-on'.

The artist who made this CD-ROM, Alexander Tsiaras, views his product as an artistic interpretation of the Visible Male's data set. His explicit purpose is to 'inform and entertain a popular audience', and he places himself in the tradition of great artists like Leonardo da Vinci, Dürer, and Rembrandt. As stated in the introduction, *Body Voyage* is the result of a perfect marriage between science and art. For the production of this CD-ROM, Tsiaras used some of the digital data provided by the CHS, yet retouched their original colours in order to create a more aesthetically pleasing digital cadaver. It is the combination of colourful cross-sections, a suspenseful plot, a 'truly' horrendous character, and morality play that warrants the success of this product. Rather than an instructional tool, this derivative of the VHP mainly echoes the Renaissance anatomy lesson's function of public spectacle. Disguised as popular science education, the CD-ROM invites the user to subject the convicted and executed prisoner, time and again, to virtual dissection.

Digital Cadavers and Virtual Dissection

By considering the *Visible Human Project* in light of the various functions of the anatomical theatre, I have argued that it represents a distinct continuation of historical anatomical practices. It should be emphasized that I do not believe that the VHP directors made a conscious effort to situate digital dissection in a European Renaissance tradition. My goal was merely to elucidate how the current practice of compiling and disseminating digital body data reflects and constructs persistent cultural norms involving age, gender, spectacle, identity, transparency, and crime and punishment, and how these various norms are historically interrelated.

Anatomical dissection, in its digital variant, may seem less inscribed with sacral symbolism and morbid connotations than conventional dissection, but as I have shown, the 'new standard of human anatomy' hardly consists of a transparent set of digital data.[33] Just as public dissections in the Renaissance reflected and constructed contemporary norms regarding the body, the design, materialization and dissemination of digital cadavers articulates our current norms with regard to the body and its transparency. The material basis of anatomical models and their representations mirror, to a large extent, contemporary standards of acceptability and aesthetic preferences for certain modes of display. The Visible Male and Female tell us as much about the history of anatomical bodies as about our contemporary cultural tastes and social norms. Virtual anatomy thus reflects the anatomical theatre of the twenty-first century, a theatre in which education, morality, and entertainment are seamlessly woven into a digital culture. It is important to realize that our knowledge of the body can never be studied separately from our knowledge of representation, the technology that mediates it, and the cultural matrix from which it arises.

José van Dijck is a Professor of Media and Culture at the University of Amsterdam and Dean of the Humanities Department. Her research areas include media and science, (digital) media technologies, and television and culture. She is the author of several books, including *Manufacturing Babies and Public Consent. Debating the New Reproductive Technologies* (New York, New York University Press, 1995); *ImagEnation. Popular Images of Genetics* (New York, New York University Press, 1998). The chapter 'Digital Cadavers' was taken from her book *The Transparent Body. A Cultural Analysis of Medical Imaging* (Seattle, University of Washington Press, 2005). Her latest book is titled *Mediated Memories. Personal Cultural Memory in the Digital Age* (Stanford University Press, 2007).

Notes

1   For a detailed explanation of the transformation of an anatomical body into a 'body of knowledge', see Sawday, 1995, chapter 1.

2   Dissections, as part of medical education, were conducted as early as the fourteenth century, but it took until the sixteenth century before medical praxis was actually based on empirical anatomical findings – knowledge that was subsequently recorded in medical atlases. See French, 1999.

3   The Center for Human Simulation's homepage provides a short overview of how the *Visible Human Project* evolved: www.nlm.nih.gov/research/visible/visible_human. html.

4   The Visible Human data sets are now available on CD-ROM: *The Complete Visible Human: The Complete high-Resolution Male and Female Anatomical Databases from the Visible Human Project*. New York, 1999. It encompasses more than 7000 cross-sections and is produced for educational use.

5   As Michael Ackerman claims in 'The Visible Human Project': 'It is hoped that this Website will serve as the prototype for revolutionary educational applications based on both the core VHP data sets and additional human imagery sources to be added later. (...) As the rapid proliferation of Web browsers and networking hardware has demonstrated, innovation and entrepreneurial spirit can sweep away decades of conventional capability in a matter of months' (Ackerman, 1999, p. 670).

6   In 1308, the body of Francesca of Foligna was cut open to see whether her heart was shaped as a cross, or whether a crown of thorns was hidden away in her intestines.

7   For an extensive description of late medieval practices of dissection, see Carlino, 1999, particularly chapter 1.

8   Vesalius was not the only one performing public dissections, but was definitely one of the most famous. The 'empirical turn', naturally, did not happen instantaneously after Vesalius took centre stage; initially, he used his observations to correct Galen's insights, yet incorporated these in the overall dominant theocentric paradigm. The empirical turn in anatomy happened gradually, but Vesalius counts as a turning point.

9   For a detailed analysis of Vesalius's techniques, see Harcourt, 1987.

10   William Harvey, in seventeenth-century Europe, was famous for his remarkable personality and the way in which he paired off rhetorical fluency with refined dissecting techniques. See Wilson, 1987.

11   Richard Satava, for instance, claims that operations of the future will be mostly computer-directed operations in so-called virtual bodies. See Satava, 1996. Thacker (1998) argues that the primary concern behind the VHP is as much about informatics as it is about anatomy.

12   Anatomical atlases and the relationship between the artist and anatomist were very much a sixteenth-century, post-Vesalian phenomenon. An example of a famous Dutch collaboration between anatomist and illustrator was that of the anatomist Albinus and illustrator Jan Wandelaar. Their differences of opinion about scientific interpretations vis-à-vis representational accuracy are well documented. See the catalogue *De volmaakte mens. De anatomische atlas van Albinus en Wandelaar*. Leiden, 1991.

13   Catherine Waldby, in her philosophical interpretation of the VHP, 'The Visible Human Project. Data into Flesh, Flesh into Data', regards the Visible Human 'not so much [as] the representation of a body in space, but as a representation of bodily

space, rendered as depth and volume which can be moved through and refigured at will' (2000, p. 33).

14 The software made on the basis of Visible Human data sets complements rather than replaces real dissection of cadavers, argues Rowe (1999).

15 As Park (1994) suggests: 'There are clear indications that anatomists sometimes eliminated the middle man by carrying out capital sentences themselves' (p. 20).

16 Practices varied from country to country. The integration of capital punishment and public dissection was not commonplace in all European countries. Italy was most reticent in this respect, England most explicit. For more details, see Carlino, 1999, p. 219, and see Edgerton, 1985.

17 This was not the case in all European cities. The anatomical theatre De Waag in Amsterdam, for instance, publicly dissected local criminals who were identified explicitly by listing their names and crimes. Britain and Italy had strict rules concerning the anonymity of the dissected corpse.

18 The cooperation between judges and anatomists is extensively described by Ferrari (1987).

19 See Carlino (1999): 'The body had to be someone who had been condemned to death (...) preferably a youthful body, in good condition, and of strong musculature, such as to permit a successful demonstration, the moral quality of the body had to be evaluated at the same time. Criminals had to be found guilty in a criminal court. Hanging was preferred, so the body was not disfigured by torture, punishment, mutilation or execution' (p. 92).

20 For a more elaborate description of the different use of female and male corpses, see Jordanova (1989).

21 Medical and other science journals published extensive correspondence between specialists on the ethics of using the cadaver of a convicted criminal for virtual anatomy. See, for instance, Wadman (1996), Waldrop (1995), and Martin (1996).

22 An interesting analysis of newspaper reactions to the Visible Male was given by Thomas Csordas in 'Computerized Cadavers: Shades of Being and Representation in Virtual Reality'. Paper presented at the conference *Biotechnology, Culture, and the Body*. Milwaukee, University of Wisconsin, April 1997.

23 Csordas (1997) cites headlines of newspapers lamenting the reanimation of Jernigan, like 'Executed Killer Reborn as Visible Man' and 'Killer Let Loose on the Internet'.

24 Besides the Visible Male and Visible Female, scientists are creating a Visible Embryo, a project supervised by the Armed Forces Institute of Pathology; the database of the Visible Embryo will use as its material basis a collection of embryos from the Carnegie Mellon Collection of Human Embryology, which was a gift to the National Museum of Health and Medicine (Washington DC) by the German embryologist Erich Blechschmidt of the University of Göttingen (Germany). See Miller (1994, p. 397) and Cohen (1996, p. 6).

25 The Visible Male database comprises 15 gigabytes, and the Visible Female, 39 gigabytes.

26 For an insightful analysis of the gender-specificity of the Visible Female, see Cartwright (1998).

27 Bologna was the first town to have an anatomical theatre, built in 1595; other cities (Padua, Leiden, Amsterdam) followed in the seventeenth century. See Ferrari (1987, p. 72).

28 On the frontispiece of Vesalius's most famous work, *De humani corporis fabrica* (1543) we can see how a large and varied crowd observes his dissection. For a detailed analysis of this frontispiece, see Carlino (1999, chapter 2).

29   Some historians have argued that there is a meaningful relationship between public dissections and the concurrent celebration of carnival. See, for instance, Ferrari (1987).

30   This detail is provided by Wilson (1987, pp. 68-69).

31   The VOXEL MAN Project has transformed the Visible Human databases into user-friendly products, such as CD-ROMs and videos, which can be used at various educational levels. The CD-ROM *Voxel Man Junior interactive Anatomy and Radiology in Virtual Reality Scenes* (1998), for instance, is a reconstruction of the Visible Male's head; the CD-ROM is suitable for students (high school), but is of little use to medical professionals.

32   *Body Voyage.* Software: Learn Technologies. Interactive Content: Alexander Tsiaras. (New York, 1997). The book accompanying this CD-ROM contains beautiful full-colour scans.

33   Simon J. Williams raises the general question of whether hyperreality may be replacing corporeality in the future, and explains digital dissection in the larger context of medical technologies, such as new reproductive technologies and telemedicine (Williams, 1997, pp. 1041-49).

References

Ackerman, M. J., 'The Visible Human Project: A Resource for Education'. In: *Academic Medicine,* 74. 1999.

Body Voyage. CD-ROM. Software: Learn Technologies. Interactive Content: Alexander Tsiaras. New York, 1997.

Carlino, A., *Books of the Body. Anatomical Ritual and Renaissance Learning.* Chicago, 1999.

Cartwright, L., 'A Cultural Anatomy of the Visible Human Project'. In: *The Visible Woman. Imaging Technologies, Gender, and Science.* P. A. Treichler, L. Cartwright and C. Penley (eds), pp. 21-43. New York, 1998.

Cohen, P., 'Tough Gestation for Virtual Embryo'. In: *New Scientist,* 152. 1996.

Csordas, T., 'Computerized Cadavers: Shades of Being and Representation in Virtual Reality'. Paper presented at the conference *Biotechnology, Culture, and the Body.* Milwaukee, University of Wisconsin, April 1997.

Edgerton, S. Y., *Pictures and Punishment: Art and Criminal Prosecution during the Florentine Renaissance.* Ithaca, 1985.

Ferrari, G., 'Public Anatomy Lessons and the Carnival: The Anatomy Theatre of Bologna'. In: *Past and Present,* 117, pp. 50-106. 1987.

French, R., *Dissection and Vivisection in the European Renaissance.* Aldershot, 1999.

Harcourt, G., 'Andreas Vesalius and the anatomy of Antique Sculpture'. In: *Representations,* 17, pp. 28-61. 1987.

Jordanova, L., *Sexual Visions. Images of Gender in Science and Medicine between the Eighteenth and Twentieth Centuries.* Madison, 1989.

Lassek, A.M., *Human Dissection. Its Drama and Struggle.* Springfield, 1958.

Martin, S., 'Concentrating the Mind.' In: *Nature,* 383, p. 381. 1996.

Miller, J.A., 'Anatomy via the Internet. Visible Human Project and Visible Embryo Project'. In: *BioScience,* 44. 1994.

Park, K., 'The Criminal and the Saintly Body: Autopsy and Dissection in Renaissance Italy'. In: *Renaissance Quarterly,* 1, pp. 1-33. 1994.

Richardson, R., *Death, Dissection and the Destitute.* London, 1987.

Rowe, P.M., 'Visible Human Project Pays Back Investment'. In: *The Lancet,* 352, p. 46. 1999.

Satava, R., 'Medical Virtual Reality: The Current State of the Future'. In: *Health Care in the Information Age.* S. J. Weghorst, H. B. Sieburg, and K. S. Morgan (eds), pp. 100-106. Amsterdam, 1996.

Sawday, J., *The Body Emblazoned: Dissection and the Human Body in Renaissance Culture.* London, 1995.

Thacker, E., 'Visible Human.html: Digital Anatomy & the Hyper-Texted Body'. In: *CTheory,* 21, no page numbers. 1998.

De volmaakte mens. De anatomische atlas van Albinus en Wandelaar. Catalogue of Museum Boerhaave. Leiden, 1991.

VOXEL MAN Project, *VOXEL MAN Junior interactive Anatomy and Radiology in Virtual Reality Scenes.* CD-ROM for educational purposes. New York, 1998.

Wadman, M., 'Ethics Worries over Execution Twist to Internet's "Visible Man"'. In: *Nature,* 382, p. 657. 1996.

Waldby, C., 'The Visible Human Project. Data into Flesh, Flesh into Data'. In: J. Marchessault and K. Sawchuk (eds), *Wild Science: Feminist Readings of Science, Medicine and the Media.* pp. 24-38. London and New York, 2000.

Waldrop, M. M., 'The Visible Man Steps Out.' In: *Science,* 269, p. 1358. 1995.

Williams, S. J., 'Modern Medicine and the Uncertain Body: From Corporeality to Hyperreality'. In: *Social Science & Medicine,* 45. 1997.

Wilson, L., 'William Harvey's "Prelectiones": The Performance of the Body in the Renaissance Theatre of Anatomy'. In: *Representations,* 17, pp. 62-95. 1987.

'Who Were You?':
The Visible and the Visceral

Ian Maxwell

In the opening pages of *The Rings of Saturn*, W.G. Sebald reflects on Rembrandt's *The Anatomy Lesson of Dr Nicolaes Tulp.* Viewing the painting at the Mauritshuis, he writes,

> We are standing precisely where those who were present at the dissection in the Waaggebouw stood, and we believe that we see what they saw then: in the foreground, the greenish, prone body of Aris Kindt, his neck broken and his chest risen terribly in rigor mortis. (Sebald, 2002, p. 13)

Sebald's first observation about the painting is a familiar one. Kindt was a thief, and the use of his body for this anatomical demonstration constituted part of the sentence he suffered for his crime. Those present at the dissection look beyond the body to an open anatomical atlas; the cadaver is a mere exemplar of a superior, abstract knowledge: mere flesh, subordinate to the ideal, as rendered material in the bound pages of a book. The art of anatomy, as exemplified in Rembrandt's painting, Sebald observes, 'was not least a way of making the reprobate body invisible' (Sebald, 2002, p. 13).

However, Sebald asks that we hold our gaze upon the materiality of Rembrandt's representation of the body itself, whereupon 'the much-admired verisimilitude of Rembrandt's picture proves on closer examination to be more apparent than real' (Sebald, 2002, p. 14). Tulp's dissection has commenced not with an evisceration of the prone to putrefaction intestines, but with the thief's offending hand. 'Now', writes Sebald,

> this hand is most peculiar. It is not only grotesquely out of proportion compared with the hand closer to us, but it is anatomically also the wrong way round: the exposed tendons, which ought to be those of the left palm, given the position of the thumb, are in fact those of the back of the right hand (…) we are faced with a transposition taken from the anatomical at-

las, evidently without further reflection, that turns this otherwise true-to-life painting (if one may so express it) into a crass misrepresentation at the exact centre point of its meaning, where the incisions are made. (Sebald, 2002, pp. 16-17)

For Sebald, it is inconceivable that Rembrandt has made a mistake. Instead, he reads in this flaw a deliberate intent:

> That unshapely hand signifies the violence that has been done to Aris Kindt. It is with him, the victim, not the Guild that gave Rembrandt his commission, that the painter identifies. His gaze alone is free of Cartesian rigidity. He alone sees that greenish annihilated body, and he alone sees the shadow in the half-open mouth and over the dead man's eyes. (Sebald, 2002, p. 17)

Here, in Rembrandt's famous painting, the very acme of the anatomical theatre as visual-aesthetic spectacle, Sebald is suggesting that something else is going on ... something perhaps that eludes the surety of vision ... something seen and unseen, something known and not known, hovering in the darkness of Aris Kindt's open, unbreathing mouth.

An empty frame, except for an upright human figure in the middle distance, on the far right of the screen; just discernible: some kind of wire and steel apparatus from which the figure is suspended. The figure is back-lit: a crisp, silver arc defines the crown of its head, outlining both shoulders, defining the outside of the right arm and, spilling, is caught in a slight fuzz of chest hair. The face, turned slightly upwards, is covered in white plaster: a death mask of sorts. Otherwise, the hanging body is a sallow pink-grey, its posture preternaturally erect as the weight of torso and limbs stretches its neck. The uniform toneless pallor of the corpse is broken only by the dark outline of genitals: it is male.

Almost immediately another figure moves into the frame, moving across the proximal plane from the left of screen. He wears a black fedora, round, wire-framed spectacles, and a vivid azure surgical coat over an open-necked shirt. His gaze is initially directed towards the back of the frame, towards the hanging corpse. The man turns to address the camera — you — and the depth of field contracts; we track in, slightly, cropping the fedora, drawn towards green eyes framed by thin-rimmed lenses, highlights flashing in the glare of studio lights, the ruddy glow of healthy skin stretched across a somewhat skeletal visage: broad forehead, a large space between upper lip and nose, the plastic tubing of an earpiece distorting the cartilaginous tangle of his left ear. As he starts to speak, the man's eyebrows arch upwards, his eyes flare wide. The contrast with the pallid, mute, faceless body looming over his left shoulder — the colours, the animation, the intensity of vigorous life — could not be more pronounced. The man speaks in a slightly sibilant, clipped, German-accented English:

> A 55-year-old man who made an extraordinary wish before he died: that his remains be used, by me, to educate people about human anatomy.

> I met him several times. He was passionate about science and the enlightenment of lay people.

> Tonight I will dissect him, and unravel the mysteries below his skin.[1]

This is the anatomical theatre of the twenty-first century. The speaker is Gunther von Hagens, introducing the first episode of the four-part Firefly-Channel 4 television series *Anatomy for Beginners*, featuring what the accompanying website describes as 'spontaneous' and 'real' dissections of human cadavers ('live and uncut', reads a deadpan sticker on the DVD packaging). We learn nothing more of the 55-year-old man, the mysteries of whose body are to be unravelled for our enlightenment; but in a sense, the show is not really about him at all.

Von Hagens is unabashedly a showman. Throughout the series, he appears in his trademark costume, embodying a cultivated eccentricity — a brooding, somewhat mysterious appearance — that bears more than a passing resemblance to that of another German performance artist, Joseph Beuys, albeit favouring iridescent blue over Beuys's earthier smocks of felt and fur. The set-pieces to camera are slightly overwrought, to the point of clumsiness. Introducing the episode titled 'Reproduction', for example, Von Hagens approaches a *tableau vivant* — an attractive young couple locked, lip-to-lip, limb through limb, atop a sculpted rock — and strikes a hand-on-hip pose, gesturing at the young man's buttocks:

> A man and a woman in love. They embrace. In 40 weeks she will give birth to their child. In 40 minutes he will [slight pause; lift of eyebrows] ejaculate. His sperm will travel a total distance of 40 centimetres from his testes to her ovaries. Tonight I will dissect a man and a woman to show you that epic journey.[2]

It is breathless, melodramatic, and just a bit salacious. And you get the sense that Von Hagens has muddled his lines, reversing the escalatory poetics of all those '40s', distracted, or perhaps seduced, by the theatricality of it all.

As if to temper the performativity — the almost histrionic excess — of Von Hagens, there is a straightman: a white-gowned, well-spoken Englishman, subtitled as 'Professor John A. Lee, Professor of Pathology at the Hull York Medical School and consultant histopathologist at Rotherham General Hospital', who lends an air of respectful gravitas to proceedings. Lee provides a metacommentary as counterpoint to Von Hagens's own 'play-by-play' narration of each dissection. The video editor has chosen to cut away to Professor Lee every now and then: at these moments, he is the very model of the restrained, careful overseer, the embodiment of a pure, disinterested man of science, craning his neck to peer into an eviscerated body cavity, nodding approval, casting a wary eye over the entire affair. It is pure theatre: titillating, mocking transgression.

We shouldn't be too quick to condemn this exercise, however, as mere entertainment, or as a betrayal of science to a theatrical populism. That it is showbiz is undeniably the case. The studio set-up — with its dramatic lighting, flatscreen video panels and displays of various anatomical sections and renderings, the studio-audience (to which, again, the editor cuts to capture key expressions: grins full of wonder, guilty smirks, overt delight) on three sides, the black-clad camera crews skating around the various dissection tables and paraphernalia — is slick and tightly packaged. Remarkable animations are projected onto live models; the cameras plunge us deep into the harrowed-out body cavities of the dissectees, capturing every fold and glistening crevice. But the science is good — very, very good — and Von Hagens is clearly very accomplished both with the technicalities of dissection, and as an educator.

Indeed, as Jane Goodall has convincingly argued, science and entertainment have long enjoyed a somewhat co-dependent, if often uncomfortable, relationship, particularly during the nineteenth century. Goodall writes of a range of performance practices, from ethnological displays to freak shows, that did not simply parody, pass comment upon or otherwise stand separately from the 'scientific' debates of the day. Rather, these performances, she argues, were a forum within which those debates were, in a real sense, played out, both in the imaginations and visceral responses of popular audiences, but in the broader public sphere. 'This is not to suggest,' Goodall qualifies, 'that such performances were theory driven, but rather that they reveal how popular curiosity often operates in the same areas as scientific study' (Goodall, 2002, p. 2).

Drawing upon the arguments developed by Richard Altick — that 'scientific' exhibitions themselves were a form of showbusiness — Goodall carefully dismantles any clear demarcation between performances such as those staged by the circus-master P.T. Barnum, and those of the burgeoning natural sciences of the nineteenth century, destabilizing any naturalized narrative of the march of positivism. 'Science' and 'showmanship' are to be understood, on this account, as locked not so much in a dialectical embrace, but chiasmatically intertwined in a struggle for the real, for the potential to tell a story about the world.

Barnum, to whose extraordinary life and exploits Goodall devotes a sizeable proportion of her book, was, she argues, no less systematic a scientist than the gentleman explorer assembling his collection along the (false?) certainty of a proto-Linnean typology; conversely, science established its audience through its capacity to mobilize the kind of performative engagement more convention-ally associated with the fairground. Goodall writes colourfully of the delicate and not-so-delicate negotiations of showmanship in which museums, compet-ing for their audience market share, were required to indulge. Indeed, she charts the complexity of Barnum's relationship to 'the march of science', noting Bar-num's 'envy of seriousness and science' and resentment at being dismissed as the 'Prince of Humbugs'. 'One of his most important gestures to posterity,' she continues, 'was the endowment of the Barnum Museum of Natural History at Tufts College in Massachusetts' (Goodall, 2002, p. 219). Goodall's closing para-graphs sketch the dimensions of the 'Darwin industry' of our own time and the tendency to hyperbolize the status of a thinker who was, after all, one of many theorists of evolution: 'Darwin,' she writes, 'has become Barnum, with more than a little humbug in the promotional mix' (Goodall, 2002, p. 220).

Perhaps we can see Von Hagens, in the self-consciously performative fram-ing of his populist pedagogic aspiration, as a throwback to or continuation of this nineteenth-century tradition, like any good sideshow spruiker, evoking and simultaneously trading upon the illicit, transgressive frisson of his practice. The lesson from Goodall is that there is no necessary shame in this; that sci-ence needs its popularizers not only to assure its own audience but, as it were, to take direction from the curiosity of humanity-at-large: to be reminded of its obligation, if not to the marketplace as construed by economists, then to the agora-as-public sphere. Goodall is suggesting that such practices, straddling the disinterest of science and market-driven populism, are in fact significant sites of the negotiation of science in its ethical relation to society in general.

Anatomy for Beginners is, of course, a spin-off from Von Hagens's main proj-ect: the *Body Worlds* exhibitions and touring shows which feature the display of 'plastinated' bodies in various states of dissection. 'Plastination', the process Von Hagens claims to have invented to preserve cadavers for public display, is a multi-step process involving the replacement of water and fats from the bodily tissue of recently deceased volunteers with various silicon polymers (Body Worlds, 'The Plastination Process'). This allows Von Hagens, in his words,

> to prepare an unrivalled collection of durable anatomical exhibits of great educational value and aesthetic quality (...). (Body Worlds, 'The Plastina-tion Process')

The plastinates, the website explains, travel the world 'with the aim of allowing ordinary people to see the wonders of anatomy for themselves' (Body Worlds, 'Demonstrators'). This same site claims over 15 million visitors to the exhibitions, the popularity of which the website attributes 'partly to the[ir] educational value'. Von Hagens and his collaborators, however, claim more than simply an educational value for their work.

> The beauty and intricacy of the human body is laid bare in a sophisticated modern version of a tradition that extends back to the middle ages and beyond [in the service of] the democratisation of anatomy. (Body Worlds, 'Home')

What might be dismissed as mere populism is reframed as the very acme of the enlightenment project: the democratization of knowledge. Perhaps unsurprisingly, given both the medium and the historical antecedents of the practice of dissection, democratization maps neatly onto visibility; in turn, one of the guarantors for the epistemological status of visibility is an idea of aesthetic beauty. For Von Hagens, visibility is inherently democratic; more, visibility is itself conflated with an aesthetic idealism: the transcendent beauty that he is able to reveal for everyone constitutes the justification for his work.

> Human anatomy is worth studying for its own intrinsic beauty and interest (...) a glimpse of the amazing complexity of our inner world – so close, yet usually so hidden from view. (Body Worlds, 'Introduction')

The price to be paid for these universalizing aspirations is, perforce, the effacement of the revealed bodies as the bodies of individual humans. Recall Von Hagens's rather peremptory introduction of the 55-year-old whose body was to be dissected: he is evoked as having made a personal sacrifice for the greater good; that is, he is allowed only so much humanity to justify his abrogation of that humanity in the name of science. The plastinates, too, enjoy a complex relationship with their own humanity: stripped of life, they are no longer the people that they were and instead are asked to function as exemplars, as *everymen*.[3] At the same time, Von Hagens makes a rather extraordinary argument about individuality:

> the exhibitions are targeted mainly at a lay audience to open up the opportunity to better understand the human body and its functions. The exhibits help the visitors to once again become aware of the naturalness of their bodies and to recognize the individuality and anatomical beauty inside of them.

> The authenticity of the specimens on display is essential for such insight. Every human being is unique. Humans reveal their individuality not only through the visible exterior, but also through the interior of their bodies, as each body is distinctly different from any other. Position, size, shape, and structure of skeleton, muscles, nerves, and organs determine our 'interior face'. It would be impossible to convey this anatomical individuality with models, for a model is nothing more than an interpretation. All models look alike and are, essentially, simplified versions of the real thing. The authenticity of the specimens, however, is fascinating and enables the observer to experience the marvel of the real human body. The exhibitions are thus dedicated to the individual interior face. (Body Worlds, 'Mission of the Exhibitions')

The transient, moral-bound individuality of the human subject is supplanted or displaced in order to effect the display of an erstwhile hidden, interior face, the site of an authentic individuality. This is made possible by a forgetting of the body in question as ever having lived.

The epistemological hegemony of visibility is as explicit, if not more so, in another anatomical project, the subject of José van Dijck in her keynote address to *The Anatomical Theatre Revisited* conference. The *Visible Human Project* (VHP) of the US National Library of Medicine is, Van Dijck argued, 'a distinct continuation of age-old anatomical practices':

> The VHP is firmly rooted in historical conceptions of the body and its representation, of crime and punishment, and of physiology and art (...) a renaissance of public anatomy lessons. (Van Dijck, 2006)

The VHP involves the production of a digital data set from MRI and CT scans of, in the first instance, a male cadaver sliced into millimetre-thick sections. The Visible Human Male data set, released in November 1994 consists of '1,871 cross-sections for both CT and anatomical images. The complete male data set is approximately 15 gigabytes.'[4]

Here, visibility is attested to by the sheer quantity of data, and the sense of wonder (and, again, a slightly prurient wonder generated by the prospect of such a finely-honed violence enacted on a human body in the name of science). But even a millimetre-thick section does not guarantee a sufficient visibility. When a female counterpart to the Visible Man was produced in 1995,

> the axial anatomical images were obtained at 0.33 mm intervals (...). There are 5,189 anatomical images in the Visible Human Female data set. The data set size is approximately 40 gigabytes. (NLM, 2006)

Six years after the first data set was published,

> [h]igher resolution axial anatomical images of the male data set were made
> available (…). Seventy-millimeter still photographs taken during the cryo-
> sectioning procedure were digitized at a pixel resolution of 4096 pixels by
> 2700 pixels. These images, each approximately 32 megabytes in size, are
> available for all 1,871 male color cryosections. (NLM, 2006)

The horizon of visibility is pushed back even further as the project drives towards ever-finer analogue and digital grains. The sheer mass of figures here
affirms the positivist credentials of the project: visibility is, effectively, quanti-
fied. We see more and more, courtesy of breath-taking technological bravura,
although we may start wondering just what it is that we are seeing and, by extension, *knowing*. For even as we (digitally) slice and dice to the quantum limits of
perception, other forms of knowledge are displaced.

Although not entirely. From the floor of the conference come questions,
framed a little awkwardly (for fear, perhaps, that the questioner might reveal
what must surely be interpreted as a prurient interest): whose bodies are —
were — these? Against the weight of the positivist construction of these bodies
as visibles, as data, the subjective questioning of the *who* recurs. Science's response is to reframe such questions as legalistic or moral issues, or else in terms
of the matter of typicality. (Much of the discussion following Van Dijck's paper
turned on this particular issue: how *typical* are these digital bodies, one that
of a convicted felon, the other that of a suburban 'housewife'? What are we to
make of the tacit claim to typicality in the definite articles used for each?) Yet
such responses do not exhaust or quench our desire to reach out to the bodies
themselves. To put it another way, there appears to be relationships of concern,
of care, which lead us to wonder about these people, which are more or less
entirely marginalized in the positivist enthusiasm for a democratic visibility.

This concern as to whose body might be recast as a reaching towards a more
fundamental relationship between bodies — between our own bodies as we
approach these other bodies, even if only in discourse and thought — bodies
that seem to resist our efforts to render them simply as data, as (merely) visible stuff. The possibility of knowing these bodies as data is not sufficient, no
matter how finely we slice them, how perfectly we preserve them for didactic
eternity, whether we mask their faces with plaster casts.

The afternoon following Van Dijck's presentation, Bozhena M. Czarnecka-Anastassiades presented her paper '"Holding the Mirror up to Nature": Bodies Anatomized, Bodies Mirrored in Pietro da Cortona' (Czarnecka-Anastassiades, 2006).
As she started her presentation, Czarnecka-Anastassiades issued a pre-emptive

apology: the images she was about to show us, she explained, were not nearly as impressive as those presented in the paper immediately beforehand. These first images were high-quality digital photographs of Von Hagens's plastinates: vivid colours in high resolution; glossy surfaced and distinct systems laid open for clarity and impact. They are startling, dramatic, wondrous, bearing out Von Hagens's own aspiration to evoke a wonder born of the fusion of science and aesthetics.

The images that Czarnecka-Anastassiades then went on to project for us were, by comparison, decidedly low-tech: plates from Pietro da Cortona's *Tabulae anatomicae*, first published in 1741.[5] These are a series of engravings made of Da Cortona's original drawings, created a century earlier. The majority of the 21 plates of Da Cortona's series illustrate a human figure in a life-like pose (just as Von Hagens's plastinates are staged 'in action'; indeed, some of Von Hagens's tableaux quote Da Cortona directly), each body partly dis-assembled: muscles curl away from bones; incisions gape, revealing layers of tissue and tightly packed coils of viscera. Czarnecka-Anastassiades called them 'the flayed bodies'.

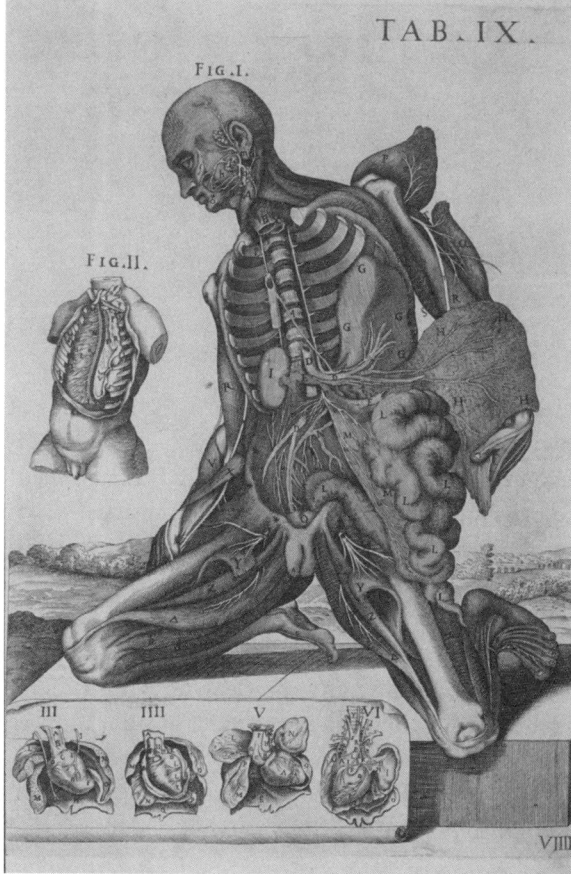

Pietro da Cortona, *Tabulae Anatomicae* 1741. Plate IX. Courtesy of John Martin Rare Book Room, University of Iowa.

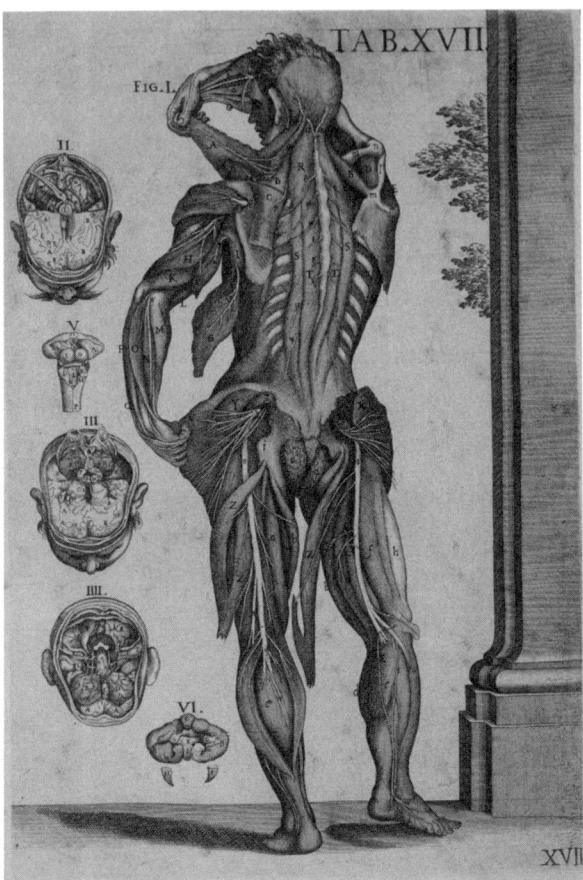

Pietro da Cortona, *Tabulae Anatomicae* 1741. Plate XVII. Courtesy of John Martin Rare Book Room, University of Iowa.

Aside from the almost absurdist/comical effect — my favourite is the image of the fellow peeling back his own trapezius muscles — two things are immediately striking about these images. First, the complex relationship Da Cortona illustrates between interior and exterior; second, the visibility of the artist's own hand in the careful rendering of depth, volume, and tangibility of the various elements of the illustrated body.

Visibility, in Da Cortona, does not partake of a simple correspondence to and with knowledge. Inside and outside are not juxtaposed in a simple opposition; his bodies are layered, recursive, folding and interleaving within themselves. The bodies do not so much reveal their inner mysteries as offer hints as to the spongy densities and interdependencies constituting body-as-organism. Viewed as a series, the images suggest dissection as a process, and a puzzling, strange process at that, rather than presenting the sanitized and triumphal products of that process.

The flayed bodies do not shrink from dissection as an act of violence, but intriguingly hold out the possibility of a violence undertaken with *care*; this much is suggested by the intensity with which the cadavers themselves partake in and observe their own dismemberment. Bodies, Da Cortona seems to suggest, only reluctantly reveal themselves, and even then the revelation is partial, complicated, unfinished.

More, looking at Da Cortona, our nascent understanding — our apprehension or grasp (the metaphor is advised, for it is grasp, touching and holding that is at stake) — of the pulsing, weighty, engorged gibbosity of the lower intestine is given by the careful shading and cross-hatching that yields their depth and liquid solidity. These representations, explicitly recanting any aspiration to 'the real', instead draw us into a sensorium — a tangibility — of the body that is not dependent upon a pure, spectacular visibility.[6] The images resist a laying-out under the rubric of a democratizing ocular centrism. The cross-hatchings and fecund darknesses remind us of the conditions of their creation as images; our relation to the work is not that of an abstract, pure aesthetic, but a profoundly human one: there is us looking, there is the artist, and there are the bodies being depicted. I am struck by the idea that these images stand to Von Hagens's plastinates as erotica stands to pornography.

At the same time, revisiting Von Hagens's performance of dissection, this tangibility, this calling out of the body to touch and flesh, is just as striking. I am watching, again, the episode titled 'Digestion'. The scraping sound of scalpel peeling away skin and fat is accompanied by Von Hagens's commentary. He is crouching, the rim of his fedora brushing the top of the open body cavity: 'Marius take your finger away (…) careful [cut-away shot to smiling audience member against a ripple of laughter]; large knife, large knife, yes', he calls to an assistant:

> and now I can take the whole abdominal specimen…[slight pause for breath as he tears the material free from the body; his voice cracks with the effort on the next word] … *down* …[7]

Here he stands, clearing his throat, in order to grasp the alimentary tract with both hands.

> We should be able to take out the last part of the [long pause to concentrate on tugging; his slightly laboured breath concusses against his lapel mike, drawing us closer to the materiality of his own embodiment] large intestine… knife…[8]

A long pause, as he saws at the last tatters of tissue connecting the anus to the muscles of the sphincter: 'so!' The viscera spills forward from the vacated body cavity (all the while, the hollowed-out body frame, freed of its weighty cargo, jiggles and flops, rag-doll-like, above him; an assistant, standing behind the cadaver, grasps both its — her — elbows to keep her — it — steady), and Von Hagens lunges to grasp it. 'Absolutely gorgeous,' he exclaims, cradling the bruised-brown lobes of the liver. He looks like a midwife nursing a newborn; a newborn that weighs, he remarks, some 15 kilograms. Registering the weight, he grunts: 'Unngghh', and flops the flaccid bundle onto the polished steel of an adjacent table. He pauses, blowing out breaths – 'phew... ungh... ahh' – as droplets of gore fall from his gloves. A nervous, tension-relieving ripple of laughter from the audience again; upstage, in the back of the shot, an assistant steadies the cadaver, placing a hand under each armpit, walking it back out of the way.

The scene is mesmerizing, theatrical, unsettling; and yet, strangely dispassionate: divorced from, or void of, life. The identity of the cadaver has been, again, pre-emptively addressed through legal disclaimer and a handful of plaster. The evisceration takes on the form of butchery; once her/its innards are secured – *delivered* – the body is carefully walked out of the picture, to stand, gutted, mute, in the background. Von Hagens uses the oldest of actor's tricks – the dramatic pause, complete with laboured breath – to pull focus, and to allow the audience to relieve its awkwardness through laughter. In this anatomical theatre, the question of life-as-lived is inadmissible: the body on the slab is pure *Körper*; of that there is no question.

By contrast, the humanity of the flayed bodies drew from Czarnecka-Anastassiades's listeners the same question posed about the Visible Humans: a question *about* those particular bodies, a question again framed apologetically, as if anticipating the accusation of prurience that it might enjoin: 'this may seem like a funny question, but (...) whose bodies were they?'

The question is unanswered and unanswerable. Nonetheless, the represented bodies lead us to their animating principle through the revelation of the care of the artist's hand as he *realizes* the weight, curve, and pulse of their being, as much as through the confounding intertwining of *Körper* and *Leib*, the living and the dead, in the form in which they are represented. In so doing, these images draw us into an ethic of care. Where Von Hagens's plastinates and dissectees contractually renounce that which made them *them*, legally ceding the right of access to their own bodies as lived, in the name of a disinterested science – a science that demands not to know about those lives, that rules those lives out of the equation – Da Cortona's bodies refuse to relinquish their hold on life. And so, they look absurd.

So far in this essay I have tried to enact a tension between ideas about visibility, through which human bodies yield knowledge in an aestheticized, putatively democratized display, and an idea about alternative, perhaps coexisting, if challenging knowledge derived from more tangible, performative, embodied graspings of those same bodies. I have pointed to moments in my witnessing of Von Hagens's postmortem dissections, or of Da Cortona's drawings, in which the kinds of knowledges of human bodies to which I am awakened defy the simple logics of beauty and demonstrable, empirical truth, and lead me towards complex, unsettling and uncomfortable territories. At stake, I am suggesting, is a certain *reaching out* (literal, rather than figurative), enacted between the stuff of my own corporeality and that of the cadavers being revealed to me, that exceeds the epistemological sureties — indeed, the epistemological hegemony — of vision and sight, in the kinds of scientistic discourses exemplified by Von Hagens's website, quoted above.

In *The Absent Body*, Drew Leder writes precisely at the point where visibility and tangibility intersect. In an extraordinary chapter titled 'The Recessive Body', Leder develops a phenomenological account of that aspect of embodiment that most defies the access not only of scopocentric knowledge, but of the individual body's capacity to feel itself. The body, writes Leder, has 'intrinsic tendencies toward self-concealment' (Leder, 1990, p. 3):

> [t]he invisibility of the eye within its own visual field, the diaphanous embodiment of language, the inaccessibility of the visceral organs: these all exhibit their own principles of absence, which can only be teased apart by a careful investigation. (Leder, 1990, p. 2)

Phenomenological studies of embodiment, including those of Merleau-Ponty, Leder argues, have primarily revolved around 'themes of perception and motility':

> Yet such functions arise within a series of impersonal horizons: the embryonic body prior to birth, the autonomous rhythms of breathing and circulation, the stilled body of sleep, *the mystery of the corpse*. (Leder, 1990, p. 2; emphasis IM)

Leder's argument is that Merleau-Ponty's account of embodiment — and in particular his figuring of the ontological notion of 'flesh' as the primal element out of which both the lived subject and the world are born, in its account of this flesh as an intertwining of the visible and the invisible through which I am given being in the world — is itself overly reliant upon, and limited by, an understanding of the lived body as both the source of, and the object of, perception. For Merleau-Ponty, the intertwining between the body as perceiver and perceived and, as perceived, as partaking of a radical continuity with the world-as-perceived is the essence of embodiment. For Merleau-Ponty, writes Leder,

> the notion of flesh remains, in the broadest sense, an ontologizing of perception. It includes the intertwining of perceiver and perceived, the synergic crossing of different perceptual modalities, the reversibility of my perception with that of another, the fleshing out of perception with ideality and language. Another name Merleau-Ponty offers for the flesh is 'Visibility' (…). It is the body surface, visioning and visible, that is taken as the *exemplar sensible* of flesh. (Leder, 1990, p. 64)

What, however, of those dimensions of one's own embodiment that defy perception? Merleau-Ponty's version of embodiment, suggests Leder, 'still bears a distant resemblance to its Cartesian predecessor, never fully fleshed out with bone and guts' (Leder, 1990, p. 36):

> my surface powers rely upon deeper vegetative processes (…) [m]ore than just a 'cluster of consciousnesses,' [Merleau-Ponty's phrase] my body is a chiasm of conscious and unconscious levels, a visero-esthesiological being. (Leder, 1990, p. 65)

Those dimensions of our bodies that are 'neither the agents nor objects of sensibility', Leder suggests, might be characterized less in terms of a logic of intertwined visibility and invisibility, than in terms of what he calls 'Viscerality':

> Like the Visible, the Visceral cannot be properly said to belong to the subject; it is a power that traverses me, granting me life in ways I have never fully willed nor comprehended. (Leder, 1990, p. 65)

It is this viscerality to which we are exposed when confronted by the anatomical body; it is this viscerality, as much as the spectacle of the body's interior, that confronts us. In no sense is viscerality reducible to visibility: even when rendered visible — and even when visibility is understood as chiasmatically intertwined with invisibility, as it is in Merleau-Ponty's ontology — the visceral defies the logics of visibility. This is what is so unsettling about the experience of the anatomical theatre: the epistemological promise made in the name of visibility cannot be delivered upon. It is this incommensurability that is registered in Rembrandt's painting and in Da Cortona; and it is this incommensurability that Von Hagens attempts, with the rhetoric of aesthetics and democracy, to sweep to one side.

To be sure, the rendering of that which is generally hidden in the cold light of the surgical lamp (or those of the television studio) constitutes a sharp break with the contours of our everyday experience. It is, writes Leder,

> quite rare for the viscera to be exposed in life. This can happen, as in surgery, wartime injury, or violent accidents, yet these are pathological and dangerous occasions. Most commonly, the direct exposure of the inner organs implies or threatens death. (Leder, 1990, p. 44)

Life is, itself, 'allied to a certain concealment, a withdrawal and protection of its vital center' (Leder, 1990, p. 45). But key to Leder's figuring of viscerality is the disjuncture between the visible and the visceral: the irreducibility of the latter to the former, and, indeed, the conditions of emergence of the former *in* the latter.

> This visceral circuit is intertwined, an identity-in-difference with the visible body (...). I can imagine the red, textured spectacle that awaits the surgeon who opens up. Conversely, my powers of vision are installed in Viscerality, shaped and sustained by anonymous life. The eye lives only by virtue of the stomach's labour (...). (Leder, 1990, p. 65)

The world is 'installed within me', writes Leder; 'I arose out of viscerality'; viscerality is the condition for the possibility of emergence of perception. Viscerality is that which reaches out to us from Da Cortona's drawings; it is what, as a fundamental of being, overflows Von Hagens's earnest entreaties for us to treat the phenomena of his public dissections as aesthetic spectacle (Leder, 1990, pp. 66-67). It is what draws us to ask: whose body is that?

And at stake, of course, is death. For just as visibility and invisibility entwine to create the possibility of knowing in perception, viscerality is shot through with the conditions of its negation:

> Where yesterday I cavorted with a living person, today I confront the physicality of the corpse. It lies there, strangely unmoving, unseeing flesh, no longer a play of absences and reference. Body qua body now emerges, freezing my gaze within its boundaries as the lived body never could. (Leder, 1990, p. 146)

For Leder, in the apprehension of the anatomized body, 'my own corpse is experienced in an anticipatory fashion, residing implicitly within my living body (...). The corpse is always approaching from within' (Leder, 1990, p. 144).

The visceral reaches across to us, even as we are invited to imagine that we are merely watching, and that this mere watching need not, should not, cannot unsettle us. The watching, far from being neutral, aesthetically mollifying, or democratizing, however, always betrays the synaesthetic grounds of watching's own possibility: even as I merely watch, I touch, I smell, I hear, feel and sense, not merely that which, once invisible, is now rendered visible; I *intuit* the breadth, depth and implacability of the visceral. The visceral demands of me a relationship with the cadaver that cannot be exhausted by legal caveat, or enlightenment nicety. A being, a life, lies on the slab, and demands that I ask of it: who were you?

Ian Maxwell is Chair of the Department of Performance Studies at the University of Sydney, Australia. He is a graduate of the Victorian College of the Arts, where he majored in Theatre Directing, before completing his PhD, an ethnography of hip hop culture in suburban Australia. He has written extensively about youth culture and popular music. His current research interests include sport and nationalism, and a comparative study of actor training and sports coaching.

Notes

1   My transcription from *Anatomy for Beginners*, 'Episode 1: Movement', produced in 2005, and released on DVD by Madman Entertainment, first screened in Australia on SBS-TV (Special Broadcast Service — Australia's multicultural and multilingual public broadcaster) in July 2006, three months after *The Anatomical Theatre Revisited* conference.

2   My transcription from *Anatomy for Beginners*, 'Episode 4: Reproduction'.

3   Most of the exhibited plastinates are male bodies. The FAQ page on the website explains why: 'Sensitive to perceived community concerns, Dr. Von Hagens did not want to appear voyeuristic in revealing too many female bodies. Further, he sees himself in the tradition of Renaissance anatomists, whose works traditionally included far more masculine than feminine bodies, since all but the reproductive systems are essentially the same. The musculature of male bodies is generally more pronounced and illustrates more aspects of the muscle system. The organs on display come primarily from the female body donors' (Body Worlds, Questions & Anwers).

4   The data sets generated by the VHP are available upon application at www.nlm.nih. gov/research/visible/getting_data.html. Accessed November 17, 2006. 'A single License Agreement covering use of both the male and female Visible Human Project® datasets is available, as either a text file or a WordPerfect file. Please make two copies of the agreement and have both signed as originals by your appropriate officials. The agreement requires that you include a brief statement explaining your

intended use of the dataset. Send both signed copies of the agreement and the statement of how you intend to use the data.' An extraordinary set of samples is available at www.nlm.nih.gov/research/visible/visible_gallery.htm. Accessed November 17, 2006.

5   The plates of Da Cortona's *Tabulae anatomicae* may be viewed and downloaded at www.lib.uiowa.edu/hardin/rbr/imaging/cortona/. Accessed November 17, 2006.

6   But maybe more than just 'grasp'; David Michael Kleinberg-Levin writes: 'If our gestures were to correspond appropriately to their ontological appropriation, they would need to relate to the being of the beings we touch and handle with a tactfulness that leaves their being intact, while also letting their transience, their perishability, and their intangible relation to nothingness become manifest' (Kleinberg-Levin, 2005, p. 252). Perhaps the Da Cortonas call out for us to stroke, hold, and caress those bodies, yielding to them in passivity, rather than simply in the seizing of that is a grasp. Thank you to Jeff Stewart for this observation.

7   My transcription from *Anatomy for Beginners*, 'Episode: Digestion'.

8   Ibid.

References

Body Worlds website,
   'The Plastination Process', www.koerperwelten.com/en/plastination/plastination_process.html.
   'Bodyworlds: Mission of the Exhibitions', www.koerperwelten.com/en/exhibitions/mission_exhibitions.html.
   'Questions & Answers', www.koerperwelten.com/en/exhibitions/questions_answers.html. Accessed November 17, 2006.

Channel 4, 'Introduction', 'Demonstrators', and 'Home' at website Anatomy for Beginners. www.channel4.com/science/microsites/A/anatomy/intro.html. Accessed November 17, 2006.

Czarnecka-Anastassiades, B. M., '"Holding the Mirror up to Nature": Bodies Anatomized, Bodies Mirrored in Pietro da Cortona'. Paper presented at *The Anatomical Theatre Revisited* conference, University of Amsterdam, April 6, 2006.

Dijck, J. van, 'The Virtual Anatomical Theatre: The Visible Human Project'. Paper presented at *The Anatomical Theatre Revisited* conference, University of Amsterdam, April 5, 2006.

Firefly-Channel 4, *Anatomy for Beginners*. Television series, 2005.

Goodall, J. R., *Performance and Evolution in the Age of Darwin: Out of the Natural Order*. London and New York, 2002.

Kleinberg-Levin, D. M., *Gestures of Ethical Life: Reading Hölderlin's Question of Measure after Heidegger*. Stanford, 2005.

Leder, D., *The Absent Body*. Chicago and London, 1990.

National Library of Medicine (NLM), Factsheet the *Visible Human Project*.

www.nlm.nih.gov/pubs/factsheets/visible_human.html.
Last updated: May 28, 2004. First published: January 1, 1996.
Accessed November 17, 2006.

Sebald, W.G., *The Rings of Saturn.* London, 2002 [1995].

Performance Documentation 2:
Excavations: Fresh but Rotten

The creation of the perfect imperfect

A physician told Marijs Boulogne how he fell into a depression for years after having suffered the loss of his newborn baby. 'How can it be that he, as a physician, does not have an answer to that?' Boulogne wondered. 'How come he has so much trouble finding ways to deal with this event?' His account made her notice the lack of narratives around this topic. It made her decide to create a story about it herself.

She began by asking herself: 'What would I do if it happened to me? In what way could I prepare myself for such an event? How would I be able to find consolation?' In reaction to these questions, she started to make a dress

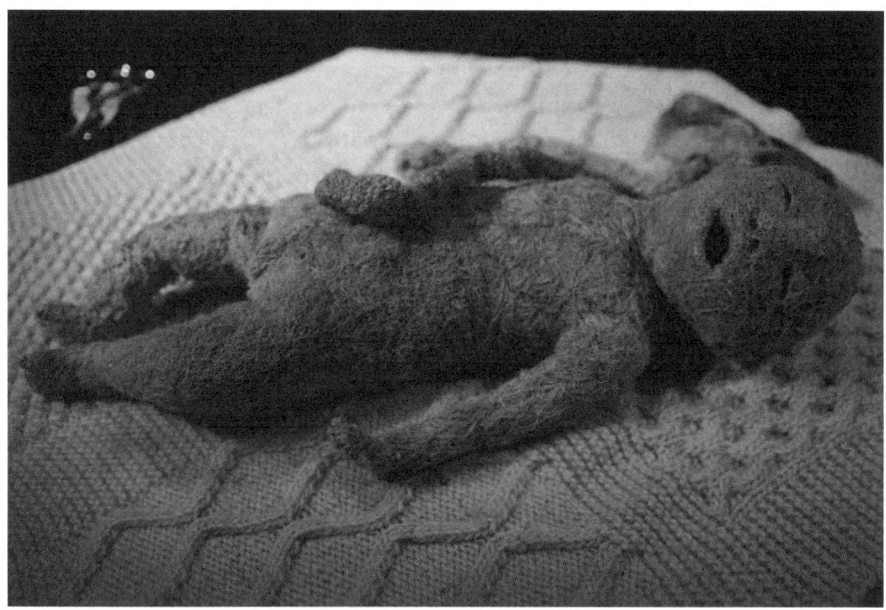

Excavations: Fresh but Rotten by Marijs Boulogne (2006). Photo: Giannina Urmeneta Ottiker.

that, in case it DID happen to her, she would be able to put on her own baby. She spent three months working on the dress, driven by the colours she was using for the embroidery. By the time she had the finished dress, it occurred to her that this was only the beginning. She decided to create the baby as well.

The preparation of this project took a couple of years. Boulogne experimented with imitating little pieces of skin and organs. The process was slow and very expensive: she soon ran out of money and material. But then she accidentally inherited piles of embroidery thread and crewel from a woman at whose deathbed she sat for months and from her grandmother, who was losing her sight. The thousand colours of this new material encouraged her decision to really start with her project, which she named *Excavations*.

Boulogne made an enormous effort to create all the baby's organs in full anatomical detail, and to correctly shape its little bones out of salt dough. For more than a year she studied anatomical manuals and read accounts of surgeons to learn about the organs she was imitating, and to become acquainted with the vocabulary of the medical discourse. Travelling frequently, she kept working on the baby. She made the placenta in Copenhagen, the kidneys in Italy, and continued her work on the intestines in Sydney. As the features of the baby began to grow, she started to get inquiring looks when screening her baggage at customs.

After ten months of work, when she finished the head and attached it to the body, she was herself astonished. The baby was beautiful. But it was also the saddest thing she had ever seen. The positive reactions of audiences to the *Excavations* performances, which she had begun to stage during the creation process, convinced her that this anatomical embroidery could nevertheless enable her to address the questions she had set out to ask: 'How to cope with the event of a stillborn baby? How to deal with the perfect imperfect?'

In *Fresh but Rotten*, the fifth phase of the *Excavations* project, Marijs Boulogne, as 'Moedere Hein' (Mother Hein) carries the baby on stage, wrapped in her arms.[1] 'This is the body of a new born baby. It is a girl. I called her Pas. But she cannot live. I made her in more than ten months. And that is way too long.'[2] On a table in the centre of the stage, she tenderly washes the baby, and subsequently examines the different colours of the baby's skin, explaining their meanings to the audience. Through a hand-held camera that is employed by the 'image nurse' Julia Clever, the details of the embroideries are shown on a big screen behind the table. Moedere Hein's examination soon moves beyond the baby's skin. 'But today I want to know. My baby is old already. Today I want to enter, and to look straight into the lungs, because I want to find out whether she has breathed.' With a scalpel, she makes a 'Y'-shaped incision, over the chest and the length of the torso. Subsequently, she displays the various, brightly-coloured organs of the baby, alternately filming them in close-up with the hand-held camera or a rigid endoscope, which results in a kind of fantastic medical imagery on the screen. After this autopsy, she puts the organs back in the body and puts a brightly embroidered dress on the baby.

The grotesque quality of an embroidered baby

Excavations presents a dissection of an embroidered baby. The prohibition of the transgression of the natural borders of the body can be regarded as a cultural law in our society, violated in the act of dissection. In medical practice, the dissection of human bodies is an everyday activity. It has often been argued that the violation of the body in medical practice is disguised by the authoritarian status of this discourse. In discussing the body in medicine, Katharine Young makes a similar statement. She argues that medicine is an aristocratic discourse, using its high status and sacralized vocabulary to hide the grotesque quality of the dissected body (Young, 1997). According to Young, the act of dissection implies a destruction of the conventional order of the body and therefore features the defining quality of what Mikhail Bakhtin has called 'the grotesque' (Bakhtin, 1984). The acknowledgment of the grotesque quality of the baby in *Excavations* offers an interesting perspective on this theatre performance. The actions of turning things upside down, inside out, and transgressing the boundaries between various discourses characterizes *Excavations*, especially in the playful approach toward the 'high' medical discourse, and in the presentation of the corpse as a vital and fertile substance.

In performing the role of Moedere Hein, Marijs Boulogne represents both the mother of the baby and the pathologist who is conducting the autopsy. The combination of these roles in one actor's character has a complex effect, due to their contrasting qualities. On the one hand, the pathologist with the scalpel, who commands the anatomical vocabulary, represents the authoritative medical discourse. Young observed that during an autopsy '[t]he particularity, the possible personhood, of the corpse is elided by the passive voice, which not only banishes agent and perceiver but also objectifies the object of perception' (Young, 1997, p. 116). On the other hand, the maternal nature of the alternative side of the character Boulogne performs seems to partially thwart this effect. Our awareness of the mother and child relationship between the pathologist and the dissected baby shifts our experience of the autopsy. It is no longer fully possible to objectify our perception of the baby or to disregard its 'possible personhood'. This surprising transgression, using two such widely different discourses, intensifies both our perception of the intimacy between mother and baby, and the violent nature of the dissection. By creating this double character, Boulogne challenges the emotional detachment that is usually associated with medical practice.

Although Moedere Hein starts with the objective to find medical evidence of life in the body, the primary function of the autopsy seems to be to bring the beauty of the baby to the fore. The hand-held camera and the endoscope used in this process function not so much as medical, but as theatrical tools. The body is not only opened to the external world through its natural orifices, the organs are lifted out and held up to be admired. In addition, the endoscope offers up even the smallest details to public view. Despite the taboo against the act of explicitly showing the body interior, the double-layered character of Moedere Hein creates a private sphere for the spectators, one in which they can admire the beauty of what is shown, rather than feeling like an uninvolved onlooker at a controversial or intimidating spectacle.

This intimate spectacle continues when the autopsy has ended. After Moedere Hein has dressed the baby, she begins piling grey, brown, green, yellow and white skeins, and yarns of different textures, onto the small body. It takes a while for the audience to realize that the process of dressing the baby at this point is transforming into the mimesis of the rotting process of the dead body. This subtle, but at the same time radical transition not only once again

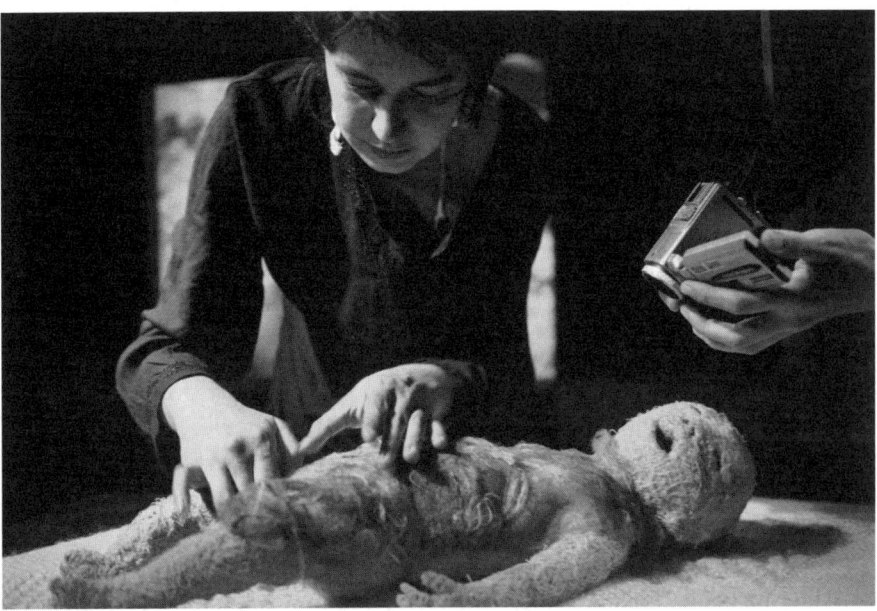

Excavations: Fresh but Rotten by Marijs Boulogne (2006). Photo: Giannina Urmeneta Ottiker.

draws attention to the beauty of the body, but also demonstrates the vital quality of the dead material.

During the autopsy the skin is cut open, and afterwards the mould starts to seep and to grow through it. This erasure of the boundary of the baby's skin emphasizes the grotesque quality of the body. The cloth skin disappears as a discrete boundary, resulting in a blurring of the distinction between the inside and outside of our conventional body orientation. Apart from its imitation of this biological process, this scene also has a strong ritual quality. As Moedere Hein starts the performance by putting the dress on the baby, this later act of covering the baby with colourful layers can be interpreted as a ritual act of decoration, which helps her to mark and cope with her loss.

When the baby is completely covered with the colourful and mouldy textures, caterpillars and snails, made out of pieces of cloth and salt dough, slowly conquer the body, making it their playground. Moedere Hein creates a miniature paradise for the small creatures, by placing a white skein of milk coming out of the baby's mouth: 'These are the places of milk and honey, there is plenty for everyone, and everything is beautiful, and tasty, and free.' The caterpillars mumble happily in reply: 'We can stay and live here! We can hide here forever. We are free. We can enter and exit, and play anywhere we want.' The hand-held camera close-ups of the animals playing hide-and-seek between

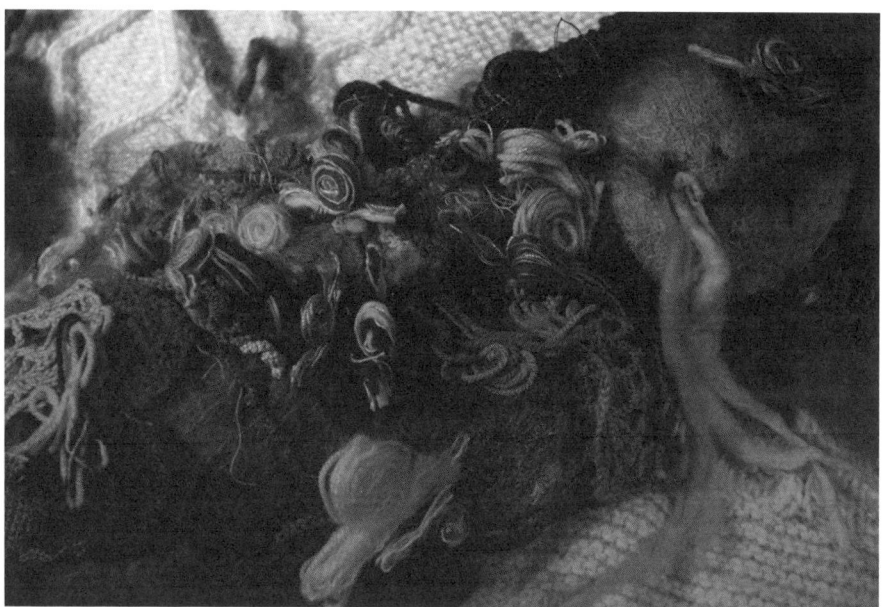

Excavations: Fresh but Rotten by Marijs Boulogne (2006). Photo: Giannina Urmeneta Ottiker.

the fantastic cloth structures emphasize that the baby has transformed into a wondrous landscape or microcosm. It has become a small fantastic universe, reminiscent of the anatomical cabinets created by seventeenth-century Dutch anatomist Frederik Ruysch (1638-1731). Ruysch was a pioneer in preserving techniques of bodily organs and tissue and made artistic tableaux using baby skeletons and injected and coloured veins and arteries to suggest a botanical environment.[3]

The vitality and fertility of dead material that is displayed stresses once more the grotesque quality of *Excavations's* imagery. The 'conventional view of the corpse as absence, barrenness, and stillness' is fully denied by this playful, dynamic scene (Young, 1997, p. 114). Then, all of a sudden, two birds that look like two golden stork-shaped scissors appear in the air above Pas. They scream: 'Feast! Feast! Feast!' diving down to devour the caterpillars, the snails, and the soft, tasty tissues the small creatures were playing in. When the festive dinner of the birds is over, Moedere Hein wraps all the animals, together with the baby, in a white cloth and takes the loose bundle back into her arms. 'Hear, the birds are singing for us, and the butterflies have come out.' As the lights fade, she carries Pas offstage. A hint of silhouettes of butterflies can be perceived, and the chirping birds continue.

Text by *Laura Karreman*

The Belgian performer **Marijs Boulogne** (1978) studied theatre direction at the Kunsthogeschool RITS in Brussels. With Manah Depauw and Bart Capelle she founded the group Buelens Paulina. *Endless Medication*, the graduation project created by Boulogne and Depauw, was staged at the KunstenFESTI-VALdesArts 2003 in Brussels. In her second graduation project Boulogne made an installation, *Fuck me dead / Foreplay*, with a doll and a dress, in which she combined embroidery, performance, and video for the first time, working together with Julia Clever.

Laura Karreman is currently finishing her RMA in Art Studies with a major in Theatre Studies at the University of Amsterdam.

Performance Data

The *Excavations* project was first presented in 2004. Since then the following phases have been staged: *Pregnancy, Excavation, Episcopy, In Memories, Fresh but Rotten*, *Report*, and *Pas(*)*. The project was first performed in Belgium and the Netherlands. The French-language version premiered at Belluard Bollwerk International 2006 in Fribourg (Switzerland). The first English-language version is due to be performed in 2007, in Oslo (Norway).

More information about this performance project and Marijs Boulogne can be found at www.excavations.be and www.buelens-paulina.be.

Concept and embroidery: Marijs Boulogne
Video: Julia Clever
Performers: Marijs Boulogne, Julia Clever, Tom de Roy, Jan Philips, Paulti Taes and
    Wilfrieda Stroobants
Production: Buelens Paulina a.s.b.s. and Vicky Vermoezen
Dramaturgy and coaching: Marianne van Kerkhoven and Lotte van den Berg
Thanks to: Kaaitheater, Kc Stuk, Time Festival 2005, Kc nOna, Stad in Vrouwen-
    handen, Beursschouwburg, Vooruit, Huis aan de Werf Utrecht and the Flemish
    Community – a special thank you to Thomas Anklin (Anklin AG) and Eugeen
    Steurs.

Notes

1   This documentation is based on the particular phase of the *Excavations* project shown
     in the Huis aan de Werf during Festival aan de Werf 2006, in Utrecht, the Netherlands,
     May 18-27, 2006.
2   All quotes are my translations from the unpublished Dutch script for this phase of
     Excavations, written by Marijs Boulogne: *Pas maar al rot. Tragedie van Handen.* (*Fresh
     but Rotten. Tragedy of Hands*).
3   Some examples of etchings of Ruysch's work can be found at the Dream Anatomy
     Gallery of the US National Library of Medicine. See for example www.nlm.nih.gov/
     exhibition/dreamanatomy/da_g_I-C-1-09.html.

References

Bakhtin, M., *Rabelais and his World*. (Trans. Helene Iswolsky) Blooming-
    ton, 1984.
Boulogne, M., 'Pas maar al rot. Tragedie van Handen.' Unpublished script,
    2007.
Young, K., 'Still Life With Corpse: Pathology'. In: K. Young, *Presence in the Flesh.
    The Body in Medicine*. pp. 108-129. Cambridge, Mass. and London, 1997.

The Anatomy Lesson of Professor Moxham

Karen Ingham

If you were to enter a theatre of anatomy, what would you expect to see? A musty old museum perhaps, replete with pickled specimens, deformed skeletons, and faded anatomical atlases? Or you may be anticipating a tour of the architectural splendours of the Vesalian Teatro Anatomico in Padua, where executed

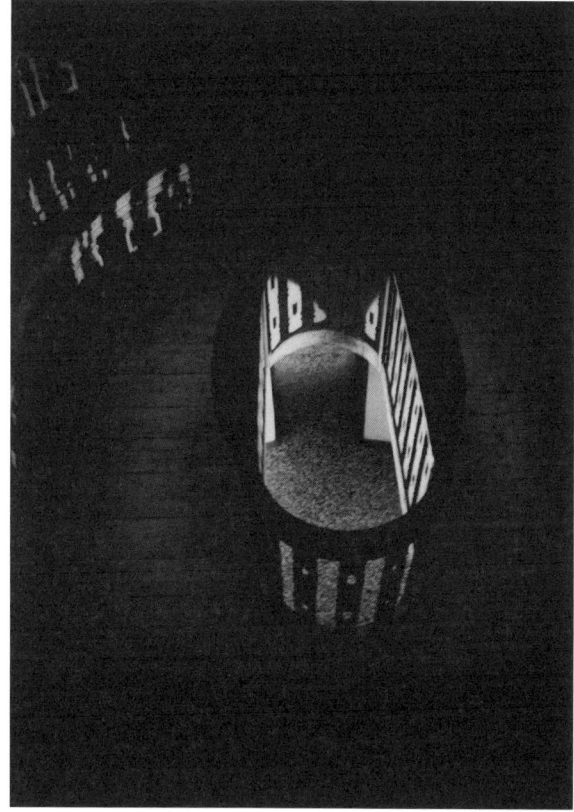

Teatro Anatomico, Padua.
Photo: Karen Ingham.
Reproduced with permission
of the photographer.

criminals had their bodies publicly dissected by the master anatomist for the edification of a paying audience of the great and the good. Perhaps, you expect to glimpse these bodies, their skin pinned back by alphabetical markers like so much loose cloth on a lifeless mannequin? Or are you of the opinion that these spectacles and specimens should remain off-limits to all but staff and students of the medical schools? But what if I were to tell you that from the comfort of your own home, you too may become a spectator in the theatre of the dead, and that the digital body of an executed criminal may be downloaded onto your computer at the flick of a switch,[1] just as his real body was extinguished when the executioner threw the switch on his 'electric chair'.

Or perhaps you were under the impression that it was only metaphysical mavericks like René Descartes that searched for the soul in the seat of the brain, labouring under the illusion that the 'mind's eye' could, in a fashion, perceive images and sense pain and pleasure through the flow of 'pineal spirits' as he suggested in his complex and ultimately flawed *La Dioptrique* of 1637.[2] Descartes's probing fingers were simply too blunt an instrument with which to decode that most complex of organs, the brain, but had he had access to a twenty-first-century fMRI scanner, he would indeed have proved his point that it is possible to 'read' the mind and to render (digitally) what pain and pleasure look like.[3] It may also surprise you to learn that you may not be so very different from that Vesalian spectator peering over vertiginous Renaissance balconies gawping at the subject made object, only your viewing is restricted to the television screen or computer monitor, or perhaps as a 'ringside' spectator at one of the infamous Gunther von Hagens's 'live' autopsies.[4] Otherwise, you are no doubt happy to leave the *real* process of death and degeneration to the experts, placing your trust in high-tech medical scanners that have made the surgeon's eye all but obsolete (see Kember, 1998, p. 55). Ah, but the mastery of the surgeon's hand lives on, you may say. But even this great metaphor of human endeavour and achievement may in time be replaced with nanotechnology that operates from *within* the diseased and damaged body, leaving the scalpel rusting on the tray while the hand gestures pointlessly.

Meanwhile, the process of death and dying goes on, and palliative carers and undertakers are thriving, and should you elect to be one of the few who donate their bodies to science, you will find yourself being taken apart by would-be surgeons whose understanding of human anatomy is not yet wholly defined by computer simulations where dissection is performed not with a scalpel but with a mouse. And beyond digital simulacra that may yet make the body redundant, what then? For as this essay posits, the epistemic positioning of the body in the anatomo-clinical[5] theatre is not a purely historic project, and even if it is perceived thus, history, like science, is discontinuous, progressively re-inventing its terms of reference. The theatre of anatomy, and the body dissected therein, is not moribund and mothballed but is, conversely, dynamic and evolving.

I am proposing that far from being a relic of the past assigned to the realms of museology, the anatomy theatre is flourishing under new surgical and digital façades. As will become apparent, I am also suggesting that contemporary collaborations between art and bioscience are re-appropriating and re-vitalizing the anatomical theatre, and the collaborative anatomical artworks of the Renaissance and the Baroque, stimulating new discourses on the nature of subjectivity and vision in an era of rapidly changing digital medical technology and genetic transformation. It will be evident in the artworks I discuss that lens-based imaging, and photography in particular, are vital components of this field of creative and scientific endeavour, as the phenomenological authority of the photograph is deeply embedded in our understanding of the anatomo-clinical body and its spaces.[6] My arguments are based in part on the observations and insights I have acquired from working as a cultural producer in what is commonly referred to as 'sciart' collaboration (creative and intellectual partnerships between the arts and sciences). My research is also influenced by arguments for the interdependence of theory and practice and by my interest in the role of the artist as simultaneous cultural and textual producer.

In my practice-based research I have collaborated with anatomists, surgeons and bio-scientists. Correspondingly, the spaces I am excavating, namely the anatomical theatre and its evolution to operating theatre and subsequently to the high-tech laboratories of the digital body, reference the history of these spaces and how these architectures of power influenced the performance of the anatomo-clinical body. Although I refer to the anatomical artworks of the Renaissance and the Baroque, I do not wish to dwell on the history of anatomical representation in these periods, but rather explore how and why the anatomical art produced at that time (which engendered some of the most enduring and inventive visual representations of the human body) continues to exert such a powerful fascination for contemporary artists questioning bodily representation and subjectivity.

I suggest that the hybridity and polysemicism of Renaissance and Baroque anatomo-art collaboration are illustrative of a time when anatomy, art, astronomy and even alchemy could happily interconnect rather than remain the discrete disciplines they are today. This trans-disciplinarity has a particular resonance with contemporary artists who are re-invigorating notions of the Baroque, not as a specific chronological period, but as a scopic regime that encompasses what Christine Buci-Glucksmann has suggestively called 'the madness of vision', a vision which leans towards more open and allegorical expressions of meaning (Buci-Glucksmann, 1986, 1994). The notion of allegory is becoming more prevalent in contemporary arts practice where allegory is perceived as constituting something 'other than itself (...) one text read through another' (Berger et al., 1989). Particularly in photographic practice, an allegorical intent in the production of visual meaning is becoming increasingly attractive in a society saturated with visual imagery, a society that is no longer persuaded by photography's guarantee of unproblematic mimetic realities.

The anatomical theatre, historical and contemporary, is a space suffused with allegory, from the Vesalian image of the *Fabrica* with the dissected female cadaver whose womb comes to represent the Copernican universe – the 'matrix' or womb of meaning[7] – to the sterile high-tech labs of the *Human Genome Project* where digital DNA fragments hang suspended in an electronic matrix. The architecture and metaphysics of the anatomical theatre influenced and continue to influence the way the anatomo-clinical body is located within particular hierarchies of power and surveillance, and we know this, in part, through anatomical collaborations that have produced artworks which provoke, stimulate and question the very notion of what it is to be human; images which seek to tell a story and teach a lesson.

The Anatomy Lesson

Rembrandt's *The Anatomy Lesson of Dr Nicolaes Tulp* (1632), suggestive as it is of the great suite of Dutch anatomy lesson paintings, is a crucial image in terms of understanding the epistemic structures and scopic regimes of the anatomical body and its theatre. The reading and interpretation of Rembrandt's image is discussed in detail in the work of Jonathan Sawday (1995) and Francis Barker (1995), both of whom bring the theatre of anatomy and its representation well and truly to light in their eloquent and incisive analysis of the Renaissance and Enlightenment cadaver and its entourage.[8] The performativity of the dead body and the hierarchy of 'players' surrounding the publicly displayed corpse was enacted on the dissecting slabs of leading European theatres of anatomy, where the opening of the body by 'star' anatomists was publicly performed as an allegory of supremacy and revelation.

Having exhibited in the very building in which Rembrandt's painting was hung (Amsterdam's Waag), the painting holds a particular significance and is central to my practice.[9] The sign in Rembrandt's painting that is perhaps most visible (and the subject of much academic discussion) is that of Tulp's gesturing hand demonstrating the physiological mechanism of the corpse's hand. The hand is a central metaphor for anatomical progress and understanding, and is a particularly visible component of the Baroque suite of anatomy lesson paintings.[10] Martin Kemp and Marina Wallace note that: 'For artists the hand was a communicative device second only in eloquence to the face. The refined motions of Tulp's own left hand precisely demonstrate the subtlety of this intricate piece of bodily design' (Kemp and Wallace, 2000, p. 28). But the real complexity of the hands within the painting becomes apparent in Barker's analysis where he observes that although Tulp's forceps seem to be the ideal instrument with which to epistemically process and reconstitute the criminal body of Aris Kindt[11] (and I use the term criminal here in its historic not judicial sense as Kindt was little more than a petty thief hardly deserving of execution), they are in fact gesturing towards a fictitious and anomalous anatomy 'lesson'. Not only would an anatomist never begin the process of anatomy with the hand, being compelled by necessity in the days of pre-refrigeration and chemical embalming to open the abdomen and extract and dispose of the already putrefying viscera first, but, according to Barker's contentious argument, the tendons in the palm of Kindt's left hand belong in fact to the back of the right hand (Barker, 1995, p. 71). But the technical minutiae of the hand argument is misleading, for what is at stake here is not realism but symbolism; the painting is not a 'lesson' but an allegorical story of its time. As an allegory the painting can be read on many different levels, its layers of meaning peeled back like loose skin. But herein lies the problem, for where an artist or cultural theorist will eschew absolutism and pedantry, likely components of an actual anatomy lesson, for the anatomist the staging of the body in the anatomical theatre represents a journey from superstition to science, and any detour from realism to relativism is a perilous one. That is why the comparatively recent rapprochement between artists and anatomists is so important in re-establishing what was once a thriving and inventive collaborative partnership. As an example of this process, I want to look at a contemporary photographic tableau that directly corresponds to Rembrandt's *Tulp*, and to analyse this and several other contemporary artworks within a broader framework of medical-arts collaboration in the anatomical theatre. *The Anatomy Lesson of Professor Bernard Moxham* is an example from my own sciart practice of a contemporary photographic tableau that re-appropriates Rembrandt's iconic Tulp painting, right down to the detail in the flayed hand of the subject, which is also reversed albeit the reversal was made with pixels rather than paint.

Pixels or paint, the point remains the same; the anatomy lesson paintings are not about the portrayal of medical reality even if the aesthetic employed is one of realism, but are far more densely constructed in terms of allegorical intent and dramatic suspension. Shot in the University of Cardiff dissecting rooms, the Professor and his staff (who like Tulp and his colleagues are practising anatomists) pose in painterly fashion by the subject of their dissective practice, a seated male figure whose hand has been skilfully flayed and taken back to its skeletal form. This *tableau vivant* pays homage to Rembrandt's *Tulp*, by re-appropriating the visual grammar of the original painting with the exception that

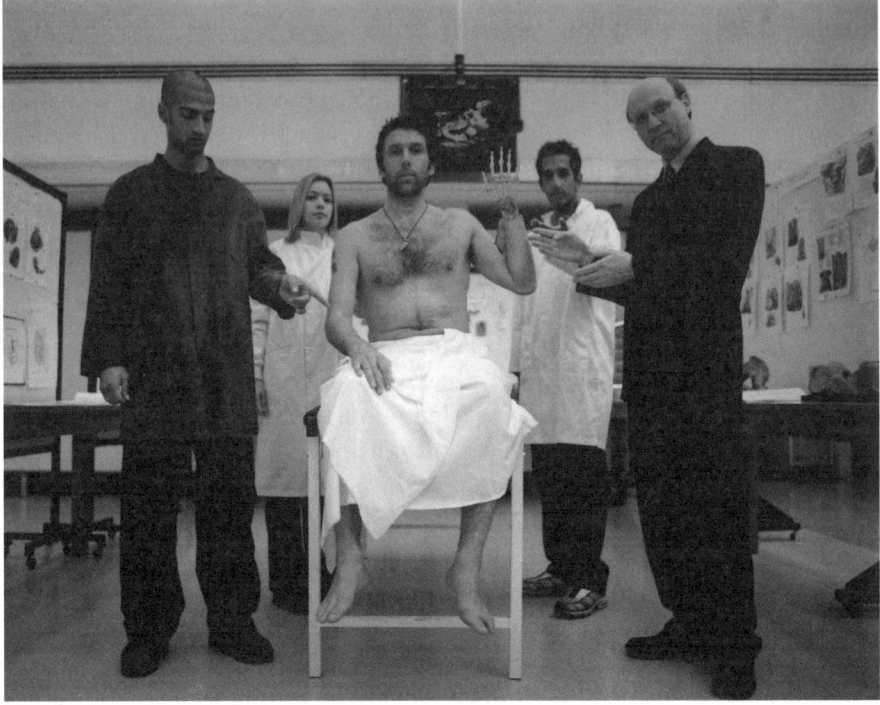

The Anatomy Lesson of Professor Bernard Moxham by Karen Ingham. Reproduced with permission of the artist.

in Moxham's anatomy lesson the instruments of dissection are digital, not surgical. Conversely, on the nearby teaching monitor a 'real' image of re-constructive hand surgery can be seen, implying that in order to successfully *re*-construct the body, we must acknowledge the anatomist's maxim 'know thyself' by first *de*-constructing the human form. Where the original anatomy lesson paintings used the medium of their time, paint, I have incorporated contemporary digital technologies, and yet the results are much the same, only now the bodies are donor bodies not those of executed criminals, and a woman is included as an active member of the medical fraternity.

One of the other key objectives of my practice-based research was the public exhibition of the artworks back in their site of origin, the actual dissecting room or anatomy museum, thus enabling the public to experience first hand the drama and latent theatricality of these normally exclusive domains (see Ingham, 2004, pp. 9-10). It is a complex and lengthy process to negotiate the staging of anatomical artworks in functioning pathology and anatomy labs due to the strict regulations regarding health and safety, confidentiality, and, in Britain at least, the 1832 Anatomy Act which is still on the statute books. The members of the public who visited the *Anatomy Lessons* exhibitions in 2003-5 were greeted by the pungent whiff of formaldehyde and working anatomists acted as their 'gallery guides'.

Yet, even anatomy theatres and labs that are no longer operational can be used to powerful effect as Amsterdam's SMART Project Space demonstrated with its 2007 exhibition *Fumus Fugiens*[12] which evoked their building's origins as a pathological anatomy lab. The Waag's Theatrum Anatomicum, though redundant for centuries as a functional anatomy theatre, frequently invites the public into this exceptional space, inscribed with the resonant traces of its bloody past, to witness new performances and artworks that re-position the anatomical body. The Waag's partnerships are evidence of the growing academic interest in the anatomical theatre from performance and theatre studies researchers.[13] This is a welcome development given the relative paucity of material for a subject that is so crucial not only to our understanding of medical epistemology and subjectivity, but also to our knowledge of how the design and performativity of a space significantly influences the nature of the acts that occur within – a kind of ergonomics of anatomy.

The development of the anatomical theatre had a profound effect not only on the evolution of our modern-day operating theatres, but also on the structures and hierarchies of learning implicit in our educational systems, with present-day universities still following the time-honoured hierarchy of professor, reader, lecturer, demonstrator, and technician, first established in the European anatomical theatres of the sixteenth and seventeenth centuries. The 'etiquette' of the anatomical theatre influenced the hierarchical seating plan and performance of the life drawing class, which was modelled on the elliptical dissecting theatres like Padua and Leiden, as evinced in Francois Salle's painting *The Anatomy Lesson at the Ecole des Beaux-Arts, Paris* (1888). In the life classes at revered art institutions such as The Royal Academy, the model took the place of the cadaver, and artists were seated closer according to experience and social status.

Following the Second World War, artists began to abandon traditional art forms such as figurative painting and drawing in favour of abstraction and new forms of modern art. When medical imaging technologies such as MRI, CAT scans, and powerful electron scanning microscopy came onto the scene, artists were attracted to this new form of bodily abstraction, and the historical relationship of the artist to the nude and to life drawing transformed into a fascination with 'the body'[14], and in particular the medical and postmortem body. Maura Flannery has commented that: 'It is ironic that when twentieth-century artists broke away from realism they grasped at elements of another realism: that of the microscopic level' (Flannery, 1998, p. 201). That the anatomo-clinical theatre is of such interest to artists comes as no surprise when we consider the array of imaging technologies that contemporary bioscience has at its disposal, or the rich and layered history of anatomical representation that artists can draw on. How beneficial sciart collaboration is to the *scientist* is another question altogether, and not one which can be brokered here, but a question I have discussed elsewhere.[15] But what is not in question is that with an informed and speculative collaboration between bio-anatomical science and art, be it textual, visual or performative, the most profound and evocative results sometimes occur.

Performing Allegories in the Theatre of Anatomy

The artist Helen Chadwick[16] engaged eloquently and poignantly with the complexities of death and disease. She frequently used allegory in her work as evinced in her installation *Unnatural Selection*, the result of Chadwick's residency at the IVF unit at King's College Hospital London. Following the artist's unexpected and sudden death, the installation was exhibited posthumously, emphasizing the *memento mori* associations of the artwork. A series of gem-like, cibachrome photographs set in clear perspex, *Unnatural Selection* is highly suggestive of the allegorized womb (think again of the Vesalian womb in *Fabrica*) integrating actual fertilized human eggs discarded by the IVF unit due to possible flaws, creating the most profound 'still life'. Chadwick used her residency at King's to learn first-hand how to locate and extract the eggs needed for her artworks, and in the process of doing so she pushed the boundaries of the emerging sciart discourse. Andrea Duncan describes the artist's engagement with the process of making the work:

> Poignantly, in some of the 'frozen' animation within the formalin, Chadwick caught the sperm still trying to enter the protective outer membranes of the fertilized and dividing egg. From these discarded eggs Chadwick created the series of photo pieces, which include works such as *Opal, Moonstrance* and *Nebula*. (Duncan, 2000, pp. 153-4)

The use of irony and allegorical intent was already established in Chadwick's work prior to *Unnatural Selection*, and her earlier works played visibly with Baroque allusions to death and the body. The sense of staging, metaphor and allegorical intent that is evident in the photographic artworks of artists like Chadwick are self-consciously authored appropriations from art historical modes of representation located in the paintings of the Renaissance and the Baroque, with their staged tableaux of the dead and their mediators.

Video artist Andrew Kotting's[17] work draws heavily on these tableaux and on the Dutch suite of anatomy lesson paintings which differ significantly from other anatomical representations in that they are concerned not so much with the physical act of dissection but with the metaphysical staging of the star anatomists reading the body as text within a heightened dramatic space – the anatomy theatre as theatre proper (as Barker and Sawday postulate). The anatomy lesson paintings make full use of the visual grammar and drama of the theatre, from Aert Pietersz's *The Anatomy Lesson of Dr. Sebastiaen Egbertsz* (1603) in which the body is barely visible, such is the throng of surgeons posturing for posterity, to the surreal *Anatomy Lesson of Dr. Frederik Ruysch* which depicts Ruysch's young son holding the skeleton of a toddler while his father dissects a stillborn infant still attached to its umbilical cord. In Adriaen Backer's *Anatomy Lesson of Dr. Frederik Ruysch* (1670), the background resembles a staged backdrop, and the impression created is that of a layered, constructed scenario where the only thing that looks alive is, perversely, the cadaver. It is this staging of the pathological body as an allegorical act of disclosure that is alluded to in Kotting's video work and publication *Mapping Perception* (2002) made in collaboration with neurophysiologist Dr. Mark Lythgoe.

At the heart of the project is an exploration of altered perception through brain dysfunction, as experienced by Kotting's teenage daughter Eden (also a participant in the project), who was born in 1988 with Joubert Syndrome, a rare genetic disorder that profoundly impairs normal neurological functioning. In one of the production's key scenes, Eden is seen lying in a darkened theatre surrounded by what appear to be Dutch anatomists straight out of the anatomy lessons suite. Beautifully lit and staged, the scene of the male anatomists scrutinizing the inert body of the teenage Eden is a profound reminder of the role medicine played in perpetuating positivist notions of difference in terms of the dichotomy between able and disabled, and how we perceive the disabled and they themselves. But what Kotting's work also reminds us of is the role medicine has played in creating male hierarchies of power and knowledge, reducing the female body to little more than a cipher or fetish, primed for de-coding and display as an allegory of the mastery of male science.

Kotting is one of a number of contemporary artists who are using allegory and metaphor to explore contemporary issues of bodily difference in the anatomo-clinical theatre, the work of Alexa Wright being another notable example. Wright is perhaps best known for her photographic tableaux of limb-impaired subjects in her 1998-9 series 'I'. This profoundly challenging and conceptually and visually layered body of work reflects many important issues: the authenticity of the body; the definition and authoring of otherness, particularly in relation to the female body; the use of new technologies to create empowering virtual realities.

In 'I' Wright creates seductive photographic images that challenge conventions of normality and acceptance in relation to the disabled body. In all but one instance Wright carefully juxtaposes her own face onto the disabled body of the sitter. In one of the most widely published images from the series, Wright's virtual and limb-impaired body is located within a baroque setting that plays on the Venus de Milo beautification of the limbless female torso.

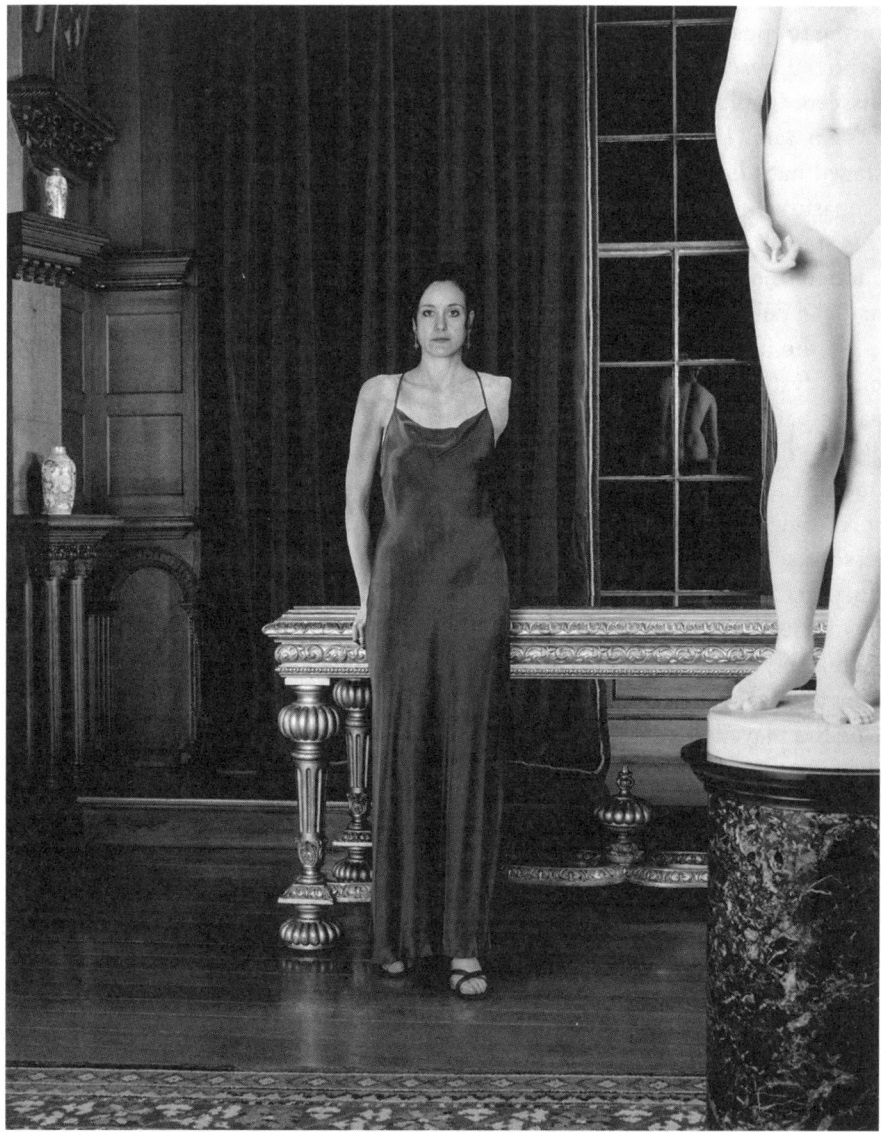

'I' by Alexa Wright. Reproduced with permission of the artist.

Rachel Gear suggests that:

> [t]he interplay between bodies is particularly important – the head and
> one arm of the statue remain outside the frame. The reflection in the win-
> dow hovers between the human figure and the statue to create a shifting
> sense of wholeness and fragmentation (...) [T]he sitter in this case, Cathe-
> rine Long, felt able to identify with the image as her own body (...) [T]he
> fact that the sitter, on viewing the image, felt that her shoulder belonged to
> another body is profound. (Gear, 2003, p. 110)

Through negotiation and collaboration, Wright turns what at first glance appears to be a troubling and potentially exploitative situation (Wright herself is
not disabled and is thus in a questionable position in representing disability)
into an empowering dialogue between able-bodied artist and disabled collaborator, and beyond to the unseen viewer. Collaboration is at the heart of Wright's
photographic artworks, and 'I' was a development from the artist's previous
collaborative project *After Image* (1997), which was informed by dialogue with
neuropsychologist Peter Halligan and neurologist John Kew. Working in close
collaboration with her limb-impaired subjects, the project helped the amputees
come to terms with the phenomena of phantom limb loss. Since 2001 Wright
has been a regular collaborator with medical physicist Alf Linney, teaming up
to create a number of art and bio-science interactions such as *Face Value* (2001),
Alter Ego (2005) and most recently *Conversation Piece* (2007).

   Wright's working practice is very similar to my own, seeking inventive collaborations through sciart funding agencies, which encourage innovation and
engagement with complex biomedical issues. Her work is concerned with questioning notions of normality (and in this sense it could be said to be a visual
expression of Georges Canguilhem's 1943 work on the normal and the pathological) and in rupturing society's accepted view of the body.

   The artist Neal White also utilizes digital imaging and diagnostic technologies in his work. The first artist in residence at the *Human Genome Mapping
Project* (HGMP) near Cambridge, White's aptly entitled *Inheritance* (1999) was,
like Wright's practice, the result of lengthy collaboration and discussion with
his scientific collaborators. The environment at HGMP is sterile and intensely
clinical as befits a scientific project using state-of-the-art computer technology
to map and analyse complex genetic data, but for an artist, the sterility of such
an environment can be visually daunting. White's response to this predicament
was to work more conceptually on the notion of genetic identity and inheritance, a task that was made somewhat easier for him through his knowledge
of computing and digital technology. In *Inheritance 3* White presents us with
a pixelated self-portrait that refers to the process of genetic markers. Sian Ede,

Arts Director of the Calouste Gulbenkian Foundation (the funder of White's residency) describes the image as corresponding:

> (...) directly to the number of markers contained within the artist's geno-type, which was established after a blood sample was refined to pure DNA and marked by HGMP researchers. As a controlling computer causes the pixels to become illuminated one by one, the genotype is gradually revea-led, made human as a photo-image of the artist's face. (Ede, 2000, p. 27)

But I suggest this pixelated 'genetic' face is less an expression of inheritance and individuality (for indeed, its very lack of definition renders it a generaliza-tion) than an allegory of anatomy. In its most basic form human anatomy is the systemic analysis of the form, structure, and most especially the internal structure of the body. The aim of the anatomist, put simply, is to deconstruct and disassemble the body in order that we may know it better. However, there are obvious dangers in deconstructing something to the point of erasure, as is possible in the context of digital bodies[18] or in looking so closely at the in-terior mechanics of a body that it ceases to exist as a holistic subject, as is the case in the Cartesian machine-body scenario. If you look too closely at Neal White's *Inheritance 3*, you will see only fragments, chaotic and seemingly ran-dom. But step back to view the picture as a whole, and the pixels acquire new form and meaning, and the smiling and reassuring face of the artist comes into focus. Looking closer does not necessarily guarantee greater truth and clarity (although the scientist would argue looking closer does precisely that), and truth is a precarious illusion, as Plato eloquently demonstrated with his oft-appropriated metaphor of the darkened cave with the flickering firelight casting shadowy spectres on the wall.[19]

In our digital age, Plato's cave is a valid metaphor for the theatre of the simu-lacrum. That the body can now be anatomized 'live' and 'performing' (again the reference to 'staging' the body in the theatre of anatomy) through the processes of non-invasive medical imaging technologies implies that we have reached a stage where we no longer require the practice of dissection in the search for medical knowledge. And yet it was the very knowledge that accrued from the act of dissec-tion, and the subsequent advances in medicine, that contributed to the develop-ment of Western medicine (and indeed, many aspects of Western philosophy and Western art) as we know it today. But as the interest in 'virtual body' projects sug-gests, in our celebrity-saturated, youth- and perfection-obsessed society, we have become a culture where death is eschewed, and the 'real' is disavowed in favour of its representation. Bojana Kunst argues in *Impossible Becomes Possible* that we have already reached the stage where the anatomical has become obsolete:

> If the theory is tenable and the relation between the ideal and real body has
> been the determining factor in the aesthetic representation of the body, then,
> at the end of the second millennium, we actually seem to be confronted with
> none other than 'impossible' bodies – evasive artificial structures, with their
> 'real' bodies becoming unnecessary and obsolete. (Kunst, 1999, p. 49)

Kunst's words are premonitory, since impossible bodies and the digital technology that produces and reproduces them (from the anatomical theatre to the
digital camera) can only exist as fragments of dissected particle, returning us to
the notion of a body without organs, a virtual palimpsest, continually erased
and inscribed anew through the act of dissection and decoding. In this regard,
Kunst reinforces Maaike Bleeker's argument that virtual cadaver projects such
as the *Visible Human Project* are simply more technologically advanced Enlightenment metaphors of the Cartesian machine-body. Bleeker suggests that:

> Deploying a rhetoric which evokes memories of a historical understan-
> ding of photography, the representatives of the Visible Human Project
> claim that 'their' bodies are beyond representation. Stressing the continu-
> ity between the physical body and the electronic images, they claim that
> these computer simulations are direct and complete mechanical inscripti-
> ons of real human bodies without the gaps or lacks that characterize other
> representational techniques, and without the distortions that result from
> human subjective intervention. (Bleeker, 1999, p. 5)

The notion of digital technology being closer to 'reality' than traditional means
of representation and rendering will be familiar to historians and theorists of
photography, where debates about the veracity of the digital medium have been
comprehensively rehearsed. But I am positing that virtual 'realities' no more
guarantee truth, objectivity, and control than do non-digital means of investi-
gation and representation. Despite the 'virtual' anxiety that digital technology
seems to induce, I would argue that even the most extravagant forms of technological and genetic exploration are not yet sophisticated enough to compete
with, let alone supersede, the complexity and individuality of an organ as intricate and exquisite as the human brain, which can now be 'seen' to perform
within its own theatre of flesh and bone. As theatres of anatomy are mothballed
as sites of museology or destroyed in order to make room for more computer
workstations, it may seem that the theatre of anatomy is less about the drama
of life and death than the downloading of digital bytes of frozen cadavers that
only exist as particles of light or pixels of digital encoding. But as the sciart
practice of artists like Alexa Wright and Neal White demonstrates, the theatre
of the body is still a space suffused with excitement and anticipation, a space

where power and knowledge continue to be brokered and negotiated, and a space where art and bioscience may find a creative dialogue that furthers our understanding of what it is to be human.

Dr. Karen Ingham is Head of the Centre for Lens-Based Arts (theory & practice) at the Dynevor Centre for Art, Design and Media at Swansea Institute, Wales, UK. She is a practising artist and writer on the anatomical theatre and the *Vanitas* memento mori. Her research focuses on creative and provocative dialogues between art, bioscience, philosophy and technology. Her publications include *Death's Witness* (2000), *Anatomy Lessons* (2004), *Seeds of Memory: art, neuroscience and botany* (2006) and the essays 'A Dark Adapted Eye: Photography and the Vanitas Still Life' in *Stilled* (2006) and 'Palimpsest' in *Fumus Fugiens* (2007).

Notes

1   Downloading the digital body at 'the flick of a switch' refers to the 1994 US National Library of Medicine (NLM) initiative the *Visible Human Project*, an electronic, biological imaging archive which enables the viewer to navigate, in intricate detail, the entire human body in 3D. The aims and objectives of the NLM's project were to create a complete visual archive of the male and female human body that could be readily accessed and downloaded via the Internet for reference in medical and bio-scientific research. The project used the latest medical imaging technology to produce longitudinal scans of a freshly deceased corpse, with the codename of Adam, via magnetic resonance imaging (MRI) and computer tomography (CT). The corpse was then deep frozen to minus seventy degrees centigrade, and rescanned before being cut into quarters (reminiscent of the historical punishment meted out to prisoners in Roman and medieval times who were frequently hung and 'quartered'), and put through an industrial planer before scanning each 'slice'. The reference to the 'quartering' of prisoners is more than incidental, as the real life body behind the code name Adam was indeed a criminal, a death-row inmate by the name of J.P. Jernigan. Jernigan was a murderer, executed in Texas in 1993 after first agreeing to donate his body to NLM's the *Visible Human Project*. (The precise means of Jernigan's execution was in fact via lethal injection rather than the literal switch of the electric chair.) For more on the *Visible Human Project*, see Sarah Kember (1998), Maaike Bleeker (1999) and José van Dijck's contribution to this volume (pp. 29-47).

2   In his translation of Descartes's writing, John Cottingham suggests that Descartes was not literally suggesting that the mind could see 'as if there were yet other eyes within our brain', but that the brain, as being ordained by God as the seat of the soul, was somehow able to inspect or 'institute' the images the eye receives independently. See John Cottingham et al. (1985). Descartes's notion of 'the mind's eye' led to what became known as the 'Cartesian Theatre', a term allegedly coined by the philosopher Daniel Dennett (1991). Gen Doy has also written fluently on the subject of the Cartesian Theatre. See Gen Doy (2005).

3   Contemporary neurologists and neuropsychologists use functional magnetic reso-
     nance imaging (fMRI) to 'see' deep within the cerebral cortex, creating biological
     images which appear to show sensations of pain and pleasure and even memory itself
     in the process of forming and consolidating. See Karen Ingham et al. (2006).

4   Described by the media as Britain's first public autopsy for 170 years, Gunther von
     Hagens's 'event anatomy', as he describes it, at the Atlantis Gallery in London in 2002
     was, I would argue, more of a carnival sideshow than serious public engagement with
     science. See also Ian Maxwell's contribution to this volume (pp. 49-66).

5   Throughout this essay I refer to the body in the theatre of anatomy as the 'anatomo-
     clinical' body, a phrase used by Michel Foucault throughout his seminal *The Birth of
     the Clinic* (1963). I extend the phrase to the actual anatomical theatre itself, the anato-
     mo-clinical theatre, as the theatre of anatomy has many forms and guises, historical,
     clinical and allegorical.

6   For more on the phenomenological authority of photography in the representation of
     the clinical and postmortem body, see Chris Townsend (1998).

7   The theory of the womb as the matrix of knowledge can be read in chapter seven of
     Jonathan Sawday (1995).

8   Francis Barker explores the relationship of the theatre of anatomy to the seventeenth-
     century-theatre of tragedy in his immensely engaging *The Tremulous Private Body:
     Essays on Subjection* (1995). Also see Sawday (1995, p. 45) where he discusses the play
     The Anatomist within the dissective culture of the period.

9   The multimedia still-life installation and webstream *Vanitas* was staged at the Waag
     Theatrum Anatomicum in April 2005 as part of my artist's residency with the Waag.
     The installation referenced the Waag's history of death and execution, a history which
     I posited was inscribed in the very fabric of the building.

10   For more on the agency of the hand, see pp. 57-65 in William Schupbach (1982).

11   The history of the judicio-anatomical body and the body's evolution from executed
     cadaver to an epistemic 'body of knowledge' can be found in Sawday's and Barker's
     work, and in Ruth Richardson (2001). Barker's work explores in detail the identity
     and 'crime' of Aris Kindt.

12   *Fumus Fugiens* was a group exhibition in Amsterdam's SMART Project Space, a pro-
     duction space for contemporary art. The exhibition was a site-specific response to the
     building's former function as a pathological anatomical laboratory built in the 1930s.

13   The international *Theatres of Science* conference at the University of Glamorgan in the
     UK (2004) attracted a wide variety of papers, many of which were from disciplines
     like theatre and drama studies, and the international conference *The Anatomical The-
     atre Revisited* at the University of Amsterdam (2006) focused on the anatomical the-
     atre, and the anatomical body therein, as a performative space and concept. See also
     Performance Documentation 5 *sensing presence no. 1*, pp. 165-168 in this volume.

14   *The Artist's Body*, by Tracey Warr and Amelia Jones, provides a comprehensive view of
     how modern and contemporary artists use the body as a site of practice.

15   I discussed this question in my paper 'Descartes Eye: theorizing the art and science
     of observation' presented at the conference *New Constellations: Art, Science and So-
     ciety* at the Museum of Contemporary Art in Sydney (2006). See also Ingham et al.
     (2006).

16   It was particularly as an installation artist (working at a time when the term installation
     was itself largely undefined) that the British artist Helen Chadwick (1953-96) came to
     prominence, working across a range of media and methods of which photography fea-
     tured prominently. Chadwick's unexpected death, at the age of 42 from heart failure, de-

prived the art world of a rare visionary. Chadwick influenced a generation of artists, par-ticularly through her work focusing on the body and notions of interiority and sexuality, and for her Baroque staging of those works. Mark Sladen, curator for the 2004 Barbican exhibition *Helen Chadwick: A Retrospective*, speaks of how the artist set out to defy mod-ern oppositions between mind and body, self and other, stating: 'The Cartesian division between the self and the world is an opposition that Chadwick examines in much of her work' (Sladen, 2004, p. 16). It is this oppositional stance that Chadwick pioneered, work-ing against the assumed binaries of body/mind, female/male, science/art, and that has subsequently led to a culture of collaboration between bioscience and the arts in Britain.

17   Andrew Kotting's film was accompanied by a book and CD-Rom, titled *Mapping Per-ception* (2002).

18   In the context of this essay, my definition for a digital body is that used by Harald Begusch in 'Shells that Matter: The Digital Body as Aesthetic/Political Representa-tion' when he states that 'a digital body usually refers to a mathematically computed optical representation which is constructed of grids, pixels and calculated areas and can be associated with the image of a "living" body"' (Begusch, 1999, p. 30).

19   The notion of Plato's cave, from Plato's *The Republic*, has been a recurring motif in discussions on photographic representation and vision, and continues to be cited in relation not only to the history of photographic vision and veracity, but also to the notion of the simulacrum (something that resembles or mimics truth or reality but is in fact a copy).

References

Barker, F., *The Tremulous Private Body: Essays on Subjection*. Michigan, 1995.

Begusch, H., 'Shells that Matter: The Digital Body as Aesthetic/Political Rep-resentation'. In: *Performance Research*, Vol. 4, No. 2, pp. 30-33. London and New York, 1999.

Berger, John X. et al., *Other Than Itself: Writing Photography*. Manchester, 1989.

Bleeker, M., 'Death, Digitalization and Dys-appearance: Staging the Body of Science'. In: *Performance Research*, Vol. 4, No. 2, pp. 1-8. London and New York, 1999.

Buci-Glucksmann, C., *La folie du voir: de l'esthetique baroque*. Paris, 1986.

Buci-Glucksmann, C., *Baroque Reason: The Aesthetics of Modernity*. London, 1994.

Canguilhem, G., *On the Normal and the Pathological*. Dordrecht, 1978.

Cottingham, J. et al., *The Philosophical Writings of Descartes (Volume I)*. Cam-bridge, 1985.

Dennett, D., *Consciousness Explained*. New York, 1991.

Doy, G., *Picturing the Self: Changing Views of the Subject in Visual Culture*. Lon-don and New York, 2005.

Duncan, A., 'Inside-Outside – Permutation: Science and The Body in Contem-porary Art'. In: *Strange and Charmed: Science and the Contemporary Visual Arts*. Ede, S. (ed.). London, 2000.

Ede, S. (ed.), *Strange and Charmed: Science and the Contemporary Visual Arts.* London, 2000.

Flannery, M., 'Images of the Cell in Twentieth-Century Art and Science'. In: *Leonardo*, Vol. 31, No. 3, pp. 195-204. 1998.

Foucault, M., *The Birth of the Clinic.* London, 2003. First edition (1963) *Naissance de la Clinique,* Paris.

Gear, R., 'Beyond the Frame: Narratives of Otherness'. In: *Masquerade: Women's Contemporary Portrait Photography.* Newton, K. (ed.). Cardiff, 2003.

Ingham, K., *Anatomy Lessons.* Manchester, 2004.

Ingham, K. et al., *Seeds of Memory*: *art, neuroscience and botany.* Cardiff and Swansea, 2006.

Kember, S., *Virtual Anxiety: Photography, New Technologies and Subjectivity.* Manchester, 1998.

Kemp, M. and M. Wallace, *Spectacular Bodies: The Art and Science of the Human Body from Leonardo to Now.* London, 2000.

Kotting, A. et al., *Mapping Perception.* London, 2002.

Kunst, B., 'Impossible Becomes Possible'. In: *Performance Research*, Vol. 4, No. 2, pp. 47-52. London and New York, 1999.

Richardson, R., *Death, Dissection and the Destitute.* Chicago, 2001.

Sawday, J., *The Body Emblazoned: Dissection and the Human Body in Renaissance Culture.* London and New York, 1995.

Schupbach, W., *The Paradox of Rembrandt's 'Anatomy of Dr. Tulp'.* London, 1982.

Sladen, M., *Helen Chadwick.* London, 2004.

Townsend, C., *Vile Bodies: Photography and the Crisis of Looking.* Munich and New York, 1998.

Warr, T. and A. Jones, *The Artist's Body.* London, 2000.

'Be not faithless but believing': Illusion and Doubt in the Anatomy Theatre

Gianna Bouchard

Michelangelo Caravaggio's painting of 1603, titled *The Incredulity of Saint Thomas*[1], depicts one scene from the New Testament biblical narrative concerned with the resurrection of Christ, described in detail in the Gospel of John. Following his crucifixion, Christ appears to the disciples and reveals the wounds of the crucifixion as proof of his identity, death and resurrection. For reasons not articulated in the narrative, Thomas, another disciple, was not amongst them for this visitation. Unable to accept on faith what his fellow apostles describe, Thomas demands proof of his own before acknowledging the truth of the resurrection: 'Except I shall see in his hands the print of the nails, and put my finger into the place of the nails, and put my hand into his side, I will not believe' (John 20:25). He desires to touch and explore Christ's wounds and only by thus invading the body interior, by mimicking the trajectories of the penetrating objects through firstly vision and then tactility, will Thomas concede the miracle of the resurrection. For Thomas at least, seeing is not fully believing.

Some eight days later, Christ again appears to the disciples, and Thomas, this time amongst their number, is invited by Christ to dispel his scepticism: 'Put in thy finger hither, and see my hands. And bring hither thy hand, and put it into my side: and be not faithless but believing' (John 20:27). Here, there is a strange aporia in the text, for it is not clear whether or not Thomas does touch any of the wounds or whether the sight of the dead Christ embodied is simply enough to dispel his doubt. He moves instantaneously from seeking tactile empirical evidence to articulating a rhetoric of belief: 'My Lord and my God' is his only reply, according to the narrative (John 20:28). In religious iconography of the scene, however, the aporia in the text is often negated in favour of a Thomas who is compelled to make contact with the wound. Caravaggio likewise makes no bones about the aporia – Thomas impinges upon the marks of the crucifixion by plunging his finger into the spear wound on Christ's torso, guided there by the touch of the resurrected man himself and embedded in the flesh.

Thomas invades this particular wound, located within the painted image, for the purpose of interrogation: it will be a conversion of thought and belief from one path to another through testing the evidence of the body before him. Proof of the resurrection is here, supposedly, verified by sight of the wound and an intimate tactile penetration of its boundaries. There is, arguably, more at stake in this wound and its representation, however, than a simple showing of an ideological shift from doubt to belief for the sceptical disciple via these sensory experiences. Firstly, it is not altogether clear that this transposition is materialized in the painting, with several elements working within the representation to unhinge that surety and produce certain problematics. In effect, instead of pronouncing Thomas's belief in the resurrection, the image manages to raise more questions and yields uncertainty.

This potential subversion in the representation is concentrated around the presence of the wound, a traumatic opening into the carnal body that allows the interior to be explored. Thus, the exposed viscus is foregrounded as the means of providing truth about the status of the body and of offering verifiable knowledge, as in the anatomy theatre. Within this scene, Thomas is explicitly constructed as the exemplary empirical and rational scientist who, paradoxically, demands proof of the material reality of the metaphysical restoration of Christ. Medical and scientific discourse enters the image not only at this level of content but also through certain representational tactics in operation here, such as perspective and the depiction of the body. The mode of representation employed by Caravaggio, which is that of realism, is itself underpinned by illusion as a founding principle. The opened body within the image, constructed through such painterly illusion but also metaphorically tested as an illusion by Thomas, produces certain instabilities and fissures in representation.

The painting is a staged representation that utilizes painterly tactics of illusion, as well as depicting illusion as its subject matter. Caravaggio's use of realism signifies a desire to manipulate the two-dimensional image into an illusion of three-dimensionality that appears then to be a more accurate representation of the world and its phenomena. Volumetric space is necessarily depicted in order to substantiate this illusion, through conjuring mass and embodied presence. The illusion is then reinforced by other painterly conventions operating in the scene, such as that of proportion, equivalence and the use of linear perspective. The illusion is of three-dimensional space that extends through the materiality of surface to a distant horizon deep within the representation. Providing this impression of an interior space within the frame, perspective neatly situates the wound of Christ inside the scene, whilst the wound that is the tear in Christ's body apparently opens into another illusory interior, that of the resurrected man. This wound then reinforces the pretence of three-dimensional space on a two-dimensional plane whilst also playfully raising the

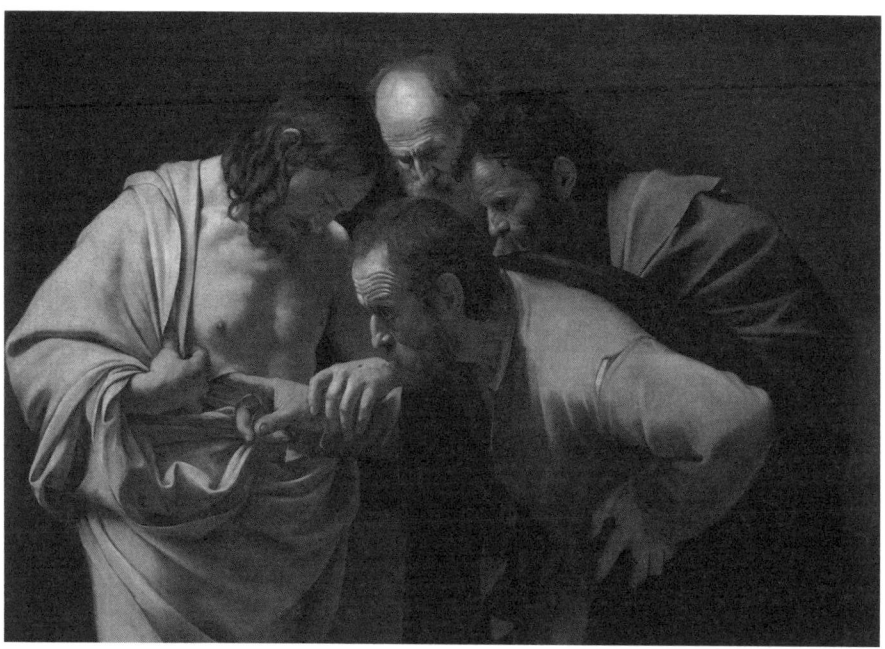

The Incredulity of Saint Thomas, Michelangelo Caravaggio (1603). Courtesy Stiftung Preußische Schlösser und Gärten Berlin-Brandenburg.

spectre of what illusions this body might contain. The revived dead body confounds normative expectations and understandings, so what could possibly be inside this body? What does Thomas actually locate with his finger inside the wound? Does he find the illusory infinity of the vanishing point, held within an illusion of embodied flesh?

Connections between illusion, depth, focus and spectatorship in the operations of perspective make it easy to align with theatrical practice in sharing similar concerns. Usually conceived of as a pictorial technique, perspective is addressed by performance studies academic Peggy Phelan, as she interrogates this same picture for resonances with theatre theory and practice (Phelan, 1997, pp. 23-43). Phelan describes perspective as a 'theatrical technology and a technology of theatre' because it 'supports the economy of substitution that drives Western theatre itself'. For Phelan, 'the 'as if', the illusionary indicative that theatre animates, allows for the construction of depth, for the 'invention' of physical interiority and psychic subjectivity' (ibid, p. 27). Associating this optical invention with its concomitant notions of depth and interiority, Phelan neatly makes a connection, both philosophical and historical, between perspective and the study of anatomy at this time that sought knowledge through revelation of corporeal depth and the internal, and the study of psychology. Through establishing the illusion of perspective in representation, the quest for knowledge of all interiors was perhaps initiated, coalescing around the vanishing point or punctum at the centre of an apparently distant horizon. Ironically, then, the illusion of perspective is suggested as the foundational technology to inaugurate a resolutely non-illusory field of knowledge, that of anatomical science.

Thomas tests the potential illusion of the resurrection by plunging his finger into the space of the wound, but is he not also testing the illusion of representation by trying to access its interior? The spectator's belief in the illusion depends upon such a test that can manifest this resurrected body as having substance and presence. By inserting his finger into the represented wound, Thomas also accesses the supportive mechanisms of illusion at work in the image that appear to provide interiority for this body. He confirms the illusion of perspective in this move that suggests volumetric space on a two-dimensional plane. I want to suggest that Thomas's finger prevents the dissolution of this illusion by plugging the wound and denying full, unmediated sight of it, for what would it reveal if it were offered to sight? In the painting, one can only get a glimpse of the blackness within its parameters, the insinuation of an emptiness that would radically destabilize meaning if made fully visible. Its flat blackness, the blank of the void, would signify pure absence inside the representation, capable of destroying illusion and offering only a hole in the body and the image. If representation may come undone by the hole at its figurative centre, so too might belief in the resurrected Christ. The image creates doubt, even as its narrative supposedly negates it, by presenting a wound that is suspiciously capable of manifesting absence within the resurrected body, where such loss could not be recuperated by the representation.

The narrative of the life of Christ and his role as Saviour depends upon his death, resurrection and return to God, the Father, in Heaven. His embodied return after death is a necessary prerequisite to the disciples' faith in his message and their future ability to continue the mission of disseminating Christianity. It is not clear what constitutes the reclaimed body, but it must act as a prop for the persuasion of men into religious faith. In other words, the body needs to be made present to sight, bear the proofs of untimely death and appear more substantial than a metaphysical entity. Luke's Gospel goes into some detail about this displayed body when Jesus appears in Jerusalem to a gathering of the disciples. They instantly mistake him for a 'spirit', but Christ reasons that a 'spirit hath not flesh and bones' (Luke 24:39). Still apparently unconvinced by this vision, Jesus says: 'Have you anything to eat? / And they offered him a piece of a broiled fish and a honeycomb. / And when he had eaten before them, taking the remains, he gave to them' (Luke 24:41-43). At this point, the disciples do concede the miracle of the resurrection and are converted to belief. These acts all apparently substantiate this body as a definite presence and make it an object of display for rhetorical ends, a persuasive prop, through the overcoming of various tests that materialize the body of Christ in an acceptable and convincing manner.

Thomas is subsequently delivered to belief, in a separate episode from the scene described above, through an act of persuasion that appropriates two main methods – demonstration and crediting. Belief in the resurrection is encouraged through the availability of Christ's body to sight and touch, a manifest demonstration of this body's thwarting of death. Crediting comes initially through the vision of Christ but more significantly via the touch of the wound where its reality is tested in the moment of tactile contact. Christ's 'body' can be interpreted as the prop, through which persuasion operates to dispel scepticism in the metaphysics of resurrection. The body as prop, identified as the site/sight for the production of certain knowledges, reverberates around the anatomy theatre and the theatre itself, where bodies are likewise materialized for specific epistemological ends. Although such bodies and the arenas in which they appear are ideologically different in many ways, they share this desire to make the body present in order to create meaning and 'show' various things. In each case, the body is animated and performed in order to persuade and convey knowledge, or certain 'truths'.

To suggest that performing bodies, the corpse on the dissecting table and the resurrected Christ, in these discrete instances, are all definable as props is to read them, to some extent, as theatrical objects with material presence in the moment of performance or display. They are located within their own spectatorial arenas (for all these bodies are looked at in the first instance), to be acted upon and variously animated to enable the establishment of particular discursive structures and narratives within their own economies. The idea that these bodies are animated or energized by functioning as props in their own fields will be developed here through a reading of Andrew Sofer's work, *The Stage Life of Props*, in which he suggests that props 'take on a life of their own in performance' (Sofer, 2003, p. 2). Sofer's rhetoric of animation and vitality seems particularly pertinent to these bodies that are on the cusp of such activity and are clearly much closer to metaphorical animation than objects.

For Sofer, the prop exists in a 'state of suspended animation' when noted in a text, from where it 'demands actual embodiment and motion (...) in order to spring to imaginative life' (ibid, p. 3). What then constitutes a prop and differentiates it from other stage scenery and furniture is Sofer's criterion of 'manipulation', whereby an actor must intervene in the object by moving it or altering it in some way, thus animating its presence (ibid, p. 12).

The corpse to be dissected within the theatre of anatomy is fundamentally a pedagogical prop, utilized by medical science to educate and elucidate through visual elaboration and proof. Through these demonstrations, the body, as a knowable, biological entity with distinguishable parts and functions, becomes revealed and visible to the spectator. Unable to display itself, the cadaver is anatomized and manipulated by the dissector, who intervenes in the flesh in order to make its significant features visible and persuade spectators of the knowledge embodied therein. Following Sofer, the corpse is here altered from being a mere dead body to the repository of anatomical knowledge and authority in the medical arena through the work of the anatomist. Metaphorically, the cadaver is activated by these procedures that transfigure it into a useful and valuable source of information.

Christ's embodied presence as a resurrected body may also be conceived as a theatrical prop, engaged with by the disciples within the scene of revelation and supposed conversion. His body and consciousness persuade the disciples of the truth of the return through sight and then by undertaking certain activities that dismiss its possibility of being ghostly, rather than corporeal, such as talking and eating. Staged by Caravaggio in this painting, Christ's restored body is not enough for Thomas, the sceptic. He finds its presence insufficient and requires touch as the final guarantor of returning from death, and thereby animates the body through his own intervention. Manipulating this body, like Sofer's theatrical props, in order to test its materiality, Thomas, figuratively, gives Christ a life of his own by setting the body into motion in time and space. The penetrative finger into the body rouses its position within the frame from a mere questionable representation to something more vital and substantial. Persuading and convincing through its presence and solidity, the body simultaneously props up the Christian faith and its key tenet in the narrative of resurrection. Detached from the flesh, because dead, and yet in the flesh somehow, Christ is an ambiguous figure, troubling representation because of his liminality.

Part of the subversive nature of this image is whether Thomas's intervention and animation of this body does convince him and, in turn, the spectator, of resurrection. What exactly does get animated here, except more doubt? By interrogating the interior of the body, it seems that the wound itself is stimulated to produce destabilizing effects within representation and the structure of belief explored here. To what end is the flesh manipulated? Sofer mentions the notion of the 'recalcitrant prop', the one that 'goes awry and eludes (…) the actor's control' (Sofer, 2003, p. 24). This is the theatrical prop that does not behave as it should, either intentionally or not, and is especially applicable to the corporeal examples being discussed here. To some extent, all of these bodies, whether corpses in the anatomy theatre, Christ's resurrected body or the theatrical corpse to be considered next, are recalcitrant in their ability to undermine the operations of illusion and representation that they are positioned within. The anatomy theatre corpse is refractory in its allegiance to the processes of death and decomposition that always circumscribe the dissector's actions. The prop must be engaged with in certain ways and order so that its recalcitrance is negated as far as possible; the abdomen was dissected first, then the head and finally the limbs, following the order of putrefaction and therefore allowing the anatomist to stay ahead of decay that would otherwise render the body useless. Caravaggio has established Christ's body as similarly recalcitrant in that it does not deliver what one might expect of it.

Theatrically, the corpse is usually represented by an actor behaving as if dead, mimicking the stillness and flaccidness of the cadaver on stage. As such, the body becomes a theatrical prop, animated by the other performers who circulate around it, perhaps move it and often address it through rhetorical speech. The theatrical illusion sometimes requires the present-absent in the scene in order to put flesh on the bones of the illusory. The insubstantial and intangible made manifest in the representation may have the ability to stabilize and perpetuate the illusion. Of course, there is another paradox here in that representation requires the spectre, corpse and the resurrected to be physically realized. Caravaggio's Christ is as substantial as the disciples around him, while the corpse must be 'played' by actors in all their fleshy presence. The illusion of insubstantiality must somehow be sustained, for these figures are not wraiths but made of flesh and blood. Hence the need in theatre for them to become objects of proof and persuasion, where their paradoxical nature can be circumvented in order to deliver something else – the illusion of death and resurrection, materiality and wounding. Theatre is the site and sight of the imagined scene. It does not exist, except as a construction and representation of the imagined artefact or figure as an embodied thing. It materializes subjects and objects, fleetingly in time and space, and the spectator witnesses both the illusion and a 'certain kind of *actual*, of having something before one's vision' (States, 1985, p. 46). The troubling body in theatrical representation, that is the one that is pretending to be dead, appears to test the manifestation of the theatrical.

The bodies being interrogated here are all problematized by their status as in-between figures: between resurrection and ascension for Christ; between representational death and actual life for the actor playing dead; and between death and entering medical discourse for the anatomized corpse. They are all in the process of crossing or switching from one state to another in their theatricalized scenes. This transit is partly between history and mythology, whereby figures become transformed by and within representation and, to some extent, are in excess of themselves through the process. For instance, Caravaggio's Christ, Thomas and disciples were life models, painted to depict biblical, even divine, figures by standing in as these icons to uphold the narrative; their representations shifting between their personal, everyday histories and Christian mythology. Likewise, the corpse on the anatomy table in the early modern period was the body of a newly executed criminal, whose punishment was thought to continue beyond death. This transgressive body, marked by capital punishment for its crimes, was transformed by medico-scientific discourse into a demonstrative prop, capable of showing universal anatomical truths and standards. The marginalized and socially rejected criminal became the privileged centre of attention and knowledge through anatomization, standing in as an appropriate and acceptable representative of all men (for these were, invariably, male bodies). These transgressive bodies become imbued with power in certain ideological arenas, where their bodies signify in excess of their materiality and normal social status. As Babcock argues, 'what is socially peripheral is often symbolically central' within cultural processes of 'symbolic inversion' (Babcock, 1978, p. 32).

A similar notion of the stand-in or substitute pervades Caravaggio's painting, as it does the very concept of theatre. Theatre is predicated on the appearance of the disappeared through substitution within the theatrical frame: the actor for the person, the costume for clothes, and make-up for the ravages of old age. Jesus stands in for God in the biblical narrative, as his incarnation in human form, able to live as a man amongst men but still divine in essence (Phelan, 1997, p. 25). Doubting Thomas stands in for those who might be sceptical of the religious story, especially the notion of resurrection. He tests the body of Christ as no one else in the text is permitted to, and his resultant conversion should persuade the reader to have faith also. Thomas is a stand-in, but there is more at stake here than simple substitution. These figures do not merely stand in for others as substitutes, but more complexly, they also behave as intermediaries, acting between subjects. Christ is the intermediary between God and man, whilst Thomas acts between the spectator and the object of doubt. Unable to see and touch for ourselves, Thomas is our interpolator in this discourse.

The wound in Caravaggio's painting is, arguably, both a stand-in and an intermediary. It is the intermediary of belief, operating between Thomas and his ideological structures, the most direct route to conversion, in the biblical narrative at least. It also substitutes for a more traumatic version of a wound, more in keeping with the horror of crucifixion. Caravaggio establishes a wound extraordinary in its physiological accuracy aligned with its surprising lack of evidential trauma. As Thomas pushes his finger into the opening, the skin above it creases as though it is not big enough to accommodate this intrusion and is forced to stretch at the margins. This veracity is simultaneously challenged by the absolute negation of injury pathology around the wound – there is no bruising, no swelling, and no detritus. Its most startling absence though is that of blood. All signs of body fluid contamination have been omitted to leave the wound sanitized and visible to an unnatural degree.

Following the anatomical work of Vesalius and the publication of his seminal text, *De humani corporis fabrica libri septem* in 1543, anatomy texts and illustrations went through something of a revolution, according to Martin Kemp (Kemp, 1993, p. 85). Anatomical subjects began to be illustrated through a 'new technique of naturalistic representation' during the early modern period (ibid, p. 85). Similarly to Caravaggio's wound, these images also erase all extraneous matter and fluids, substituting instead an ideal, aestheticized wound and viscera. The wound is an intermediary between inside and outside and as such is the in-between object of an unstable partition. These images, predicated on realism, reconstitute these boundaries by eliminating traces of abjection around the object. They seemingly cannot afford to leak at their borders, or display an excess of substance and so take on anti-realist representational strategies.

Such a statement is clearly paradoxical, as the visceral is always messy and excessive and to show this authentically would mean incorporating all of its disorder. So, the alleged realism of these pictures involves aestheticizing the body and draining it of fluids and superfluous matter. At the moment of representation, abundance and leakage are halted and negated, action is denied, and time is halted. The realism that these images are predicated on contains within its operations the rupture of anti-realism, in order to maintain the illusion. The representation of truth, supposedly the foundation of realism, is usurped at its very heart by the idealized wound. In this state, it is apparently able to intermediate between Thomas and Christ, between structures of belief and between embodied understandings, but it resolutely fails to deliver final meaning. The wound's aestheticization disconnects it from both normal, temporal relations and any normative pathological functioning, so that the body is thrown into flux. It renders the body ambiguous as it seems dead and alive, conscious but not entirely biologically animate.

Theatrically, the wound appears on-stage in various guises, but in realism it is most often simulated with fake blood and the pretence of trauma. It might be evoked through rhetorical devices and made the subject of the narrative, where language describes its presence, standing in for its messiness and abjection. Wounds are simulated and constructed through various means, and the spectator is duly expected to willingly suspend their disbelief in the artificiality of it all, in order to enter into the imaginary space of the theatrical. Even though manifestly pretend, they are staged, sometimes in highly convincing and complex ways, to maintain the illusion of reality being forged within the remit of realism. Alternatively, the real wound is inflicted and suffered in the uncompromising performance arena of live art, where artists incise their own bodies, and the spectator witnesses blood, trauma and pain that is authentic and, at times, brutal. Between the two modes, of pretence and reality, rests a wound such as the one found in Italian theatre company Socìetas Raffaello Sanzio's 2001 production of *Giulio Cesare*, that troubles in its intermediate position and will act as a final case study.

The production of *Giulio Cesare* by Socìetas Raffaello Sanzio stages various bodies that should not be there. Extraordinary, transgressive bodies substitute for normative ones in the casting, which then challenge representational systems and discursive structures within the text by their very presence on stage. Inevitably, these bodies also confront the spectator with their unexpected and unusual conditions. Given significance and marked, in some cases, by medico-science, they disrupt the theatrical frame by coming into public and being on the stage. Their otherness is offered by director Romeo Castellucci as a literal and metaphorical rendering of the narrative and its ideologies; bodies to be read in all their materiality and difficulty within the frame of Shakespeare's *Julius Caesar*.

By claiming that the bodies of the actors in the production should not be there, I am making reference to their anomalous presences on the stage. Nick Ridout, analyzing the use of animals and children in the work of Socìetas Raffaello Sanzio, articulates the problem thus:

> We know whom we expect to see on stage. We expect to see actors. This needs saying: we do not even expect to see human beings, in all their diversity, but, as their representatives, a kind of group apart, more beautiful perhaps, more agile, more powerful and subtle of voice. Creatures who have been chosen on the basis of some initially desirable attributes, which they have subsequently honed and refined by means of professional training. So when we get something else, it appears as an anomaly, and a worrying one at that. (Ridout, 2004, p. 58)

Castellucci has employed bodies in *Giulio Cesare* that are other than what is expected of actors, thus drawing attention to the materiality and physicality of those bodies in a very explicit manner. They are entered into systems of representation that cannot deny their 'irreducible materiality', but instead they offer a direct challenge to them, failing to be totally taken into those representational economies (ibid, p. 60).

Julius Caesar, in this production, is played by a fragile and physically decrepit old man who is weak and disturbingly still on the stage. The other actors appear to nurse him and care for him, as one would a patient in a hospital. In his nakedness there is a vulnerability to his presence that is shocking, and which undermines not only the supposed physical presence of Caesar but also his ideological position as ruler of a great empire.

Cassius and Brutus are played by two males in Act One but are then replaced by two females in the Second Act, both of whom are anorexic and obviously so. Their bodies are wasted and skeletal, painful to observe as they appear also too fragile and vulnerable for the work of the theatre and the parts they have to play. They perform within a stage space that is a reconstruction of a devastated theatre auditorium, with ruined drapes and burnt-out seating, and somehow match that wasteland with their own disintegration and echo of loss. Metaphorically, they carry the guilt of Caesar's murder within them, that eats away at their dignity and selfhood, and Castellucci literalizes this in their physical beings.

The final character and the most important for this analysis is that of Mark Anthony, who is played by an actor who has had a laryngectomy. This operation involves the surgical removal of all or part of the larynx. The actor has a perma-nent wound, or stoma, in his neck that is similar to the aestheticized and ideal wounds described in anatomical illustrations previously and that Caravaggio has depicted on the body of Christ. The wound's borders have been reconsti-tuted in such a way as to negate any abject substances, yet the stoma remains a direct opening into the interior of the body. On the neck of the actor, it looks like a black hole that becomes animated by the movement of the actor's throat as he 'speaks'. The actor, Dalmazio Masini, is the most unlikely figure to be cast in a role that demands so much from the voice, in terms of power, stamina, in-flection and technique.

His is a voice that must persuade through his use of language, it needs to re-gain the confidence of the crowd and incite that crowd to violence and revenge

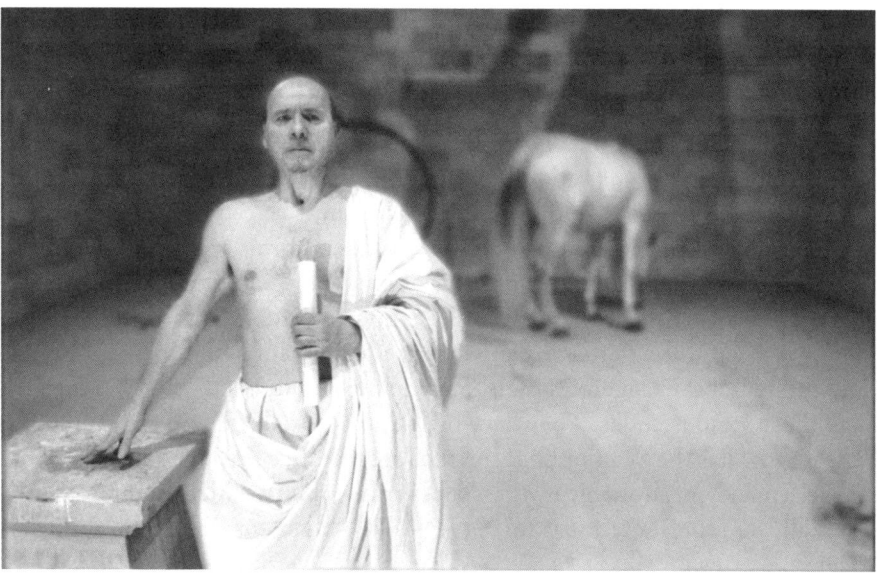

Dalmazio Masini as Mark Anthony in *Giulio Cesare* by Socìetas Raffaello Sanzio. Photo: Gabriele Pellegrini. Reproduced with permission of Socìetas Raffaello Sanzio.

on behalf of Caesar. This actor must deliver one of the most familiar speeches from Shakespearean texts and swing the tide of the play against the treachery of the murderers. The scene is set in Ancient Rome, where rhetoric and oration were highly prized and celebrated skills, learnt and practised in order to enter into the public and political arena. So, the subversion of this particular wound is twofold – it undermines the context of the narrative, and it destabilizes the work and ideology of the actor. This is speech that has been absented and then revived through a technique that requires painstaking practice. It struggles to emerge from this body and is constituted in a physical process far removed from normative techniques that only serve to draw attention to the work that is being done within the actor to make speech, an ability and expectation that the spectator takes for granted. The laryngectomy, revealed on the actor's neck, materializes and embodies the act of speaking in a stark and dramatic way. By association, however, attention is not just drawn to this particular actor's speech but to the construction of voice and sound by every actor in the production.

For De Certeau, bodies 'become bodies only by conforming to (...) codes' that are socially constructed for disciplinary ends so that our carnal beings adhere to a certain physicality and dynamic in the world (De Certeau, 1984, p. 147). Castellucci's cast overtly demonstrates such laws by breaking and confronting them; they are not contained by them but remain resistant to their power, existing outside of and somewhat distanced from their economies. These are bodies that have not capitulated to those demands; they have failed or simply cannot respond to the codes as required. They frustrate the codes and taunt them by entering the theatrical frame and making themselves public and visible.

De Certeau suggests that 'at the extreme limit of these tireless inscriptions (...) there remains only the cry', when something else escapes – 'the body's difference, alternately *in-fans* and ill-bred, intolerable in the child, the possessed, the madman or the sick' (ibid, p. 148). Perhaps these staged bodies are that cry made physical, with people who are unable to conform, or in the case of the anorexics, this is the extremity of inscription, where the physical body is exhausted and sickened by the codes. These bodies that have failed to represent society to itself through its laws and inscriptions are entered into a representational system that exaggerates their 'cry' and the fragility of the body in the face of all these various codes. They have bent to this social will and are crumbling beneath it. That they can uphold the theatrical edifice throughout the performance is made questionable by their sheer vulnerability, which might not withstand all the representational forces at work. This is theatre on the brink of collapse.

Ridout's actors, who are 'a kind of group apart', a group in excess of the normative in their beauty, stature, presence or other 'desirable attributes', have been replaced here by those at the opposite limit (Ridout, 2004, p. 58). Obviously delineated and marked by medico-scientific discourses, they are pathologized and marginalized by them: obesity, anorexia, geriatry and laryngectomies are all means of describing the body and its condition, its care and status through those specific languages and values. Each trauma or medical transgression heightens awareness in the spectator of the context of medicalization that now surrounds every body in the West. They are instantly read as bodies that are subject to medical discourse and intervention, whether they confront it or have been marked by its procedures. This is how bodies are made sense of in the late twentieth and early twenty-first century, and this perception is simultaneously challenged by the alternate understandings of the body in the narrative of the play.

Two ideologies are made to meet in the phenomenal presentation of bodies within the theatrical system. De Certeau's conception of juridical politics confronts medical politics through the text and material bodies circulating within the same representational frame (De Certeau, 1984, p. 142). This is the same juxtaposition that can be found, to a lesser extent, in the Caravaggio painting, with Thomas, the medic, opposing the body of Christ, inscribed by penal codes. The bodies are subject to these two different inscriptions of the law in *Giulio Cesare*, one metaphorically and representationally in the juridical notion of the body politic and the other physically in medical markings. Underneath this tension, however, is the sense that both systems of coding, the juridical and the medical, are intended to inscribe and circumscribe the body in particular ways, according to social codes, which allow the body to represent society to itself, in De Certeau's terms.

The characters in the Shakespeare play – Caesar, Mark Anthony, Brutus and Cassius – all represent or stand in for groups of people in relation to certain power dynamics. Caesar represents the Roman Empire; Mark Anthony represents Caesar and those who support him and, in the future, will represent Rome; whilst Cassius and Brutus represent those who conspire against that power and its embodiment within a single male figure. As such, they each represent the body politic, signifying a collective in excess of their individual bodies, and yet, they are marked in the performance by singularity, made unique by their wounds and pathologies. These anomalies draw excessive attention to themselves, and the body politic is thus circumvented by their extraordinary physical exceptions, and they remain in excess of representation, which seemingly fails to recuperate these bodies and incorporate them into its systems. They stand firm in their 'irreducible materiality' (Ridout, 2004, p. 60). This is surely the downfall of Caravaggio's painting, in which Christ's body should represent something in excess of itself that is divine and holy, yet this moment is made ambiguous by the wound, in its curious materiality that ruptures the representation.

Castellucci deliberately employs these bodies in all their specificity to embody certain ideologies underpinning the text. Dalmazio Masini's surgically altered body is used to draw attention to the creation of speech and its importance to the narrative in terms of persuading the crowd of the treachery involved in Caesar's untimely death. The wound in his neck animates this discourse by emphasizing the labour involved in vocalizing thought and language. In this way, Castellucci stages this wound as a prop to structures of rhetoric and their construction in the body. It also works to displace the locus of power from the authorial text into the actor's body, which then works to articulate the text in particular ways. The text as some transcendent and metaphysical force in the theatre is situated within this material body that struggles to speak it coherently and forcefully. The wound once again destabilizes the illusion of realism, where speech is supposed to be spontaneous and natural, by instead rupturing and making apparent the very instruments of its production. Castellucci employs this recalcitrant prop to heighten this revelation by allowing it to be made visible in the theatrical frame.

Describing the wound on Masini's neck as a recalcitrant prop refers to its unstable status that makes it the source of potentially unexpected occurrences. It may elude the actor's control at any point, and the spectator bears witness to this constant battle in the actor. He is continually striving and labouring to make the wound and the remains of his speech organs obey his desires and requirements. Speech is not guaranteed in this process, or indeed sound in any definable or recognizable pattern. The voice that emerges is strange and sounds somewhat synthesized or non-human. It is made recalcitrant by its very precarious operations that make the voice insubstantial and liable to disintegration or failure.

Recalcitrance does not simply reside in the pathologized voice of this particular actor, however, as the wound makes explicit the fragility of all voices in the theatre. They are expected to be so much 'more' than the voice of the everyday – one only need consider the range of vocal techniques and training manuals for the actor to recognize this imperative. Behind the realist façade of effortless and 'natural' speech lays a mastery of technique and intense labour that may, similarly, break down and reveal its own illusions. The voice that cracks, which cannot be heard, that runs out of breath, that becomes dysfunctional, all resonate across this wound. What is made apparent is that the articulation of text and dialogue in performance is always labourintensive for the actor and inherently unstable. Both body and voice are pushed to the extreme limit of their capabilities in Castellucci's theatre, and we fear their subsidence into stasis. The capacity for theatrical undoing is central.

It seems appropriate to consider the presence of this wound in its particular scene – that of rhetorical argument. Rhetoric is constructed to influence and

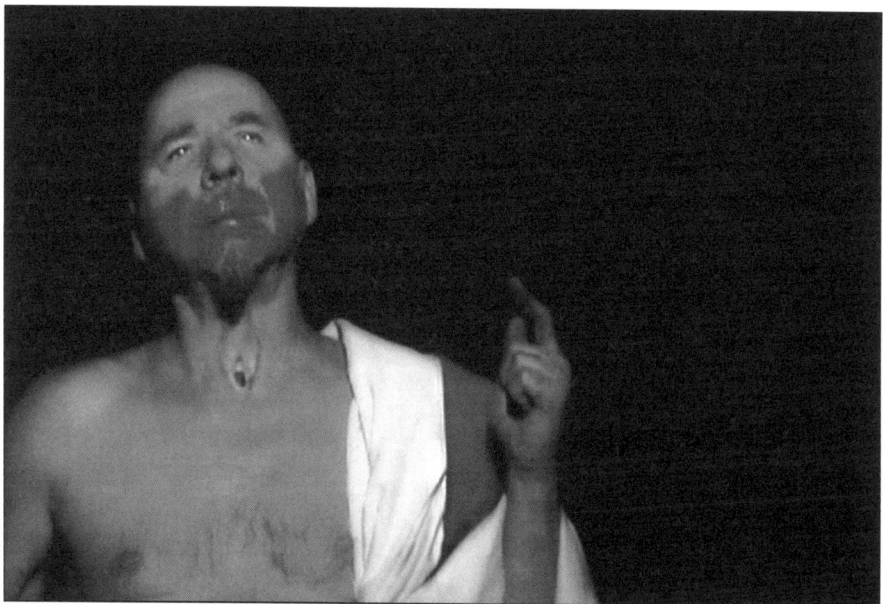

Dalmazio Masini as Mark Anthony in *Giulio Cesare* by Socìetas Raffaello Sanzio. Photo: Gabriele Pellegrini. Reproduced with permission of Socìetas Raffaello Sanzio.

convince audiences of particular opinions or knowledge. Once more then, we have a wound that is staged in a scene of doubt and persuasion. Mark Anthony must convert the crowd to belief in the injustice of Caesar's murder in order to incite them to take revenge and seek justice. He does this, as we have seen, in the play by evoking the wounds of Caesar through rhetorical language and in utilizing the body as prop to these arguments. In the performance of *Giulio Cesare*, the wounds on Caesar's body are substituted for Mark Anthony's stoma, which is made visible to all.

The substitution is heightened by blood and death being symbolically draped round Mark Anthony, as he hangs the theatre curtain over his shoulder, like a makeshift toga. Its plush redness and weight of velvet imply the imperial body and significance of Caesar, whilst the use of the curtain as part of the theatrical apparatus blurs the boundary between the real and fictional elements of the theatre. In the realist theatre, the curtain distinguishes the real world of the auditorium from the illusory space and time of the stage. It demarcates those borders and also plays a part in the revelation of the illusion, as it is raised on the scene, invoking a moment of 'lo and behold' for the spectator. It reveals the aperture through which we view the action and behind which the illusion is constructed. What usually contains and frames the illusion is deliberately drawn into the theatrical moment to become part of the representation, as if the stage can no longer hold the edges or maintain its integrity. Might the red curtain be the wound or rupture in the economy of realist theatre, aggressively bisecting fiction and reality?

The actual wound, the stoma, stands in for all the wounds on Caesar and substitutes his multiple injuries in one, permanent stoma that makes it difficult to articulate Anthony's viewpoint. It echoes with these other gaping mouths and finds it almost as difficult to speak, not through excess but through absence and loss. Loss of the larynx, loss of wholeness, loss of actorly gravitas and beauty, however, do not remain as an absence within the theatrical frame, for this body and its wound saturates representation with the actual. As an intermediary between character and actor, between Anthony and Masini, the wound produces an actor doing the work of acting in an embodied and physical manner. It destabilizes illusion by manifesting its internal, bodily constructions on the part of the performer. Drawing in the curtain, as cleaver between stage and world, puts into flux other theatrical illusions as the actor envelops himself in its folds.

Within this production we are not sure if Anthony's speeches do persuade because there is no crowd assembled on the stage to hear and react to him. Anthony and his wound, instead, confront the spectators in the auditorium by standing at the front of the stage and using direct address. Doubt is transferred elsewhere within this scene, and I would argue that it lingers with the audience through the presentation and display of this particular actor's body. This wounded, suffering body draws the spectator towards it in visceral and empathic relations, reflecting all our bodies, their frailty and eventual breakdown. Yet, these bodies are emphatically hopeful too, that such things can be overcome. This is a wound that provides relief and has become a means of replacing diseased parts, too pathologized to continue within the body. The body has been re-educated to cope with alterations in its constitution and has found a substitute for normative speech formation. The wound is both a *memento mori* and a *memento vivante*.

As in the anatomy theatre, the wounded and opened bodies laid out in this essay for analysis act as props to various acts of persuasion and demonstration. Their incisions and interiors are staged to deliver certain truths, even though they are embedded within structures of illusion that underpin their representational framings. I have argued that the opened body in these circumstances is seemingly unable to maintain the illusion and either destabilizes its operations or ruptures it, and thereby fails to deliver truth, knowledge and/or belief. Instead, the anatomized body can expose other processes at work within these moments, such as the labour of voice production in *Giulio Cesare* or the liminality of these bodies, as both transgressive and substitutable figures.

Gianna Bouchard is Senior Lecturer in Drama at Anglia Ruskin University, Cambridge, UK. She has published in *Performance Research* and is Reviews Editor for the same journal. She was awarded her PhD from the University of Surrey, Roehampton, in 2006. This project was titled *Performing the Anatomised Body* and was an interrogation of the interface between the performed body and the medicalized body, funded by the AHRC. Its focus was on representations of the wounded and opened body in art and performance. Her wider research interests include contemporary theatre and performance (particularly live art), experimental theatre and interdisciplinary art practice.

Notes

1   Michelangelo Caravaggio (1603) *The Incredulity of Saint Thomas*, Preussische Schlösser und Gärten, Berlin-Brandenburg, Potsdam, 107 x 146, oil on canvas.

References

Babcock, B., *The Reversible World: Symbolic Inversion in Art and Society*. Ithaca, 1978.

Certeau, M. de, *The Practice of Everyday Life*. (Translated by Steven Rendall.) Berkeley, Los Angeles and London, 1984.

Kemp, M., 'The Mark of Truth: Looking and Learning in Some Anatomical Illustrations from the Renaissance and Eighteenth Century'. In: *Medicine and the Five Senses*. Bynum, W.F. and R. Porter (eds). Cambridge and New York, 1993.

Phelan, P., *Mourning Sex: Performing Public Memories*. London and New York, 1997.

Ridout, N., 'Animal Labour in the Theatrical Economy'. In: *Theatre Research International*, Vol. 29, No. 1, pp. 57-65. 2004.

Sofer, A., *The Stage Life of Props*. Ann Arbor, 2003.

States, B., *Great Reckonings in Little Rooms: On the Phenomenology of Theater*. Berkeley, 1985.

Performance Documentation 3:
De Anatomische Les

De Anatomische Les (*The Anatomy Lesson*), a choreography of the American dancer and choreographer Glen Tetley, premiered January 28, 1964, in the Koninklijke Schouwburg (Royal City Theatre) of The Hague. The choreography was based on Rembrandt's *The Anatomy Lesson of Dr Nicolaes Tulp*. In *De Anatomische Les* a male body is laid on the dissection table among a group of seventeenth-century anatomists. The body suddenly revives, gets up, and starts to dance.

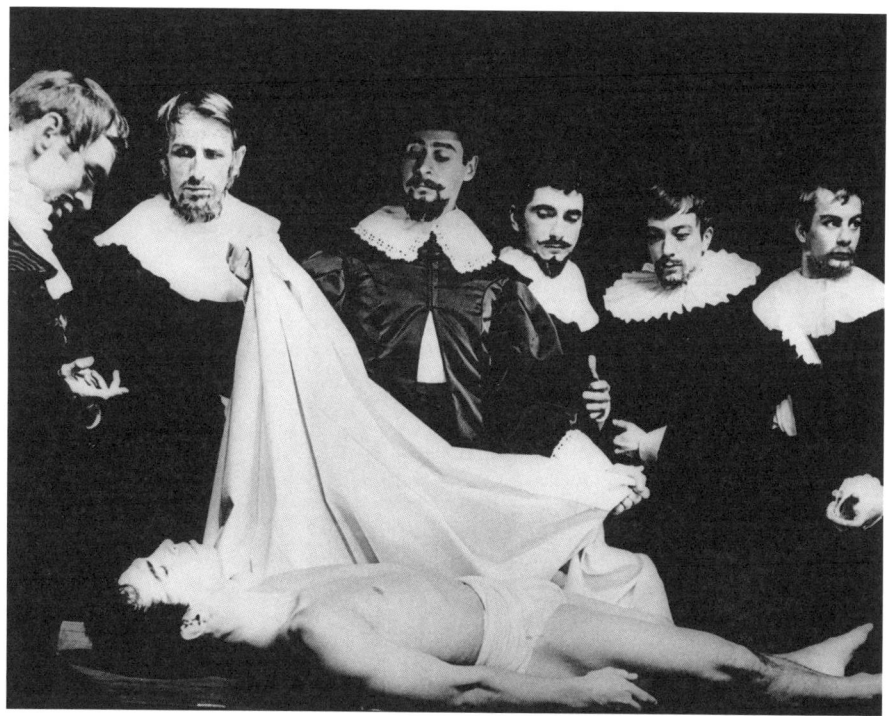

De Anatomische Les (Nederlands Dans Theater, 1964). Choreography: Glen Tetley. Photo: Ger J. van Leeuwen. Courtesy of Vivienne van Leeuwen.

Tetley (1926-2007) first studied medicine before he began his dance studies at Hanya Holm's modern dance studio in New York. Afterwards he danced with the company of Martha Graham. He joined the Nederlands Dans Theater (Netherlands Dance Theatre) as a dancer and choreographer at the beginning of the 1960s and was the artistic director of the NDT together with Hans van Manen until 1970. Just like *Pierrot Lunaire* (1962), *De Anatomische Les* belonged to Tetley's first choreographies that still had the quality of a dramatic narrative. From the end of the 1960s, his choreographies moved away from storytelling and began to show a more expressionist form of ballet.

Performance Data

Choreography: Glen Tetley
Music: Marcel Landovski
Stage design and costumes: Nicolaas Wijnberg
Performers: Jaap Flier (the man), Willy de La Bije (his mother), Alexandra Radius
    (his wife), Ger Thomas (the anatomist), Hans Knill (his assistant).

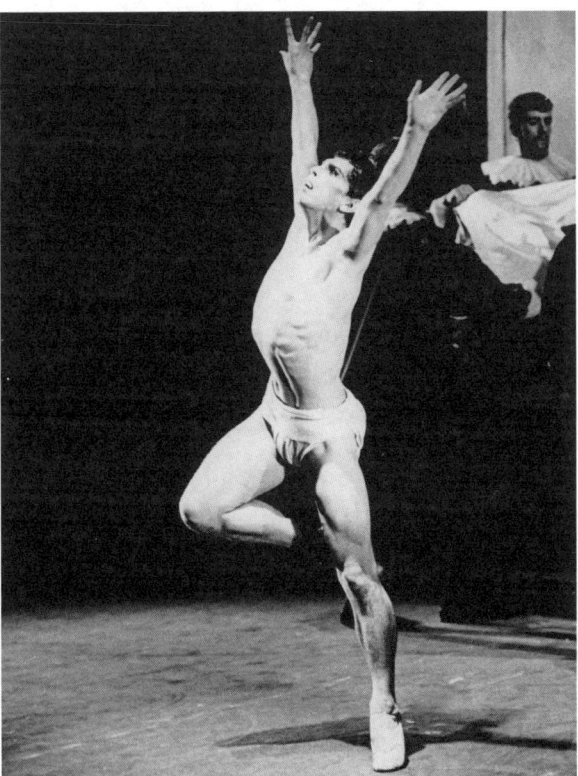

De Anatomische Les
(Nederlands Dans Theater,
1964). Choreography:
Glen Tetley.
Photo: Ger J. van Leeuwen.
Courtesy of Vivienne van
Leeuwen.

Of Dissection and Technologies of Culture in Actor Training Programs – an Example from 1960s West Germany

Anja Klöck

The Actor as Mediator between Inside and Outside: A Historical Trajectory

The practices of representing and constructing certain ways of knowing one's body in acting theories and acting programs are historically contingent as well as participating in historical long-term processes. Since early modern times, these processes have been conditioned by an interlocking of cultural practices, aesthetic forms, technical innovations, and strategies of producing and transmitting knowledge of the body. In his study of the Renaissance culture of dissection, Jonathan Sawday investigates early modern ways of knowing the body at the intersection of medical discourses, scientific procedures, representational practices, cultural conventions and an increasing emphasis on seeing as a mode of knowledge production. Focussing on the practices of dissecting and representing that which hitherto remained unseen in cultural discourse, he argues that 'the early-modern period sees the emergence of a new image of the human interior, together with a new means of studying that interior, which left its mark on all forms of cultural endeavour in the period' (Sawday, 1995, p. viii).

Not surprisingly, his study presents a large number of historical images representing different views of the various organic layers inside the human body of flesh as they were known, knowable and representable at a specific historical moment. Not only do these pictures remind us of Roland Barthes's insight that 'even and especially for your own body, you are condemned to the repertoire of its images' (Barthes, 1977, p. 36). Not only do they remind me of the impossibility of looking at my own interiority without technologies of representation such as X ray pictures or screens visualizing ultrasound waves. Not only do these images point at the fact that, within an optical space, knowledge of the interior make-up, as much as the exterior appearance of our bodies, is always already representational. The images in Sawday's book also mark a desire of stabilizing, conserving and disseminating that which is known or should be known through a set of principles by which the body's inside appears to the onlooker. What can be seen and how it becomes visible is dependent on an interplay of anatomical discourses and practices, instruments, cultural conventions, media in the narrow sense (such as etchings, engravings, drawings), aesthetic forms and historical proceedings.

In an image by Andreas Vesalius (1543), for instance, the interior of a human being is visualized by making the skin transparent in order to represent a specific physiological system, such as the nervous system; Juan Valverde de Hamusco (1560) presents the figure of a man holding the ghostly appearance of his own skin that he cut off with a knife, thereby revealing the defining strands of muscles and sinews beneath to the spectator; some etchings by Pietro Berretini da Cortona (1618-1620) show female figures in architectonically structured

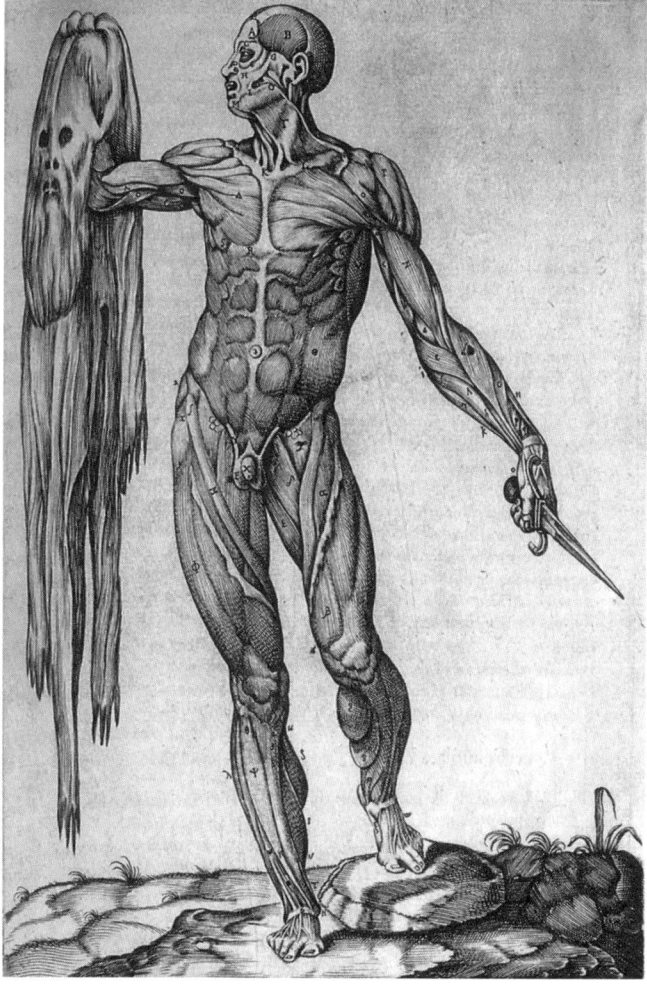

Juan Valverde de Hamusco, *Historia de la composicion del cuerpo humano* (1556), p. 64. Courtesy of the US National Library of Medicine.

interiors peeling back parts of their own skin like fabric or curtains, thereby offering a specific sight of the interior within a baroque frame of presentation; or a womb and foetus are represented as blossoming from a woman's body in an idealized landscape represented as transitory in images by Adriaan van de Spiegel (1626).[1]

Each of these images reveals different strategies engulfing the representation of dissection. Each of these images presents a different construction of the border between the interior and exterior realms of a human body, thereby marking a respectively different zone of intersection between medical discourse, dissecting practices, technologies of representation, aesthetic conventions, and strategies of knowledge production and knowledge transmission.

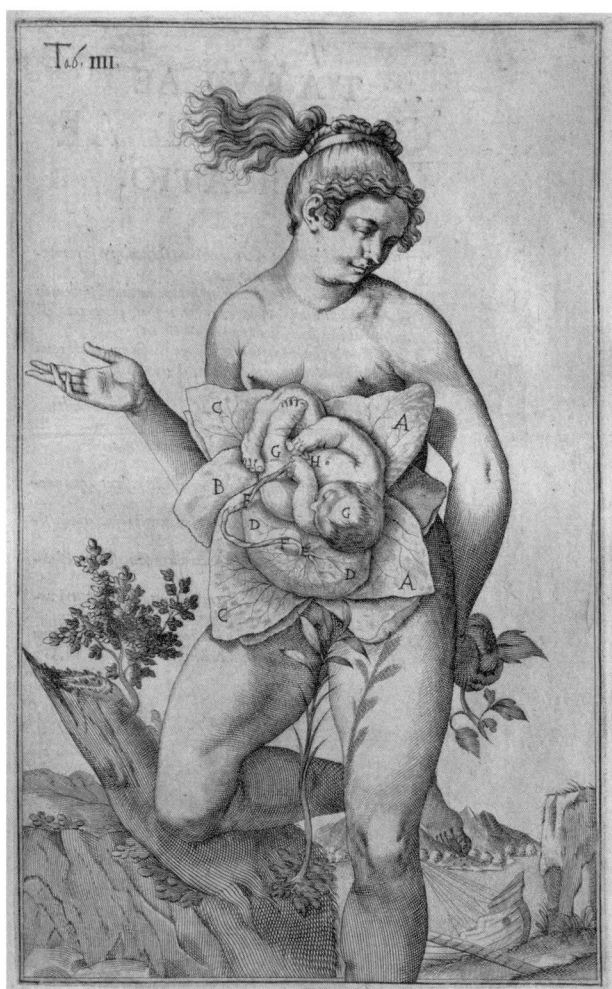

Adriaan van de Spiegel, *De formato foetu liber singularis* (1626), Table 4. Courtesy of the US National Library of Medicine.

The struggle of different regimes of knowledge over how the body's interiority could be seen, known and represented, however, did not halt at dead bodies and hence it did not solely centre on the organic material to be found underneath the skin. It also crystallized around living bodies and the question of how the living body's exteriority and interiority interrelated, how they could be re-defined and controlled in a non-theological sense. The increasing number of publications on the art of acting in the eighteenth century may be regarded as a symptom of this larger interest.[2] Much like the bodies of the dissected human figures in the images from anatomical books, the actor's body becomes a site where the relationship between the externally perceivable and the internally concealed aspects of being is explored in representation. On the actor's body, like on the anatomized dead body, different conceptions and knowledges of the human body are probed: Is the body a sensitive organism that, being part of nature, cannot and should not be controlled, or is the body a machine that functions according to certain rules that may be learned and perfected? What is the relationship between the imagination and physical excitement, the image of a passion in the mind and its manifestation in the body, how is physical af-fect transported to the spectator, and how can these techniques be learned and transmitted? Is the relationship between mind and body to be modelled after Descartes's ghost in the machine, or should mind and body both be regarded as vitalistic matter, as proposed by La Mettrie in *L'Homme Machine* (1748)?[3] These are the central questions driving the eighteenth-century discourses on acting. In his book *The Player's Passion*, Joseph Roach rationalizes this interest in the actor's body in the following way:

> The modernization of the physical sciences, their subsequent disentangle-ment from ancient authority, helped eighteenth-century theorists for the first time to interpret the actor's emotion from outside the framework of classical rhetoric. At the same time the growing secularization of enligh-tened science extricated empirical investigations of vitality from obfusca-ting issues like *soul*. (Roach, 1985, p. 12)

With the foundation of acting academies in Europe as early as Konrad Ekhof's Schweriner Akademie in 1753, this epistemologization of the relationship be-tween an actor's expressivity and his internal, invisible processes becomes ra-tionalized and institutionalized. The actor cannot physically dissect or peel off his skin in front of the spectators in order to present a deeper knowledge of hu-man interiority. But he is presenting and incorporating the *phantasma* of cross-ing the line separating us from looking at the interior space of our own bodies, a line also associated with death, social or religious taboos or an exceptional status in society. In that sense, the actor, not unlike the surgeon, occupies what

Sawday calls a 'rare cultural status as mediator between the exterior and the interior worlds' (Sawday, 1995, p. 12). However, this status is already bound to the ideology of mastering and controlling the body with certain techniques or a refinement of its instruments (such as voice, body, imagination). Ever since the institutionalization of actor training, it has been assumed that the actor may learn a technique with which to penetrate his or her own body without losing his or her integrity as a subject in everyday life. He or she is expected to do so not in order to present and accumulate knowledge for medical cures, but in order to present and accumulate knowledge of how to control the physical manifestation of affects in public representation. Within this ideology of the technical mastery of the body, the actor could be seen as the knife (instrument/technique) and the surgeon (specialized subject) as well as the body (object), as much as their representation (performance) and cultural construction (through aesthetic conventions and discursive concepts of the body). In order to reach that implied status of a mediator in Western societies, it is assumed that the actor must either learn a specific technique or otherwise be exceptionally gifted with a talent that needs to be cultivated by a certain kind of praxis. A residual fracture of the cultural practices that crystallized in a discursive construction and dissection of the border between interiority and exteriority of human bodies in the sixteenth-century anatomical theatres is being played out on the body of the so-called professional European actor or actress ever since. His or her mode of being is imagined on an always differently defined border between the always differently defined inside and outside of a human body.

A Case-Study: Actor Training in 1960s Germany

In 1967, Hans-Günther von Klöden, professor of acting in the acting program at Hannover University of Music and Theatre, Germany, writes in his book *Grundlagen der Schauspielkunst*, or *Basics of Acting*:

> Our training is training for a profession, training in a craft (...) The work on one's self that aims at genuineness is a life-threatening enterprise; there is everything to win and everything to lose; because the social role, the mask, is the shield of the human being not only from society but also from his own abyss. The task of the actor, however, is to take off this earnest mask, and to liberate himself for the transparent mask of playing.[4]

The aim of the acting method presented by Von Klöden in his book is the actor's ability to become transparent. Transparency, here, however, is not an anatomical transparency, such as in Vesalius's representation of the nervous system beneath a transparent skin. The transparency between exterior appearance and interiority demanded by Von Klöden in 1967 is sociologically defined. His methodological program of actor training crystallizes at the intersection of Johan Huizinga's play theory, Carl Jung's theory of psychological types and German studies in the field of sociology and social psychology such as P.R. Hofstätter's *Sozialpsychologie* of 1956.[5] In his seminal work *Homo ludens* (written in 1938 and translated into German in 1939), Johan Huizinga argues that all cultural systems such as politics, science, religion and law stem from playful behaviour that has been institutionalized through a process of ritualization. Through this process, play becomes serious. Once the rules of play are written in stone, they cannot be easily changed, and hence they become compulsory. Following Carl Gustav Jung's definition of 'persona', meaning 'mask' in Latin, Von Klöden calls the individual's adaptation to these social rules 'mask'. Bringing Jung's 'analytical psychology' to Huizinga's play theory, Von Klöden points at the potential of playful behaviour to change or make transparent hardened structures of social interaction, or 'role-playing'. To Huizinga, too, playing is to be equated with 'liberty of action' and freedom - it presupposes independent thinking and ethical standards.[6] Drawing on this definition of play, Von Klöden argues that the craft of the professionally trained actor lies 'in a certain state of consciousness, which is marked by freedom and by the consequences of this freedom for language and movement'.[7] In order for the acting student to achieve this freedom, his or her consciousness needs to be changed through exercises that help to move the so-called 'double consciousness' (between social mask and the liberty of playing, between objectification and identification) into 'the direction of the healthy, sound, whole' (Von Klöden, 1967, p. 24). On the level of his or her consciousness, the actor or actress is to become aware of the opposites at work in himself or herself as well as in society. The program of actor training described here aims at a kind of anatomization of the social-psychological body of the actor in order to achieve the integrity and health of his or her own social body much as the integrity and health of the onlookers, of society[8]:

> The knowledge of playing a role in everyday life fictitiously distinguishes the healthy from the pathological case. Hence one could regard the good actor as a model human being acting healthily.[9]

Interestingly, this task of negotiating the border between external, social mask and individual liberty is still associated with death and with social taboos. As mentioned above, Von Klöden calls it a 'life-threatening enterprise', because 'such freedom of changing masks borders on chaos' (Von Klöden, 1967, p. 26). At stake is not the life of and control over the organic body, but the functioning of the social body. Hence it is only logical that this definition of good acting necessitates a method by which the process of becoming socially transparent and socially 'healthy' may be learned and controlled. The method prescribed by Von Klöden is a 'two-way method', which he demands for all aspects of actor training (voice, movement, acting exercises). This two-way method may be regarded as a response to a world and a body that to Von Klöden, much as to Carl Jung, appear as bifurcated:

> The oppositional pairs form and content, conscious and unconscious, craft and intuition, diligence and talent, interior and exterior - just to mention the ones used most often in our work - govern our thinking. This is where we have to start when embarking on the journey to overcome these oppositions in order to arrive at an experience of wholeness. It is important that the students recognize these antinomies first as oppositions, then as poles of the same thing and finally strive to overcome them in a coincidentia oppositorum.[10]

In order to overcome the perceived oppositions, Von Klöden draws on the neoplatonic concept of coincidentia oppositorum - the falling together of opposites in eternity. This concept was coined by the theosophist Nicholas of Cusa in the fifteenth century as the least imperfect description of God. In the second half of the sixteenth century, Giordano Bruno (1548-1600) uses this concept in his writings in order to describe a borderless world of flowing life in constant movement. In 'Spaccio de la bestia trionfante' of 1584, for instance, Bruno describes the constant movement between opposites as a condition of constant change and the source of ethical motion, order and diversity.[11] In the infinity of animated nature, the oppositions between the corporeal and the mental, the objective and the subjective fall together, much as good and evil appear in coexistence.[12] Hence, to Giordano Bruno it is important that a wise person knows how to encounter and deal with these opposites. To his mind, only the person who allows for change is able to be conscious of these opposites and hence the only one able to deal with them productively and ethically.

In his *Basics of Acting*, Von Klöden indicates that he is deriving the concept of coincidentia oppositorum from this historical, neoplatonic trajectory:

> The coincidentia oppositorum, the falling together of opposites, which in Cusanus and in Giordano Bruno is a quality ascribed to God only, in the new perspective of natural science becomes the subject of objective observation as well as, demanded by physical matter, an ideal end of human effort.[13]

Through this mystification of natural science or rationalization of mystical unity, the least imperfect description of the One becomes the least imperfect description of the actor as an idealized, knowable, transparent human being in a democratic society. As such, he or she is supposed to integrate the antinomies listed in the table 'Pferd und Reiter' (horse and horseman): yin and yang, night and day, moon and sun, female and male, warm and cold, subjective and objective, Dionysus and Apollo, anima and animus, soul and mind, feeling and ratio, ecstasy and consciousness, imagination and design, intuitive and logical, endothyme grounding and personal superstructure, bios and logos, nature and culture. By doing so, she or he achieves harmony and wholeness in an *a priori* bifurcated existence of living chaos on the one hand and dead form on the other.

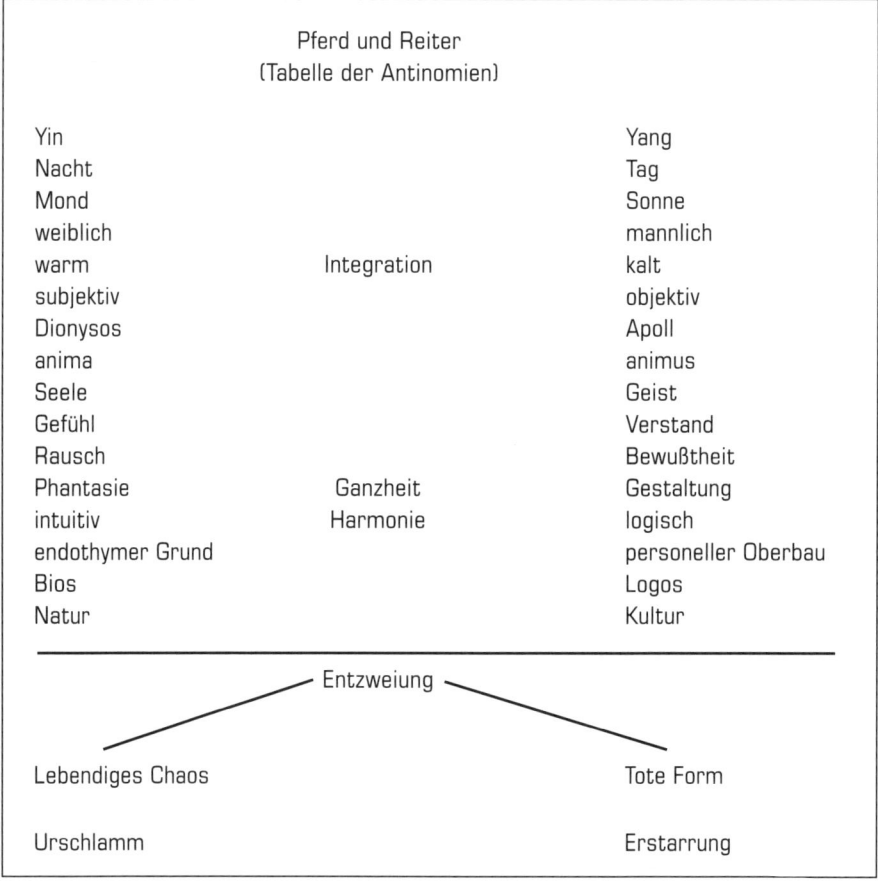

Pferd und Reiter
(Tabelle der Antinomien)

Yin		Yang
Nacht		Tag
Mond		Sonne
weiblich		mannlich
warm	Integration	kalt
subjektiv		objektiv
Dionysos		Apoll
anima		animus
Seele		Geist
Gefühl		Verstand
Rausch		Bewußtheit
Phantasie	Ganzheit	Gestaltung
intuitiv	Harmonie	logisch
endothymer Grund		personeller Oberbau
Bios		Logos
Natur		Kultur

Entzweiung

Lebendiges Chaos   Tote Form

Urschlamm   Erstarrung

Pferd und Reiter (Tabelle der Antinomien). (Horse and horseman (Table of Antinomies).) In: Hans-Günther von Klöden, *Grundlagen der Schauspielkunst II: Improvisation und Rollenstudium*, 1967, p. 25.

Key to the social transparency of the actor demanded by Von Klöden is a special consciousness that needs to be scientifically educated about these opposites and trained in the ability to oscillate between them in an eternal strife for wholeness, which can never be completed: 'The end of our way, which we will never reach, is to let the actor become how God had meant him to be.'[14]

The freedom to play with the various social roles without losing one's ability to make decisions is another important aspect of this process. The ability to make decisions and the 'double consciousness' here signify the integrity of the individual within a democratic system that is entirely dependent on its members' ability to make responsible, 'healthy' decisions.

It is not a coincidence that Von Klöden formulates this approach to acting in the Federal Republic of Germany, six years after the building of the wall, and less than a generation after the end of the Second World War. He himself had founded the Hannover acting school right at the end of the war and, like other founders of actor training programs in one of the four occupation zones in Germany at that time, developed an acting methodology according to the cultural-political program of democratizing, de-nazifying, demilitarizing, and decentralizing Germany. Von Klöden regards his book of 1967, with which he clearly demands a technique of mediation between dualistic extremes, as a reaction to the student generation of 1945:

> In the young generation of 1945 I no longer found the superficial, mendacious, technical make-believe, against which the 'method' [of Stanislavski, AK] had been thought out. On the contrary, I found a fanaticism for truth, for the sake of which all technical-formal aspects were in danger of being disdainfully left out. This did not change in the following years until this very day.[15]

In Von Klöden's rationalization of the situation after 1945, the students rejected the technical, declamatory acting style that had been prevalent on the national stages of the Third Reich and turned, in a counter-reaction, towards a search for inner truth. This search for inner truth was supported by the early writings of Stanislawski, which became available in German after 1945 through the cultural political program and publications within the Soviet occupation zone (Gaillard, 1946). Von Klöden poses his acting method as a reaction to this counter-reaction after 1945, offering an approach to acting that, while recognizing these two extremes, avoids an extremist mode of being on stage. At the same time, Von Klöden's argument for a two-way method in 1967 echoes contemporary publications in the field of sociology such as Herbert Marcuse's *One-Dimensional Man: Studies in the Ideology of Advanced Industrial Society*, published in

German in 1964, and the renaissance of the writings of Max Weber, initiated by Herbert Marcuse, among others, at the Heidelberger Soziologentag, also in 1964. In *One-Dimensional Man*, just to remind us, Marcuse warns about the pathological type of a bureaucratic one-dimensional man who can carry out genocides by patriotically paying his or her duty and obedience to the state government (Marcuse, 1978). The critique of the one-dimensional man is echoed in Von Klöden's differentiation between the 'pathological case' who cannot negotiate the encrusted 'mask' of the social role playfully, and the actor as a model human being who is liberated by his ability to decide to do so. To offer the actor as a remedy to these social and historical issues, Von Klöden has recourse to a neoplatonic concept, the aforementioned coincidentia oppositorum, in which the body is constructed as one-half of a bifurcated whole. However, whereas in Bruno the opposites fall together in the omnipresent God in nature, Von Klöden equates this eternal force with the omnipresent laws of natural science.

Dis/Continuities in Technologies of Culture

Such mystification of natural science and of actor training methods is nothing unusual in the publications coming out of those post-war German actor training programs that were founded in the occupation zones of the Western allies (French, British, American) after 1945. Actor training programs in all four occupation zones or Berlin sectors promised to break with the declamatory acting style conditioned by the national socialist cultural propaganda of the 1930s and 1940s, and strove for a continuity of 'theatre arts that were not endangered by having been influenced by the national socialist side'.[16] At the same time they also rejected the experimentations of the historical avant-garde in the 1910s and 1920s.[17] The early writings or speeches on actor training coming out of schools such as the Acting Program of the German Theatre Institute in the Soviet Occupation Zone in Weimar (opened in 1945 and institutionalized in 1947), the Falckenberg School in the American Zone in Munich (conceived in 1945/46, opened in 1947 and named after Otto Falckenberg in 1948), the Hannover School in the British occupation zone (founded by Von Klöden in 1945), the Hebbel Theatre School in the American Sector in Berlin (opened 1946) or the School associated with the Deutsches Theater in the Soviet sector in Berlin (re-opened 1946) reflect a struggle for reorientation in the name of 'truth' and a heightened awareness of the actor as a model human being in the reconstruction of German society. However, the means by which 'truthful acting' should be achieved methodologically, how truthful acting was defined, and in the service of which political system it was to operate, differed depending on the respective occupation zone or sector within which a school was situated, on the cultural and political self-understanding of each victor nation, and on the local traditions and artistic trajectories of the founding members of these schools.

In addition to all differences, the schools in the Western occupation zones tended to take recourse to a Christian value system while insisting on a clear, which is to say dualistic, differentiation between good vs. evil, true vs. false, right vs. wrong. Hans Gebhardt and Otto Falckenberg, for instance, wrote in 1948:

> For our present and future existence, it is crucial that we order our terms of value, in the way that 'evil' will be addressed and judged as evil without hesitation, and that 'good' is bound to mean good in all cases; that 'ugly' is simply ugly and nothing else and 'beautiful' will be honestly perceived as beautiful; that God and man will not be mistaken for each other and neither nature for art; that children are children and parents parents; that through no malicious art injustice may be passed as justice or lies as truth. This is what it means: 'To start anew.'[18]

Around the same time, Ernst Schröder, head of the Hebbel Theatre School in the American sector in Berlin, kept a diary together with his students, in which they used quotations from the bible and called the actor a 'tight-rope walker between drive and prayer'. Schröder demands from the actor that he or she 'must find the hidden entrance leading back to Paradise in order to give us a shimmer of the innocence of Man before the Fall'.[19]

Von Klöden's *Basics of Acting*, within the discourses and political forces of 1960s West Germany, reacts against this institutionalization of a dualistic order of the world in the aftermath of the National Socialist Regime and the Second World War and, at the same time, echoes the post-WWII search for truth and innocence in a Christian value system with his mystification of the actor as an idealized human being making good, transparent decisions within a democratic social order. The actor's body becomes a site where the border between the externally perceivable social order and the internally concealed and possibly unordered aspects of being are explored. The dualistic struggle and harmonization between body and soul, materiality and assumed immateriality, which – as Jonathan Sawday reminds us – was 'the dominant model for understanding the relationship between body and soul within western culture prior to the fifteenth century', becomes fundamental to Von Klöden's perception and construction of individuality in 1960s West German society (Sawday, 1995, p. 17). Hence he takes recourse in a pre-modern concept of being, which, combined with the increasing rationalization of knowledge in the form of 'natural science' in the Western industrialized nations after WWII, set the actor onto a never-ending methodological journey toward a paradisiacal state of a complete and free human being.

Anja Klöck is Professor of Drama at the Hochschule für Musik und Theater 'Felix Mendelssohn Bartholdi' in Leipzig, Germany. She holds a PhD from the University of Minnesota, USA, and subsequently taught at the Johannes Gutenberg University in Mainz, Germany. Her work has been published in *Theatre Journal, Theatre Research International, Performance Research*, a number of German anthologies and the series *Theater der Zeit Recherchen*. In her current research, which is funded by the German Research Foundation (DFG), she is investigating the interrelationships between actor training programs and cultural politics in Germany after 1945.

Notes

1   Nervous system in Andreas Vesalius, *De humani corporis fabrica* (1543); flayed figure in Juan Valverde de Hamusco, *Anatomia del corpo humano* (1560); dissected female figure in the *Tabulae anatomicae* of Pietro Berrettini da Cortona (1618-1620); self-demonstrating figure in Adriaan van de Spiegel and Giulio Casseri, *De formato foetu* (1627).

2   Consider, for instance, Franciscus Lang's *Dissertatio de actione scenica*, published 1727, Pierre Rémond de Sainte-Albine's *Le Comédien*, published 1747, Francesco Riccoboni's *L'Art du théâtre*, published 1750, Aaron Hill's *Essay on the Art of Acting*, published 1753, Denis Diderot's *Observation sur une brochure intitulée Garrick ou les acteurs anglais*, written in 1769/1770 and posthumously published as *Paradoxe sur le comédien* in 1830.

3   See particularly chapters 4 and 5 of René Descartes, 'Discourse on the Method of Properly Conducting One's Reason' and 'On Seeking the Truth in the Sciences' (1637) in Descartes, *Discourse on Method and other Writings*. (Trans. and with an introduction by F.E. Surcliffe.) Harmondsworth, 1968, and Julien Offray de La Mettrie, *L'homme machine = Die Maschine Mensch* (Trans. Claudia Becker.) Hamburg, 1990, p. 5 ff.

4   'Unsere Ausbildung ist Berufsausbildung, Ausbildung in einem Handwerk, und muß es bleiben. [D]ie auf Echtheit zielende "Arbeit an sich selbst" ist ein lebensgefährliches Unternehmen; es gilt hier entweder alles zu gewinnen oder alles zu verlieren; denn die Lebensrolle, die Maske, ist der Schutz des Menschen nicht nur vor der Gesellschaft, sondern auch vor den eigenen Abgründen. Für den Schauspieler gilt es aber, diese ernste Maske abzunehmen, sich frei zu machen für die durchsichtige Maske des Spiels' (Von Klöden, 1967, pp. 25-26). Unless otherwise noted, all translations are my own.

5   Johan Huizinga, *Homo ludens: Vom Ursprung der Kultur im Spiel* (1938). (Trans. H. Nachod.) Reinbek bei Hamburg, 1994 (1956); C. G. Jung, *Psychologische Typen*. Zürich, 1960 (1920); Peter R. Hofstätter, *Sozialpsychologie*. Berlin, 1956.

6   For Huizinga on play and freedom, see Huizinga, 1994, p. 16 ff., on play and ethics p. 230 ff.

7   'Und worin besteht dieses Können, dieses Handwerk? Fraglos zunächst im Sprechen-Können und in der Möglichkeit der freien Bewegung. Aber nicht nur hierin, sondern weitgehendst in einer ganz bestimmten Bewußtseinsverfassung, die einmal gekennzeichnet ist durch Freiheit und durch die Folgen, die diese Freiheit in Sprache und

Bewegung hat, aber nicht zuletzt durch eine höchst eigenartige und diskursiv kaum darstellbare Ambivalenz von Identifikation und Objektivation, die es dem Schauspieler ermöglicht, quasi gleichzeitig aus der Vorstellung des Figurseins und des In-der-Situation-Seins, das heißt aus der Phantasie intuitiv zu handeln, als auch aus dem Sich-selbst-und-seiner-Figur-Gegenüberstehen zu "gestalten" (Doppelbewußtsein)' (Von Klöden, 1967, p. 8).

8   See Sawday, 1995, p. 2: 'In medicine, too, anatomization takes place in order that the integrity and health of other bodies can be preserved.'

9   'Da das Wissen um eine Scheinhaltung beim Spielen einer Lebensrolle den gesunden vom pathologischen Fall unterscheidet, könnte man den guten Schauspieler geradezu als den vorbildlich gesund handelnden Menschen betrachten' (Von Klöden, 1967, p. 16).

10 'Die Zwei-Wege-Methode bezieht sich nicht nur auf das Gegensatzpaar Form und Inhalt, sondern durchdringt in immer neuem Zusammenhang die gesamte Schauspielererziehung. Die Welt erscheint uns dualistisch. Die Gegensätze Form und Inhalt, bewußt und unbewußt, Handwerk und Intuition, Fleiß und Begabung, Innen und Außen - um nur die in unserer Arbeit am häufigsten gebrauchten zu erwähnen - beherrschen unser Denken. Von dieser Tatsache haben wir auszugehen, wenn wir uns auf den Weg machen, diese Gegensätze zu überwinden, um zu einem Ganzheitserlebnis zu kommen. Es ist zuerst notwendig, daß die Schüler diese Antinomien zuerst als Gegensätze, dann als Pole ein und derselben Sache erkennen und sie schließlich in einer coincidentia oppositorum zu überwinden trachten' (Von Klöden, 1967, p. 26).

11 'Quello che da ciò voglio inferire, è che il principio, il mezzo ed il fine, il nascimento, l'aumento e la perfezione di quanto veggiamo, è da' contrarii, per contrarii, ne contrarii, a' contrarii: e dove è la contrarietade [contrarietà], è la azione reazione, è il moto, è la diversità, è la moltitudine, è l'ordine, son gli gradi, è la successione, è la vicissitudine. Perciò nessuno, che ben considera, giamai per l'essere ed aver presente si desmetterà o s'inalzarà d'animo, quantunque, in comparazion d'altri abiti e fortune, gli paia buon rio, peggiore o megliore' (Bruno, 1909, p. 22).

12 See Calcagno, 1998, p. 31: 'As part of this cycle of ethical change from one state to its opposing state, from love to hate and vice versa, etc., there is an assurance that we are not eternally condemned to one constant and static onto-ethical reality. We are, therefore, not absolutely bad or good, as we fluctuate between these apparent opposites.'

13 'Die coincidentia oppositorum, das Zusammenfallen der Gegensätze, die bei dem Cusaner und bei Giordano Bruno eine Eigenschaft ist, die ausschließlich Gott zugestanden werden kann, wird in der neuen Sicht durch die Naturwissenschaften sowohl Gegenstand objektiver Betrachtung, als auch, eben durch den physikalischen Gegenstand gefordert, wieder ideales Ziel menschlicher Bemühung' (Von Klöden, 1967, p. 27).

14 'Das Ziel, zu dem wir auf dem Wege sind, das wir aber nie err.eichen werden, ist, ihn wieder so werden zu lassen, "wie Gott ihn gemeint hat"' (Von Klöden, 1967, p. 24).

15 'Bei der jungen Generation von 1945 fand sich nicht mehr die oberflächliche, verlogene, technische Mache, gegen die die 'Methode' erdacht war, sondern im Gegenteil ein Wahrheitsfanatismus, dem zuliebe alle technisch-formalen Gesichtspunkte immer wieder geringschätzig über Bord geworfen zu werden drohten. Das blieb auch so bis in den folgenden Jahren auf den heutigen Tag' (Von Klöden, 1967, p. 7).

16 From Otto Falckenberg's 'report of activities' presented to the American Military Administration. Birgit Pargner, *Otto Falckenberg – Regiepoet der Münchner Kammerspiele*. Berlin, 2005, p. 208. See also Ernst Schröder's diary as head of the Hebbel

Theater School in Berlin, 1946: 'Der Mensch heute muss sich auf der Bühne an-
ders äußern als der etwa von 1939. Auch in der Darstellung eines Klassikers ertragen
wir nicht mehr den kleinsten Druck auf die Stimme, nicht mehr den Ansatz einer
zufälligen Gebärde. Die Schiller und Kleist gemäße Überhöhung ist heute nur dann
zu erreichen, wenn sich der Schauspieler *als Mensch* aufdeckt. Er darf nichts mehr
verstecken, er kann sich nicht mehr verbergen. Kein übersteigerter Ausdruck ver-
mag standzuhalten vor der Erschütterung durch unsere tatsächlichen Erlebnisse'
(Schröder, 1966, pp. 51-52).

17   See Gebhart and Falckenberg in Gebhart, 1948, p. 15: 'Wie aber – : stand nicht das
apokalyptische Geschehen des Zweiten Weltkriegs (...) im Zeichen einer Reaktion
g e g e n den Geist, die sich nicht laut genug als Vitalismus proklamieren konnte? Die
Vernichtung des Lebens geschah im Namen einer Botschaft des Lebens!'
Compare with:
'... Rußland ist sehr entschieden von diesem 'proletkultischen' und vom intellektuel-
len Regisseurtheater abgerückt. Der menschliche Realismus Stanislawskijs wurde
als eine große kulturelle Leistung des bürgerlichen Theaters anerkannt, und das
Theater der Sowjetunion knüpfte an seine fortschrittlichen Traditionen an' (Gaillard, 1946, p. 19).

18   'Es ist von äußerster Erheblichkeit in unserm jetzigen und künftigen Dasein,
beispielsweise unsere Wertbegriffe zu ordnen, – so etwa, daß 'böse' einwandfrei
und ohne Schwanken als böse angesprochen und eingeordnet wird, und daß 'gut' in
jedem Sinn verbindlich als gut gilt; daß 'häßlich' einfach häßlich und nichts weiter
ist und 'schön' ehrlich empfunden schön; daß Gott und Mensch nicht verwechselt
werden und nicht Natur und Kunst; daß Kinder Kinder sind und Eltern Eltern; daß
Unrecht durch keine Kunst der Bosheit für Recht ausgegeben werden kann und
Lüge für Wahrheit. Das heißt ungefähr: "Von vorne anfangen"' (Gebhart, 1948, p.
18).

19   Published in Schröder, 1966, pp. 25-30.

References

Barthes, R., *Roland Barthes.* (Trans. Richard Howard.) London, 1977.

Bruno, G., 'Lo Spaccio de la bestia trionfante'. In: *Le Opere Italiane* vol. II, ed.
Giovanni Gentile. Bari, 1909.

Calcagno, A., *Giordano Bruno and the Logic of Coincidence: Unity and Multiplic-
ity in the Philosophical Thought of Giordano Bruno.* New York, 1998.

Gaillard, O., *Lehrbuch der Schauspielkunst – Das Deutsche Stanislawskij-Buch.*
Zürich, 1946.

Cortona, P. da, *Tabulae anatomicae a Pietro Berretini Cortonensi et a Cajetano Pi-
etrioli Romano.* Romae: Impensis Fausti Amidei, Ex typographia Antonii
de Rubeis, 1741.

Gebhart, H., *Über die Kunst des Schauspielers – Gespräche mit Otto Falckenberg.*
München, 1948.

Huizinga, J., *Homo ludens: Vom Ursprung der Kultur im Spiel* (1938). (Trans. H.
Nachod.) Reinbek bei Hamburg, 1994 [1956].

Klöden, H.G. von, *Grundlagen der Schauspielkunst II: Improvisation und Rollen-studium*. Hannover, 1967.

La Mettrie, J.O. de., *L'homme machine = Die Maschine Mensch*. (Trans. Claudia Becker.) Hamburg, 1990.

Marcuse, H., *Der eindimensionale Mensch – Studien zur Ideologie der fortgeschrittenen Industriegesellschaft* (Trans. Alfred Schmidt.) Neuwied, 1978 [1967].

Roach, J.R., *The Player's Passion: Studies in the Science of Acting*. Newark and London, 1985.

Sawday, J., *The Body Emblazoned: Dissection and the Human Body in Renaissance Culture*. London and New York, 1995.

Schröder, E., *Die Arbeit des Schauspielers*. Zürich, 1966.

Spiegel, A. van de and G. Casseri, *De formato foetu liber singularis*. Padua: Patavii, apud Io. Bap. De Martinis, Liui u Pasquat u ... expensis eiusdem Liberalis Cremae, 1926 [1626].

Valverde de Amusco, J., *Anatomia del corpo humano*. Roma: Ant. Salamanca & Antonio Lafrerij, 1560.

Vesalius, A., *De humani corporis fabrica libri septem*. Basileae: Ex officina Ioannis Oporini, 1543.

Ocular Anatomy, Chiasm, and Theatre Architecture as a Material Phenomenology in Early Modern Europe

Pannill Camp

Husserlian phenomenology, long a critical apparatus employed by theatre and performance scholars, is already infiltrated by a theatrical mode of thought that is more or less explicit in much of Husserl's philosophy. It has chimerically incorporated the architecture of the theatre in the mode of the Western, frontally oriented, proscenium stage. Supporting such a claim requires a careful calibration of the terms of 'phenomenology' and of 'theatre architecture' as historically bounded modes of thought, each of which reflects an underlying condition of knowing, or *connaissance*[1], that is itself conditioned by history. The articulation of this *connaissance* is manifested in phenomenology's tendency to build a structural consciousness, member by member, as though it were an architectural entity. Husserlian phenomenology can be seen as constituted by and as possessor of an architectonics that is distinctly theatrical in that it adopts certain spatial attributes of theatre architecture of the Renaissance and modern era.

If it can be demonstrated that theatrical architecture as an ideal, if malleable, structure was available for more or less explicit incorporation into Husserl's project, then one wonders 1) what attributes would recommend this particular architectural model above others and 2) what genealogical factors shaped theatre architecture such that these attributes were incorporated into it in the first place. It is here that the figure of the chiasm, a crossing of positional terms over each other in space, can be found occupying a central position in every sense.

Western theatre architecture developed contemporaneously with the rationalization of ocular anatomy to geometric optics from the seventeenth century onwards, and there is reason to believe that the morphology of both types of structure manifests a grand, diffuse reorientation of mankind's relationship to the world. As vision, constituted in the emerging understanding of the eye's function, came to be a central figure for man's relationship to other things (which is to say, objectivity), theatre buildings came to model this same relationship and to embody an *isomorphism* with ocular anatomy. In each case, the relationship of the subject to the object is spatially figured by a chiasm that mediates between one and the other.

I will argue that the human oculus is taken up by theatre architecture gradually in the seventeenth and eighteenth centuries as demonstrated by the advent of the proscenium arch, which locates a chiasmic relation of auditorium as subject to stage as object-space, just as the pupil comes to signify this same relationship and locate a similar crossing of 'sightlines' between internal and external space. The conjugation of theatre architecture with ocular anatomy crystallizes in the Théâtre de Besançon of Claude-Nicolas Ledoux, whose theorization of the forestage, or *avant-scène*, the space that dwells beneath that anatomized arch, between the audience and stage proper, resonates powerfully with the figure of the protostage, or *archi-scène*, which Derrida installs as a model of temporality within Husserl's phenomenology. Finally, I will suggest that the chiasm, besides diagramming the anatomical condition of the frontal, visual encounter with the object, meaningfully articulates a modern theatrical *connaissance* by virtue of its minimal attendant temporality, one that conditions the transposition of positional terms through space. As such, theatre architecture in the mode of the proscenium arch, both as a model of an emerging mode of knowledge and as a technology of thought imported by phenomenology, will be shown to be of pivotal importance to the epistemic shift that marshals modernity into existence and is, in fact, a historical condition of phenomenological thought itself.

Renaissance Theatre Architecture and Optics as an Incipient Phenomenology

The completion of Aleotti's Teatro Farnese at Parma – with its fully articulated, permanent proscenium arch – is considered by many to be the 'prototype' of the modern theatre. Its construction coincided with the publication of *Oculus: Hoc Est*, an optical treatise by Christoph Scheiner considered to have described the eye's anatomy accurately for the first time. Thus, both the history of theatre architecture and the history of ocular science select the year 1619 to mark their passage into the modern age.[2] My argument takes this collision of history — events separated by less than one year and by roughly 250 miles — as the first indication that optics and theatre architecture share a unique relationship. I hope to show that these two discourses modernized in tandem, occasionally drawing on a common fund of discourse and spatial representations.

Theatre architecture approached by way of its history and, necessarily, its morphology offers itself up as a cultural formation whose conditions may be variously assessed. The theatre architecture of the Italian Renaissance has been read as evidence of larger social, economic and intellectual trends: the popularization of secular drama, revisions to models of state and polity, a flourishing but contested Classicism. It is commonplace to refer to the 'evolution' of theatre architecture, as though it adapted progressively towards increasingly complex and rational incarnations.[3] Unfortunately, such unqualified remarks suggest a positive evolution of cultures and further imply intercultural evolutionary differentials insofar as they presume that a rational, uniform *telos* determines architectural practices. The present intervention will posit theatre architecture as a complex of *technics*, which is to say an array of practices of organizing inorganic matter subject to the determining factors of economic need, available resources, internally and externally imposed limitations and the potential for borrowing.[4] While it is admissible within this framework to mention technical advance in developments in theatre architecture, these processes are understood to be contingent upon a variety of factors explicitly divorced from the 'genius' of a given culture and to be progressive in only the temporal sense.

The proliferation of public theatres for secular performances in the sixteenth and seventeenth centuries not only marks a sea change in modes of performance and the undercurrents of political philosophy that explicitly determined them, but also demonstrates the production of *connaissance*. Put simply, theatre architecture of the Vitruvian model served to enable novel ways of thinking about mankind in relation to the world. Foucault has argued that the 'Classical episteme' ultimately expired as the category of 'man' came to be put into doubt. Signs became separated from their referents, wealth from intrinsic value, and living things from a grand tabular hierarchy. As the seventeenth century came to a close, Foucault claims, it became possible to think of man as simultaneously sovereign and subjected, as the agent of a potentially infinite knowledge and yet conceivable himself in an empirical finitude (Foucault, 1971, pp. 3-16). As part of this process, Foucault explains, knowledge itself came to be recalibrated in new analyses:

> There are those that operate within the space of the body, and – by studying perception, sensorial mechanisms, neuro-motor diagrams, and the articulation common to things and to the organism – function as a sort of transcendental aesthetic; these led to the discovery that knowledge has anatomo-physiological conditions, that it is formed gradually within the structures of the body, that it may have a privileged place within it, but that its forms cannot be dissociated from its peculiar functioning; in short, that there is a nature of human knowledge that determines its own forms and that can be at the same time made manifest to it in its own empirical contents. (Foucault, 1971, p. 319)

A look at the application of Vitruvian theatre architecture to two radically different projects, those of Giulio Camillo's Memory Theatre and Andrea Palladio's Teatro Olimpico at Vicenza, shows that theatre architecture was appropriated to model the relationship of man to the catalogue of human knowledge in
the first case, and to articulate the problematic heterogeneity of visual perspective in the second. The stunning fact that the same architectural technique was
taken up for the purpose of modelling both the ideal position of humanity with
respect to knowledge and the contours of a generalized practice of vision both
reinforces Foucault's epistemic topology and forecasts the merging of these
two projects in the form of Claude-Nicolas Ledoux's Theatre at Besançon two
centuries later. The architectural theatre represents in each case a groping articulation of epistemological problems that prefigure notions of embodiment
and consciousness that have supported much phenomenological writing in the
twentieth century.

Giulio Camillo (1480-1544) attained remarkable fame in Europe for a creation he called his Memory Theatre. The infamous, unfinished wooden structure was seen by few and understood by perhaps none. According to accounts
of those who saw versions of the structure in Venice and in Paris, it was large
enough to fit two people within it, and the occupants of the theatre found themselves before a semi-circular array of images and boxes, across which were displayed symbols that represented all human knowledge. Camillo conceived of
this theatre as a type of memory aid or rhetorical apparatus that would empow-
er the occupant 'to discourse on any subject no less fluently than Cicero'.[5] While
a comprehensive account of the theatre and its workings does not survive, the
device was widely known, and Camillo spent decades travelling between Italy
and France hustling for financial support to bring the theatre, and a tome which
would theorize it, to fruition. Tellingly, this means that Camillo's theatre, or at
least word of it, crisscrossed the geography that would situate most of the major
innovations in theatre architecture of the sixteenth and seventeenth centuries,
fomenting intellectual curiosity as to the workings of a theatre structure vis-à-
vis human knowledge and elocution. What is more, Frances Yates emphatically
describes Camillo's structure as an incarnation and 'a distortion of the plan of
the real Vitruvian theatre' (Yates, 1966, p. 136). The circulation of this particular
model of theatre structure in Italy during the early sixteenth century may well
have prompted architects to consider their own Vitruvian revivals.

According to an orthodox historiography, a properly phenomenological
outlook — a philosophy explicitly concerned with consciousness as such — is
not possible before Descartes's *cogito*. Yet there is reason to consider Camillo's
Memory Theatre to be an early, architectural model of the fraught relationship
between man and the world available to him as knowledge, and therefore evidence of an incipient phenomenology. While the structure may be interpreted

as a tool for the enhancement of memory and elocution, it also attempts to aggregate all possible knowledge into a hierarchically-layered grid, both positing an order to knowledge as such and groping at the limits of that knowledge. Camillo, it seems, considered the theatre to be not just a model of knowledge as ordered by the form of the world, but an architectonics of the human psyche itself. According to Erasmus,

> He calls this theatre of his by many names, saying now that it is a built or constructed mind and soul, and now that it is a windowed one. He pretends that all things that the human mind can conceive and which we cannot see with the corporeal eye, after being collected together by diligent meditation may be expressed by certain corporeal signs in such a way that the beholder may at once perceive with his eyes everything that is otherwise hidden in the depths of the human mind. And it is because of this corporeal looking that he calls it a theatre. (Yates, 1966, p. 132)

That the theatre models the mind and soul, that it enables the apprehension of hidden things which can be accessed through diligent meditation, that it plumbs the depths of the human mind — all stamp Camillo as the proponent and architect of a philosophy of consciousness prematurely born. For Camillo in 1540, the eye already looms as an organ whose function is the aspiration of the theatre. Yates points out that the middle of the seven rows which arrange the store of knowledge in Camillo's theatre, 'the grade of the Theatre dealing with the "interior man", is marked with the image of the three Gorgon sisters who shared one eye between them' (Yates, 1966, p. 149). Not just 'seeing,' but the eye itself comes to be identified with the apparatus of knowing. That which cannot be seen with the eye of the body demands a wooden structure to produce another manifest vision. That is to say that Camillo's theatre is the embodiment of a *seeing* whose station and peculiar form is to produce an adequate *knowing* – in its materiality it is thought to manifest knowledge itself; the corporeal looking in the form of the theatre amounts to what Yates calls 'a new Renaissance plan of the psyche' and demonstrates the emergence of a novel regime of knowledge that depends, to some degree, on the deliverances of the senses (Yates, 1966, p. 149).

In accordance with this pattern – this practice of framing objects of knowledge – the protractedly percolating preoccupation with vision and perspective would come to be incorporated into the architecture of the theatre and expressed as an *ocular theme*. The coincidence of a reinvigoration of theatre design, the sundry perspective techniques in the visual arts, a proliferation of human anatomical knowledge and the rectification thereof with a refined understanding of light and optics produced a series of buildings that manifest clear isomorphic resonances with the human eye. In particular, the chiasmic confrontation with respect to sightlines between stage and auditorium was articulated quite early by Camillo's contemporary, Andrea Palladio.

The decades during which Camillo shuttled between Italy and France promoting and raising funds for his speculative Memory Theatre were the same ones during which Palladio was exposed to key influences, which may have included Camillo himself. Yates speculates that Camillo's enigmatic project was the subject of intense discussion in the academic halls of Italy and therefore might have been known to Palladio, who came to be the sole 'artist' charter member of the Accademia Olimpica in Vicenza, on whose premises the Teatro Olimpico was finally completed in 1580.[6] This remarkable structure, still standing with its original scenic enhancements, demonstrates a concern with embodied practices of vision of a different valence than those manifested in Camillo's Memory Theatre. While it imports a quasi-Vitruvian design for stage and auditorium (shortened into an ellipse due to site constraints), Palladio's theatre was fitted with a recessed scenic complex beyond the *scenae frons* that has marked the Teatro Olimpico as a unique venture in the genealogy of Western theatre design development. Four years after Palladio's death, Vincenzo Scamozzi and Palladio's son Silla fitted the *scenae frons* with seven perspective street scenes, five of which diverge from a nodal point on the threshold of the stage. These elaborate scenic constructions, backed by a dome painted as the sky, were designed according to the perspective-foreshortening conventions described by Sebastiano Serlio in his 1545 *Architettura*. Rather than converging in Serlian fashion, however, to a vanishing point on the sagittal line of the theatre, they fanned out dramatically across a range of axes such that 'at least one street [is] visible to each member of the audience' (Leacroft and Leacroft, 1984, pp. 46-47). The result, when seen in plan, reveals a crossing of sightlines from the outermost ranges of the auditorium over each other down opposing street perspectives. Five of the seven streets converge at the intersection of the proscenium threshold with the sagittal plane of the theatre, creating a 'nodal point' suggestive of the reference point in ocular anatomy from which light rays seem to originate as they travel to the light receptors in the retina.[7] Such a comparison implies the emergence of an ocular theme in theatre architecture, conscious or otherwise, which would not be realized explicitly until two centuries later.

Andrea and Silla Palladio and Vincenzo Scamozzi were surely less concerned with biomorphism in the design of their multiple-vista scenic constructions than with the optical conventions of perspective. The Teatro Olimpico, accordingly, is an eccentric attempt to cross the imperatives of Vitruvius's theatre model with the fashion of Serlian perspective scenery — to incorporate an optical theme based on the conventions of perspective whose concern was the geometry of space as perceived, rather than the anatomical make-up of the eye. Yet it would be hasty to assume that Palladio was not thinking of the anatomy of the body in relation to architecture. According to Ackerman, Palladio has been interpreted as an architect whose designs are guided by 'human physical and psychological make-up in their appeal to permanently valid laws of harmony and in their reference to the structure of the human body' (Ackerman, 1966, p. 185). Ackerman also points out the influence of the widely published anatomical drawings of Andreas Vesalius, who worked in Padua during Palladio's youth. Whether or not Palladio thought of his Teatro Olimpico as recapitulating natural anatomical forms, his exemplary design nonetheless marks the instantiation of a chiasm that propagated through Western theatrical architecture.

The crossing over of sightlines from the outer edges of the auditorium and the frontal encounter between spectator and spectacle determine a seam along the proscenium edge that is chiasmatically coded. In the theatre one speaks of 'stage right' interchangeably with 'house left' in reference to the point of view of actor or audience, respectively. The persistence of this terminology in fact necessarily implies the dominance of the architectural convention of bilateral symmetry, upon which depends the fact of a constant, clear 'right' and 'left'. In other words, the chiasm of sightlines made evident in the Teatro Olimpico marks the crossing over of a certain flat threshold, an instrumental perpendicular plane articulated and enforced by the architect's volition. This morphology — the perpendicular slicing and windowing of the theatre to designate conceptually opposed space — is forecast by the gaping central arch in the *frons* of Palladio's design, and manifested by the proscenium arch whose use became commonplace in permanent theatres as early as 1586, and whose installation into the stage that would be called the 'prototype of virtually all those that were to follow during the next 300 years' was countenanced in the 1619 Teatro Farnese of Giovan Battista Aleotti in Parma.[8] This landmark date in the histories of theatre building and optics occurs during an era in which published work on optics, astronomy, and the workings of the eye multiplied.

The 1604 publication in Frankfurt of Johannes Kepler's *Optics* is considered by some to 'inaugurate the modern approach to optics, with a clear understanding of how the eye works'.[9] This treatise and its illustrations, and those of Christoph Scheiner, demonstrate a detailed and intimate mapping and analysis of the eyeball as an entity with mechanical and optical features whose function allows for the manipulation of light. Optics, astronomy, and ocular anatomy were interdependent categories of knowledge since the refractions of light through the atmosphere and material of the eye itself had been identified as sources of error in the apprehension of visual phenomena. Optical and anatomical drawings in the pages of Kepler and Scheiner are highly suggestive of chiasm: both that of the crossing of light rays from an image over each other at the pupil (the *camera obscura* or pinhole effect) and the crossing implied by the convergence of lines that extend from the outer surface of the eye to distant objects. Moreover, Kepler's use of architectural metaphor suggests that an indwelling architectonic founds the rendering of the eye's anatomy. Witness the following proposition from Kepler's 'On the Foundations of Catoprics and the Place of the Image':

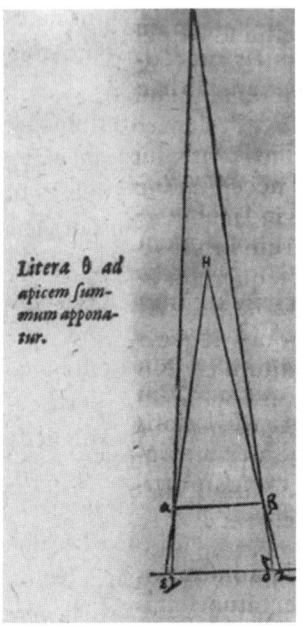

Litera θ ad apicem sum-mum appona-tur.

Now let this be taken from the senses as generally admitted: that genuine vision occurs when the folding door (valuae) or pupil of the eye is exposed most closely to the arriving ray of light. Thence it follows that vision from the direction whence the light approaches, is rendered more certain by this direction of the eye and of the entire face, which is like a support. (Kepler, 2000)

Diagram illustrating the relationship between the distance of a visible object and the breadth of the visual rays cast onto the back of the eye from Johannes Kepler, *Ad vitellionem paralipomena* (1604). Brown University Library.

Kepler here corroborates Foucault's observation that anatomical structure came to be an inextricable term in the function of certain knowledge production and suggests that this type of analysis was possible in the early seventeenth century. What is more, it demonstrates a predilection for architectural metaphor in anatomical knowledge. Kepler introduces the Latin *valuae*, a word for the large double door typically found in a temple or palace. This choice of anatomo-architectural description makes of the eye a kind of chamber, onto which adjoining space may be connected through a structure that admits opening and closure — a notion that was later adopted by Enlightenment theatre architects in France, who spoke of the proscenium as an *ouverture*, or opening onto stage space.[10]

Kepler makes passing reference to the notion of *theatrum mundi* in his preface, invoking the preferred Renaissance structuring metaphor for the world in its appearance, but the identification of theatre architecture itself with the organic conditions of knowledge would not be fully expressed for another two

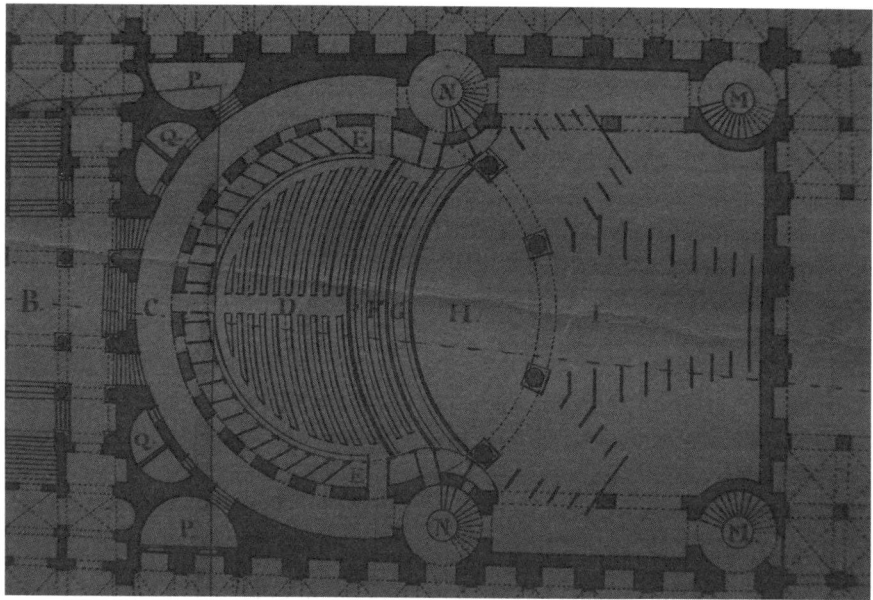

Plan drawing of a design by Charles de Wailly and Marie-Joseph Peyre for the Odéon (1770).
Archives Nationales – Paris site: Carton O1 846.

centuries. More suggestive of the convergence of ocular anatomy with theatre architecture, however, are the patterns of combined geometric figures that populate both Kepler's and other optical studies of the eye and architectural plans for theatres. The astronomer diagrams the eye with a geometric repertoire of cones, pyramids and spheres, calculating the proportions of light rays traversing the 'different coverings and humors, within and without' and their attendant refractions (Kepler, 2000, p. 79). Kepler takes on a deeply phenomenological attitude in laying out the geometry that describes the means of vision:

> But this visible world is itself concave and round, and whatever we behold of the hemisphere or the greater with a single fixed gaze, is a part of this roundness. It is therefore fitting that *the ratio of general objects to the whole hemisphere be estimated by the sense of vision, in the ratio of the entering form to the hemisphere of the eye.* (Kepler, 2000, p. 79; original emphasis)

The order of the world here is, strikingly, hemispheric for Kepler just as it was for Camillo, though in an entirely different sense. For Kepler, the hemispheric surface of the eye's interior, that anatomical contour itself — that is, its geometric form — exists in ratio not to the world itself, but to the contour of its appearance. The geometry used by Kepler and Scheiner to describe these appearances speaks to a repertoire shared with the geometry of Renaissance theatre architecture. Acute angles intersect circles symmetrically at their outermost points, or else cross over within them. Chiasm is a ubiquitous figure throughout. The hemispheric shape, common to Vitruvius, Camillo, Palladio, Kepler and Scheiner, is inevitably affixed to pairs of lines that cross each other, designating sightlines, either in the theatrical sense or in the sense of lines etched to model the passage of light rays through the body's own orbits.

Eighteen years after Scheiner's *Oculus*, Descartes gives a striking explanation justifying the inverted appearance of images projected onto the back of the eye. He explains that the eye of a cadaver, when stripped of layers of sclera at its back, reveals a screen onto which moving pictures of an overturned world could be projected, and he thought that this was not strange, but was 'just like our blind man's being able to feel, at one and the same time, the object B (to his right) by means of his left hand, and the object D (to his left) by means of his right hand' (Descartes, 1988, p. 67). The human body is in part composed of mechanisms that cross the world in front of it. The eye is inscribed with one or several chiasmic lines to make this legible. The borders of admitted light are traced across the curved surface at the back of the chamber against which light strikes. The magnitudes of distances and the extension of objects themselves were found to exist in ratio to the area of space they projected onto the retina. The eye becomes the measurer of things, a precisely functioning device that allows us to speak about the world. The optical and ocular aspects of knowledge were rectified and justified against each other; error was identified, explained, measured, and factored away in order to prepare for the emergence of a transparent reason for which vision would be the most favored sense. Proscenium arches proliferated, and auditoria cupped around them to gather their light, but the shape of the eye and that of the theatre did not consciously converge until 134 years after the death of Descartes in 1650.

Ledoux and the Conjugation of Theatre Architecture with Ocular Anatomy

In his 1804 *L'architecture considérée sous le rapport de l'art, des mœurs et de la legislation*, Claude-Nicolas Ledoux included an engraved superimposition of theatre architecture with the eye's anatomy. The frame of the engraving is filled with an eye, the iris and pupil of which appear to open onto an auditorium just like that of Ledoux's Théâtre de Besançon, which opened for the first time in 1784. The resemblances of the Théâtre de Besançon to the Teatro

Olimpico are numerous and striking. Ledoux installs a semicircular colonnade and frieze of heroic scenes highly suggestive of Palladio's Classical roots. Photographs of the auditorium of Palladio's theatre from the vantage of the central perspective vista show a similar picture through the arch of the *cavea*. Anthony Vidler has noted that plan and section drawings 'reveal a multiplication of distinctions enforced by the social codes of the town, while showing the influence of the model of Palladio's Teatro Olimpico' (Vidler, 1990, p. 170). That the rigidly compartmentalized auditorium design enforced social distinctions and made Besançon's class and rank striations legible is made clear by Vidler and corroborated by Robert Darnton's assessments of processions of dignitaries and merchants in the mid-eighteenth-century provinces (Darnton, 1999, pp. 107-144). Undoubtedly, Ledoux designed this theatre with social strata and a utopian social order in mind, and likewise he clearly drew directly from classical models, hoping to press the potentially unruly municipal scene into geometrically structured slots inspired by the renewing cultural force of antiquity.[11] Yet, at the same time, the explicit conjugation of theatre building with the anatomy of the eye — the expression of the ocular thematic in Western theatre architecture — signals Ledoux's participation in the architecturally founded techniques of the pre-phenomenological inquiry into consciousness.

Ledoux's engraving, as Vidler points out, signals the biomorphism of the theatre's rounded proscenium arch. The arch gapes across the building, spanning the width of the second tier of boxes, and vaults up in roughly semi-circular fashion, mimicking the curvature of the iris partially covered by the upper eyelid. All of the theatre's many functions as an institution, even those of arousing passions and demonstrating virtue, come to be governed by the eye. As a conduit for the senses, passions and sentiments, the Théâtre de Besançon

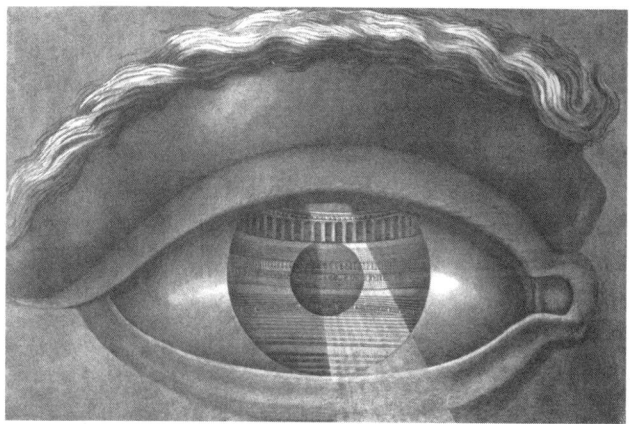

Coup d'oeil du théâtre de Besançon from Claude-Nicolas Ledoux's 1804 *L'Architecture considérée sous le rapport de l'art, des moeurs et de la législation*. Bibliothèque Nationale de France (BnF) Est. HA-MAT 1.

might provoke 'tender tears that bathe drop by drop without grimace;' it may also spur 'heartrending sobs, oppressive visions' (Ledoux, 1997, p. 373). The allegory of embodied vision so thoroughly pervades Ledoux that his emotional spasms must express themselves in lachrymal imagery. Ledoux's theatre is the eye for the consideration of pure morals and virtues: it takes itself for anatomy, for a corporeal looking in its own right, a *coup-d'œil*. While the eye remains for Ledoux a figure for the knowledge to be imparted by instructive spectacles, it also lends its shape to a project of self-effacement. In 'Théâtre de Besançon: Idées Générales', the architect suggests that the congruence of the proscenium arch with the eye's geometry causes the former to collapse into the latter, and disappear:

> What do we mean by a forestage? It is the window well, the intermediate thickness that separates the action from the outside; it is a smooth body; it is a rest during which the eye prepares itself for augmenting the pleasure of the soul, opposing the variety of situations of all types to the simplicity of the frame. I see nowhere that which is set forth; that which is called the forestage, legitimated by its usage, is nothing but the continuous line of the auditorium against the stage. (Ledoux, 1997, p. 380)

The window frame, after all, is not intended to separate the outside, but open onto it. An arch of smooth masonry, deep enough to contain boxes for seating the visiting municipal potentates, and dizzyingly wide, thought Ledoux, would only enhance and amplify access to the performance, not enforce a separation. The theatre effectively imitates the eye, which Ledoux identifies as the 'first frame', and lines up behind it, hiding it from view. Vidler calls this biomorphic arch 'the image of a view transparent to the scene itself,' calling to mind the suspensions and reductions of Husserl's philosophy, which promised access to a mode of pure knowing capable of freeing the object from presuppositions, a mode within which vision remained the most privileged sense (Vidler, 1990, p. 177).

Ledoux's other choices forecast the instantiation of a heightened viewing, free from distractions. Ledoux sunk the orchestra into a pit both to prevent the music from drowning out the voices of the actors and to obscure them from view. Furthermore, Vidler points out that the various segregations of seating (sections included four boxes for the King and Queen, Intendant and Governor of the Province, parquet, balcon, 1st and 2nd row of boxes, 1st and 2nd parterre), while enforcing a visibility that would deter 'lubricity', also prevented audience mixing which could encourage distracting chatter. Ledoux's attempt to control the atmosphere of the theatre extended to the control of odour. The outer row of the parterre was reserved for soldiers and the poorest members of the municipality so that the centre of the theatre wouldn't smell like 'people pressed into a carriage' (Vidler, 1990, p. 170). Every aspect of the auditorium and forestage was meant to effect a calm and controlled environment where 'one sees well everywhere' and where 'one is well seen' (Vidler, 1990, p. 176).

By 1784, optical concerns in theatre architecture have yielded to the ocular theme, which subsumes but does not suppress them. The modelling of sightlines still demands that the theatre building display its optical genealogy. Plans of a proposed theatre for Marseilles, much larger than the one at Besançon, bear the hashed lines of two angles, one that demonstrates the termination of seating where sightlines allow an unobstructed view of the depth of the stage and another that delimits seats that can see the forestage only. These caliper-like angles, when examined next to Kepler's demonstration of the ratio between proximity of the object and the breadth of the image projected on the retina, speak to discourses that have come to draw on overlapping fonts of geometric knowledge. Anatomical and architectural renderings, similarly dependent on Cartesian space, interpolate a grid, and find their proportions according to the observable behaviour of light. Sightlines, broadly defined, confer morphology upon the theatre, but there is no uniform ideal of theatre construction. The Théâtre de Besançon's ocular isomorphism makes legible a confluence of philosophical inquiry, social reform, and epistemological uncertainty prevalent in the seventeenth century. The conjugation of optics and theatre design at the end of the eighteenth century suggests a *connaissance* as yet unsettled in the wake of Enlightenment rationalism and empiricism. That the architect would propose to load the city into a model of the human eye in order that passions, virtues, and morals might be made apparent implies the co-immanence of theatre and a practice of interrogating the appearance of the world which would itself crystallize under the banner of phenomenology another century later.

Ledoux's Théâtre de Besançon is usually overlooked in narratives of Western theatre design, but there is evidence to suggest a genealogical link between this theatre and another building of interest to students of phenomenology. Leacroft and Leacroft posit that Ledoux's theatre, in its united and open, if still segregated, auditorium and utopian aspirations, served as an influence for Wagner and Bruckwald's Festspielhaus at Bayreuth. Ledoux's 'orchestra, set partly beneath the stage with a curved reflecting rear wall, was also taken up by Wagner'.[12] The 'mystic chasm' effected by Wagner and Bruckwald's staggered proscenia may be presaged by Ledoux's no less ideologically rendered *avant-scène*, for both articulations claim to reduce the factual world away so as to foster communality between the audience and the scene. Both Wagner's discourse of purity, of an unimpeded encounter with the world within the frame, and his 'preoccupation with the visual' serve to locate him in a line of descent from Ledoux's architectural eye (Izenour, 1977, p. 282).

The opening of Wagner's world-famous theatre in 1876 could not have escaped the attention of a young Edmund Husserl, who in that same year began his university studies in Leipzig, roughly 100 miles away. Though we can only speculate what particular theatre Husserl imagined as he penned his 1905 example of the 'illuminated theatre' in his *Phenomenology of Internal Time Consciousness*, it is beyond a doubt that he was aware of this exemplary structure, if not its kinship with certain strains of Enlightenment thought.

Chiasm as a Formal Element for the Phenomenological Encounter with the Other

In *La Voix et le Phénomène* (*Speech and Phenomena*), Derrida discovers a theatrical architectonic at the heart of Husserl's theory of signification. What is proposed by Husserl as absolute subjectivity, as a self-immanence of speech, the timeless moment of 'hearing oneself speak', is in fact always infiltrated by a negativity upon which it depends to cleave it from the empirical. *Différance*, Derrida's coinage, locates this 'non-concept' that makes concepts possible and 'produces a subject' in spatial designations of an outside and in temporal movements. Derrida finds the stage as he lays out the ramifications of *différance* for phenomenology:

> As a relation between an inside and an outside in general, an existent and a nonexistent in general, a constituting and a constituted in general, temporalization is at once the very power and limit of phenomenological reduction. Hearing oneself speak is not the inwardness of an inside that is closed in upon itself; it is the irreducible openness in the inside; it is the eye and the world within speech. *Phenomenological reduction is a scene, a theatre stage* [*La reduction phénoménologique est une scène.*] (Derrida, 1973, p. 86; original emphasis)

This is to say that what phenomenology figures as a pure space, a uniform and continuous present, is actually divided within itself. It opens onto another space that is somehow continuous but not identical with it. In order to mark this difference, something must be crossed. At this node in Derrida's argument, is the invocation of the stage, of the Greek *skēnē*, surprising? Does Derrida choose this moment to retrieve the theatrical architectonics of phenomenology as a flourish? In fact, the minimal attendant temporality of chiasmus accounts for the convergence of phenomenology and theatre architecture. The reversal of space that occurs in the theatrical model (where my right lines up with the left of the other facing me), the reversal figured in the divergent street perspectives of the Teatro Olimpico, intervenes in Derrida's phenomenology precisely because it conveys: 1) an instantiation of place within otherwise bland space, 2) a simultaneous retention and relinquishment of identity and 3) a minimal event of renewal or concatenation. Derrida's critique exploits these quintessential theatricalities, which haunt Husserl as much as the theatrical structure does. Thus, theatricality in the sense of a symbolically laden architectonics not only constitutes phenomenology, but can be seen to inhabit deconstruction as well.

In the optical treatises of the early seventeenth century, the chiasm of the *camera obscura* through the lens of the eye was not understood to exist in time. Kepler declares that '*The motion of light is not in time, but in a moment.*' Since light was without weight, 'the medium does not resist light, because light lacks matter by which resistance could occur. Therefore, the swiftness of light is infinite' (Kepler, 2000, p. 21). Yet, it does have direction, motion. It is the object of a receiving, and to it 'belongs an outflowing or projection from its origin towards a distant place' (Kepler, 2000, p. 20). The instantaneous concatenation that brings light to its destination, then, is embodied a minimal temporal unit, an asymptote of flux, and this unit would have to be retained by the chiasmic receiving of light in the eye's function. Descartes assumes the travel of light to be infinitely swift, comparing it to the way 'movement or resistance of the bodies encountered by a blind man passes to his hand by means of his stick' (Descartes, 1988, p. 58). Yet, these characterizations require flux, the condition of alterity, or else the eye could have no function in time. Chiasmus, therefore, may have lent itself to appropriation by optics, since as a rhetorical device it is defined by a simultaneous retention and relinquishment of identity. In the transition from AB to BA, order is sacrificed but combination salvaged; the self takes on the aspect of the other. This aspect, however, is only understood according to its position, the *fact* of its counterposition in space. In every frontal glance is a necessary crossing, as long as the object returns to its front side. In Camillo's mnemonic array, in the sight lines of Palladio, in Ledoux's arch, in every face-to-face encounter, the object is positioned in space.

In its peculiar brokering of spatial and temporal meaning, chiasm is cast as the formal link between the stage and phenomenology. Ledoux's *avant-scène*, just like Derrida's *archi-scène*, locates the central chiasmic locus that intervenes between the *cogito* and the object. In each case, the stage is a continuity that divides. It is a technology that enables us to encounter the present, but in precisely such a way as to separate it from ourselves. As an opening of present space onto another space whose intelligibility depends upon a certain cleavage (this is meant in the sense of a splitting as well as a clinging), theatre architecture interpolated chiasm. Forced to account for the role of the body in an ongoing articulation of the possibility of knowledge, theatre buildings adopted a shape determined not just by the usual concerns of audibility and visibility, but also by the geometry of vision itself — that of the eye. The ocular thematic in theatre architecture speaks to a recalibration of the category of human knowledge in general. The role of this architectural thematic in phenomenology's attempts to describe the structure of consciousness is only beginning to come to light.

Pannill Camp is a PhD candidate in Theatre and Performance Studies at Brown University. His articles have appeared in the *Journal of Dramatic Theory and Criticism* (Fall 2004) and *Theatre Journal* (December 2007). His dissertation project, '*Le Premier Cadre*: Theatre Architecture and Objects of Knowledge in Eighteenth-Century France', examines the appropriation of spatial representations and geometric forms from optics on the part of theatre architects near the end of the *Ancien Régime*, and argues that the spectatorial encounter cultivated by late eighteenth-century dramatic theorists and architectural reformers took on attributes of empirical philosophy's encounter with the natural world.

Notes

1   In the *Archaeology of Knowledge*, Michel Foucault employs this term to denote 'the relation of the subject to the object and the formal rules that govern it' (New York, 1972).

2   These two proclamations are, of course, contestable, but it will suffice for our argument that standard publications in each field demonstrate the coincidence. Both Oscar G. Brockett's standard textbook *History of the Theatre* 9th ed. and George C. Izenour's formidable *Theater Design* identify the Teatro Farnese as the model for the proscenium arch that would be reproduced countless times on the European continent and off during the next 300 years, though Brockett points out that this building was almost certainly not the first with a permanent proscenium arch. It is Clyde W. Oyster's *The Human Eye: Structure and Function* that confers the corresponding title on Christoph Scheiner.

3   Brockett, for example, posits without qualification that there exists an 'evolution of theatre architecture' legible in structures like the Teatro Olimpico (Brockett, 2003, p. 171). James S. Ackerman assesses this same structure as 'a poorly adapted mutant in the evolution of its species' in *Palladio* (Ackerman, 1966, p. 180). Izenour is even more doctrinaire, predicting that asymmetrical auditoria will inevitably become extinct: 'Categorically asymmetry does not work as well as symmetry for either sight lines or acoustics, because one side of the house works better than the other, simply because geometry makes it so. Like all other fads and contagious diseases it will in time pass from the scene. *Sic transit Gloria theatri*' (Izenour, 1977, p. 28).

4   See Bernard Stiegler's *Technics and Time* for a discussion of Aristotle's category of tekhnē (Stiegler, 1998, pp. 1-81).

5   Erasmus, *Epistolae*, ed. P.S. Allen and others, IX, p. 479. Quoted in Frances A. Yates, *The Art of Memory*, 1966, p. 131.

6   Yates, 1966, p. 171. See also Ackerman, 1966, p. 31, 161.

7   The 'nodal point' of the Teatro Olimpico, as discovered by tracing the central axes of the street perspectives across the proscenium, coincides roughly with the centre of the threshold between proscenium and orchestra. Izenour chooses the same point to anchor his comparisons of theatre scale in Chapter 12 of his *Theater Design* (e.g. Izenour, 1977, p. 563). For a diagram showing the approximate 'nodal point' for the study of ocular anatomy, see Oyster, 1999, p. 38.

8   See Brockett, 2003, pp. 170-173. See also Izenour, wherein the Teatro Farnese with its 'deep enclosed articulated proscenium arch' is deemed 'the final development of the Renaissance theater' (Izenour, 1977, pp. 44-46).

9   Quoted from the preface of Dana Densmore and William H. Donahue to Johannes Kepler's *Optics*, 2000, p. ix.

10   The truncation of a circle or oval by the 'ouverture' of the stage space became a common means of describing the relationship between the salle and scène in eighteenth-century French architectural descriptions. See, for example, the Chevalier de Chaumont's 'Véritable construction d'un théâtre d'Opéra à l'usage en France...' Paris, 1766, p. 10.

11   Jean-Claude Bonnet, quoted in Vidler, 1990, p. 165.

12   Leacroft and Leacroft, 1984, p. 92. See also p. 113.

References

Ackerman, J.S., *Palladio*. Harmondsworth, 1966.

Brockett, O.G., *History of the Theatre 9th ed.* Boston and New York, 2003.

Darnton, R., *The Great Cat Massacre and Other Episodes in French Cultural History*. New York, 1999.

Derrida, J., *Speech and Phenomena, and Other Essays on Husserl's Theory of Signs* (Trans. by David B. Allison.) Evanston, 1973.

Descartes, R., 'Optics'. In: *Descartes: Selected Philosophical Writings*. (Trans. J. Cottingham, R. Stoothoff, D. Murdoch.) Cambridge, 1988.

Foucault, M., *The Order of Things: an Archaeology of the Human Sciences*. New York, 1971.

Foucault, M., *Archaeology of Knowledge*. New York, 1972.

Izenour, G.C., *Theater Design*. New York, 1977.

Kepler, J., *Optics: Paralipomena to Witelo & Optical Part of Astronomy*. (Trans. William H. Donahue.) Santa Fe, 2000.

Leacroft, R. and H. Leacroft, *Theatre and Playhouse: An Illustrated Survey of Theatre Building from Ancient Greece to the Present Day*. London, 1984.

Ledoux, C., *L'architecture considérée sous le rapport de l'art, des mœurs et de la legislation*. Paris, 1997.

Oyster, C.W., *The Human Eye: Structure and Function*. Sunderland, Mass., 1999.
Stiegler, B., *Technics and Time, 1: The Fault of Epimetheus*. Stanford, 1998.
Vidler, A., *Claude-Nicolas Ledoux: Architecture and Social Reform at the End of the Ancien Régime*. Cambridge, Mass., 1990.
Yates, F. A., *The Art of Memory*. Chicago, 1966.

Performance Documentation 4:
Camillo – Memo 4.0: The Cabinet of Memories – A Tear Donnor Session

In 1998 Emil Hrvatin presented his installation *Camillo – Memo 4.0: The Cabinet of Memories – A Tear Donnor Session* at the Slovenian National Theatre Museum. Hrvatin reconceptualized the idea of the *Theatre of Memory*, as developed by Giulio Camillo. According to Hrvatin, Camillo is 'a paradigm of the free mind, the innovator of the theatre, an installation artist in the age of Renaissance, and someone who knew how to conceive the net-like, combinatory nature of communication' (Hrvatin quoted in Žerovnik, 2003, p. 126). Hrvatin's installation explored the relationships between visibility and knowledge, individuality and

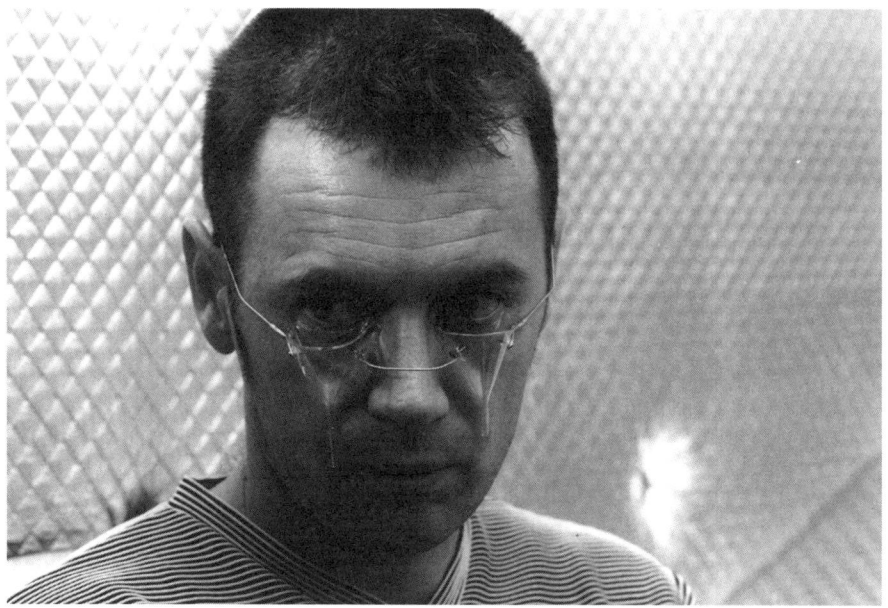

Emil Hrvatin in *Camillo – Memo 4.0: The Cabinet of Memories – A Tear Donnor Session*. Photo: Igor Delorenzo Omahen. Reproduced with permission of the artist.

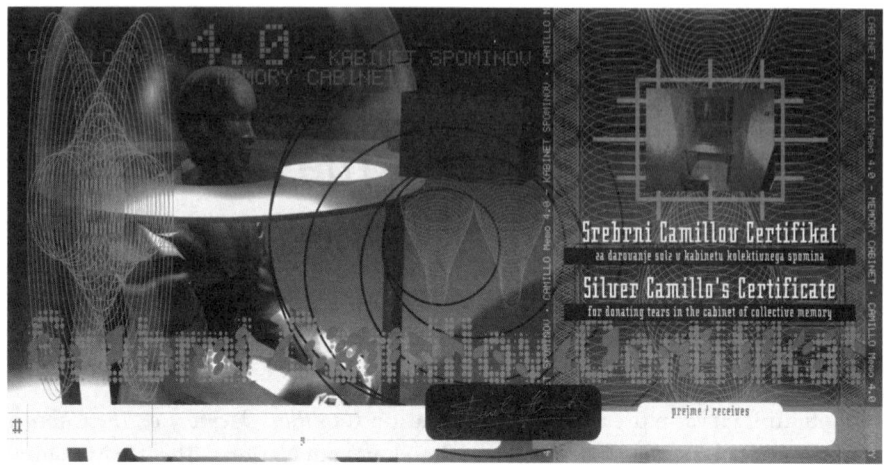

Camillo – Memo 4.0: The Cabinet of Memories – A Tear Donnor Session. Silver Certificate. Reproduced with permission of the artist.

society, and, first and foremost, the relationship between body and mind. Visitors to *The Cabinet of Memories* were kindly asked to donate their tears. This was accomplished by recalling memories — in order to materialize their memories, to embody their thoughts.

The following quotes from visitors to *The Cabinet of Memories* both describe and reflect upon the spectator's position within the installation.

'The installation/performance *Camillo Memo 4.0: The Cabinet of Memories – A Tear Donnor Session* (...) is conceived as a private tear-jerker. A tear-jerker in a very literal and direct sense, since the spectators are actually expected to donate their tears. Hrvatin built a glass tear receptacle, in which they can collect the tears that they are willing to shed. To stimulate the production of tears, the spectators are invited into one of three boxes. In the *Cabinet of Individual Memory*, they find only a mirror with which they can confront themselves with painful memories. Every spectator is invited to re-enact scenes from his or her past that could generate a stream of sorrow. If successful, they are rewarded with a Golden Certificate because, in this installation, an individual crying is understood to be the most valuable form of emotion memory. Individual spectators who have difficulty shedding tears 'on personal command' can try their luck in the *Cabinet of Collective Memory*. This cabinet is equipped with video and television screens from which the spectator can choose his or her favourite tear-jerking scene. These devices of emotional self-stimulation offer several collective "climaxes" which are supposed to make you cry for joy or bitterness. (...) If successful, you are awarded a Silver Certificate. Spectators who have still failed to shed a tear in these virtual boxes of sorrow and pity can turn to artificial aids in the third Cabinet, the *Cabinet of the Physiological Memory*. In this box, the spectator is made to cry through the use of chemical substances or simply by being exposed to the effects of chopped red onions. This is the most effective method, but, at the same time, it has the least affective value, so that the Certificate granted for the shedding of these tears only mentions that one has been a participant' (Luk van den Dries in: Žerovnik, 2003, pp. 13-15).

'Indeed, one could interpret the performance as a competition in emotion management, in which the winner is the one with the most authentic feelings. Equally it is a kind of personal test, causing members of the audience to ask: What makes me cry? Do I have an individual or a collective emotional energy? Or perhaps I have none at all? And, last but not least, it is of course a social event: the spectator is a donator and his or her donation is very personal indeed' (Van den Dries in: Žerovnik, 2003, pp. 15-16).

'In the *Cabinet of Physiological Memory* the participant transforms from user to actor. S/he is not merely a distant element or a joint structure, but an internal actant, an agent of memories that is induced to function. S/he is a kind of a robot, an artificial engine that shows clearly how our memories are constructed, manipulated, made artificial. To take a place in the spherical construction chair in the *Cabinet of Physiological Memory* means to take the position of an actor and to be the most internal element of this performance installation piece. This is a direct passage for the public from the private into the public sphere' (Marina Gržinić in: Žerovnik, 2003, pp. 36-37).

'Hrvatin's *Cabinet of Memories*, not unlike Camillo's theatre, contained material that was designed to trigger the spectator's association of images with his or her individual emotional and intellectual experiences. The spectator was invited to create an invisible performance in the spaces of his or her own memory, using the offered factual data and his own experience as the starting point' (Barbara Orel in: Žerovnik, 2003, p. 56).

'In *The Cabinet of Memories*, Hrvatin conceives of his terminal spectactor [a term introduced by Hrvatin to refer to the combination of spectator and actor in one person, FB] as Baudrillard's human subject, that is, as a terminal in the information network, as a link in the network of performative activities. The site of action is no longer the stage but rather the body of the spectator, the body with its own experiential history, memory, and consciousness, and the only spectator here is this same individual who lends his body to the theatre. The terminal spectactor is the locus of the event and, at the same time and all in one person, its own scene, performer and spectator. The spectactor is the object of looking as well as the subject of vision. The viewing position, that is, the position of the see-er, coincides with the position of the seen, and this only adds to the complexity of the relation between fiction and reality' (Orel, pp. 175-176).

Text by *Fleur Bokhoven*

Emil Hrvatin (in 2007 he changed his name to Janez Janša) is an author, per-former and director of interdisciplinary performances, e.g. MISS MOBILE, WE ARE ALL MARLENE DIETRICH FOR – *Performance for soldiers in peace-keeping missions* (together with Erna Omarsdottir) and PUPILIJA, PAPA PU-PILO AND THE PUPILCEKS - RECONSTRUCTION. He is the author of a book on Jan Fabre (*JAN FABRE - La Discipline du chaos, le chaos de la discipline*, Armand Colin, Paris 1994; published in Dutch, Italian and Slovenian) and was editor-in-chief of *MASKA, a performing arts journal*, from 1999 to 2006. He is the director of MASKA, institute for publishing, production and education, based in Ljubljana, Slovenia.

Fleur Bokhoven is currently finishing her RMA in Art Studies with a major in Theatre Studies at the University of Amsterdam.

Performance Data

Camillo – Memo 4.0: The Cabinet of Memories – A Tear Donnor Session was pre-sented for the first time in 1998 at the Slovenian Theatre Museum in Ljubljana.

References

Orel, B., 'The Question of the Point of View. The Spectator as the Melting Point of Fiction and Reality'. In: *Text & Reality / Text & Wirklichkeit*. J. Bernard, J. Fikfak and P. Grzybek (eds). Ljubljana, 2005.
Žerovnik, M. (ed.), *Memory, Privacy, Spectatorship: On Emil Hrvatin's Perfor-mances*. Ljubljana, Maska, 2003.

Martin, Massumi, and The Matrix

Maaike Bleeker

'This is anatomy that is alive,' claims Gunther von Hagens in a promotional video about his famous exhibition *Body Worlds*. *Body Worlds* presents dead bodies preserved via a technique called 'plastination' and presented in postures and configurations meant to show viewers how it is with us, in our living bodies. The exhibition thus reiterates what might be called one of the central paradoxes of anatomy, namely the use of dead bodies to teach about living ones. Von Hagens invites us to identify our living selves with these dead ones; these bodies are *real*, he claims. But what exactly is so real about them? The bodies on display are real dead human body material, complete with glass eyes, dyed to look like living tissue. They are bodies reduced to the Cartesian *res extensa*, preserved and fixed in positions that these bodies may or may not have assumed when alive. Does posing as if they are alive make them live? (Does posing as if he is Joseph Beuys make Gunther von Hagens an artist?)

What would make anatomy alive, rather than a re-staging of the dead, would be to rethink the body itself, this is *res extensa*, as the 'very stuff of subjectivity' (Grosz, 1994). To do this is to undo the deadly fixations of the Cartesian paradigm and rethink the body as that which does the thinking, knowing and understanding. The question then is not, or not only, what we imagine living bodies to look like, but also how living bodies are involved in looking, and in imagining. What are the implications of this involvement for our understanding of what it means to look, what it means to imagine, what it means to think?

A crucial question here is that of movement. In this respect, Von Hagens's project presents an interesting example. In his staging of 'anatomy that is alive', a lot of effort is invested in suggesting movement, bodily action, and activity. We see dead bodies 'playing' chess, 'throwing' a lasso. They are 'fencing', or about to walk away. They seem to be frozen in mid-movement, in poses that bring to mind artistic strategies of suggesting movement used in painting or sculpture. A horse with horseman is fixed in mid-rear. A specimen (Von Hagens's term) named 'The Runner' is shown in a running position, having the muscles of his arms and legs detached from their origin at one side and stretched out backwards, opposite to the direction this Runner is supposedly moving. The effect is not unlike that of lines indicating speed in a cartoon drawing.

Despite the abundance of signs of movement, movement itself is emphatically *absent*. These bodies, frozen and fixed, read as a neat illustration of Brian Massumi's observation that 'adding movement to stasis is about as easy as multiplying a number by zero and getting a positive product' (2002, p. 3). He makes this observation in his *Parables for the Virtual*, a book that begins with the following remark:

> When I think of my body and ask what it does to earn that name, two things stand out. It *moves*. It *feels*. In fact, it does both at the same time. It moves and it feels, and it feels itself moving. Can we think a body without this: an intrinsic connection between movement and sensation whereby each immediately summons the other? (Massumi, 2002, p. 1, italics in the text)

This intrinsic connection between movement and feeling, Massumi argues, is essential to what bodies are. This connection is also essential to how we, as bodies, engage with the world we live in, to how our bodies are involved in constituting our awareness of this world, and also to our awareness of ourselves in relation to this world. Massumi continues:

> If you start from an intrinsic connection between movement and sensation, the slightest, most literal displacement convokes a qualitative difference, because as directly as it conducts itself it beckons a feeling, and feelings have a way of folding into each other, resonating together, interfering with each other, mutually intensifying, all in unquantifiable ways apt to unfold again in action, often unpredictable. Qualitative difference: immediately the issue is change. (Massumi, 2002, p. 1)

The issue is change, and change and movement appear to be in many ways connected. Yet thinking the relationship between change and movement appears to be harder than it seems. According to Massumi, the difficulty of thinking this relationship is one of the central problems with cultural theory of the past decades. A lot of effort has been invested in theorizing bodies and change, but somehow cultural theory has missed how bodies and change are connected through movement and sensation as the two sides of an intermediate term. Movement and sensation, in their immediate connection, have been bracketed. Cultural theory has thereby failed to account for the significance of bodies and change, even though these have been of consistent concern – perhaps the central concern in the humanities.

Massumi's way of stating the problem evokes phenomenology and its use of bracketing as a means of isolating and separating. Jonathan Crary, in his seminal *Suspensions of Perception: Attention, Spectacle and Modern Culture* (1992), observes how this method of bracketing became important to the early Husserl as a means to both counter and stabilize the perceptual modulations, fusions, and resonances as they occur in the embodied observer and mutate into stable, objectively valid cognitions. That is, bracketing became important as a procedure precisely to counter movement and sensation as an aspect of embodied experience and cognition. Crary refers to Francisco Varela, who observes that:

> The irony of Husserl's procedure, then, is that although he claims to be turning philosophy toward a direct facing of experience, he was actually ignoring both the consensual aspect and the direct embodied aspect of experience. Husserl's turn towards experience and the things themselves was entirely theoretical. (Varela quoted in Crary, 1992, p. 286n16)

In this theoretical approach, movement and sensation are bracketed as continuous processes and cut up in a succession of isolated moments fixed in time and space, like in the famous late nineteenth-century photographic experiments of Muybridge. These experiments show bodies in a succession of moments of one continuous movement. The photographs illuminate the relative position of the various body parts at these isolated moments. Dissecting movement into discrete events, they provide us with a means of imagining where each part of the body is at successive moments. Thus, the photographs suggest a particular understanding of what movement is. Movement here appears as change or transformation from one position to the next. The transformation itself, however, is precisely what is put between brackets. What we see is not movement, but positions, poses. Movement is what is not in each one of them. Or, as Massumi puts it: 'When a body is in motion it does not coincide with itself. It coincides with its own transition; its own variation' (Massumi, 2002, p. 4). In Muybridge's photographs, as in the phenomenological act of bracketing, movement is what is left out, just as movement is what is absent from Von Hagens's staging of 'anatomy that is alive' in *Body Worlds*. In this sense, it seems Von Hagens's project could be called symptomatic of the cultural condition criticized by Massumi.

The practice of bracketing stages a stable relationship between an objective world and a stable point of view, a position from whence the world can be defined by means of pinning isolated phenomena down on the grid of culturally constructed significations. Massumi terms this the problem of positionality. 'The idea of positionality,' he writes, 'begins by subtracting movement from the picture. This catches the body in cultural freeze-frame' (Massumi, 2002, p.

3). Positionality describes the situation in which movement is subordinated to the positions it connects, safeguarding the position of a stable subject in relation to a stable world. Positionality involves the particular type of kinaesthetic awareness described by Susan Foster in her contribution to this volume: the kinaesthetic awareness of the observer implied within cartographic technologies such as Mercator's, in which the world appears as an object of vision by a stationary and unified subject, and is constituted according to the logic of a grid of horizontal and vertical lines. These cartographic technologies mediate in a conception of the world as a territory for survey by a static viewer who can see it all as it is, objectively.

Foster characterizes the subject of the vision provided by these maps in terms of a particular kinaesthetic awareness, rather than the absence or lack of kinaesthetic awareness. This is a significant choice that points to the need to conceive of positionality in terms of a duality. Positionality is neither about the grid nor about the static viewing position but about the perceptual-cognitive practices from which both emerge in relation to one another. Positionality, therefore, is not a denial of movement but a denial of movement as qualitative transformation. Positionality involves a denial of movement/sensation as constitutive of the way in which the world appears to us as an object of cognitive perception. These perceptual-cognitive practices are the subject of this text, and I will approach them through dance. At first sight, dance, as a practice in which movement plays such an important part, may seem to be at odds with positionality. However, I will argue that positionality is in fact deeply engrained in how dance, especially ballet, is traditionally understood.

Knowing Ballet

Imagine a little girl, twelve years old, devoted to ballet. She has been doing ballet ever since she was four. Ballet fascinates her, and she spends a lot of time in the studio. She loves going to ballet class, the various exercises she is asked to perform, and she is able to perform these quite well. Yet, she is not a dancer. Not in the sense that she is not a professional dancer. It is not about being professional. It is about movement. It is about her complicated relationship with movement. How is it possible that she feels at home in a ballet class but uncomfortable moving?

On her thirteenth birthday, one of her presents is a book about the technique of academic ballet. The book (in Dutch) is titled *Klassieke Ballettechniek. De techniek en de terminologie van het akademische ballet* (in English: *Classical Ballet Technique. The technique and terminology of academic ballet)*. The book explains ballet: what it is, and how it is done, much of which the little girl al-

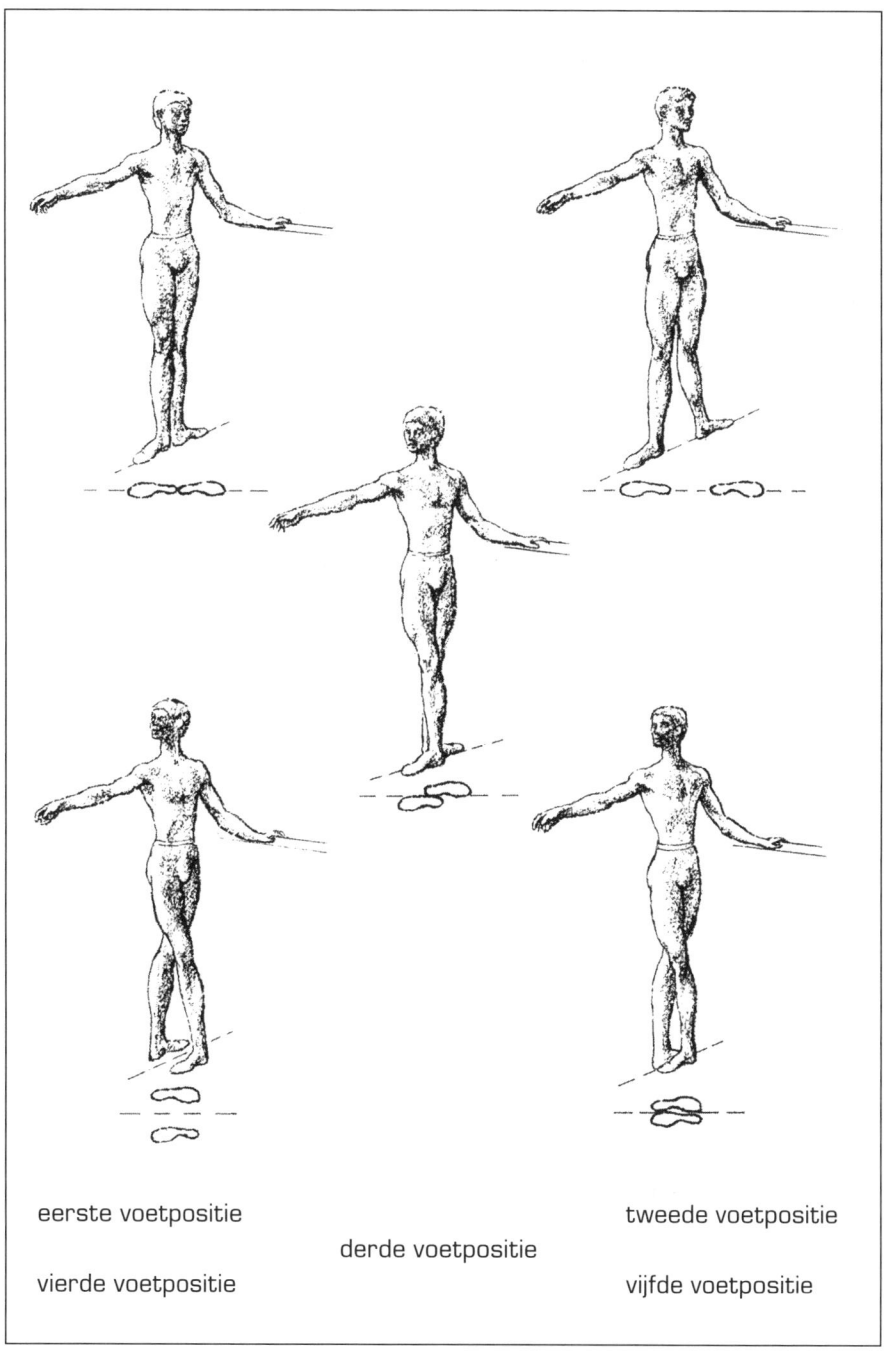

eerste voetpositie

derde voetpositie

tweede voetpositie

vierde voetpositie

vijfde voetpositie

Positions of the feet by Toer van Schaijk. From: René Vincent, *Klassieke Ballettechniek* (1982), p. 16. Courtesy of Walburg Pers. Reproduced with permission of the artist.

ready knows. The book starts with the five basic positions of the feet. These are followed by more positions of the feet, of the legs, of the arms, of the head, of the upper body, the *grand poses* like *attitude* and *arabesque*. Then follow *ports de bras*, exercises *à la barre* and *au milieu*. Each exercise is accompanied and explicated through drawings that dissect the movement into a series of successive moments, illuminating the relative position of various body parts at these successive moments.

How is it possible that a book devoted to the technique of classical ballet does not address the question of how to move?

Maybe I am exaggerating. Of course I am. The book does contain descriptions of how to move. But typically, movement is only introduced after all possible poses and positions have been described and depicted. Only then is movement introduced (literally) as that which connects these positions. Movement thus appears as merely a means of going from one position to the next. Like the photographs by Muybridge, books like this one represent ballet in terms of a succession of fixed poses that the body is supposed to pass through while moving. An important difference, however, is that for Muybridge, freezing bodies in movement through photography was a means of analyzing the relative position of body parts in successive stages of a particular movement. The result is not a manual for *how* to move, which is precisely what the ballet manual does claim to be. The successions of poses shown on the page are presented as a way to understand how ballet is done. The images of the moving body, reduced to its positions, are used as a means of transferring dance, a means of transferring understanding of what movement in ballet is, and how movement is executed.

Whatever the (implicit or explicit) claims of books like this one may be, in actual performance ballet cannot be reduced to assuming, or connecting, a series of poses and positions. This is what the little girl was struggling with in her ballet class. She knew ballet and what she knew was confirmed by the book. But this did not make her a dancer. So, instead, she opted for the book. For books. Until, many years later, these books brought her back to dance. That was when she started reading John Martin's *Introduction to the Dance* (1965, [1939]).

Like Massumi, Martin observes a close connection between movement and feeling. This connection becomes all the more important in the developments in modern dance in the early twentieth century, the time at which he was writing. The great pioneers of modern dance, among them Martin's much admired Martha Graham, rejected the conventions and techniques of academic ballet in favour of new types of movements that were understood to be the direct expression of inner feelings. Martin, in his turn, comes up with a theory to explain the impact these dances make on their audiences, and on him, which is also based

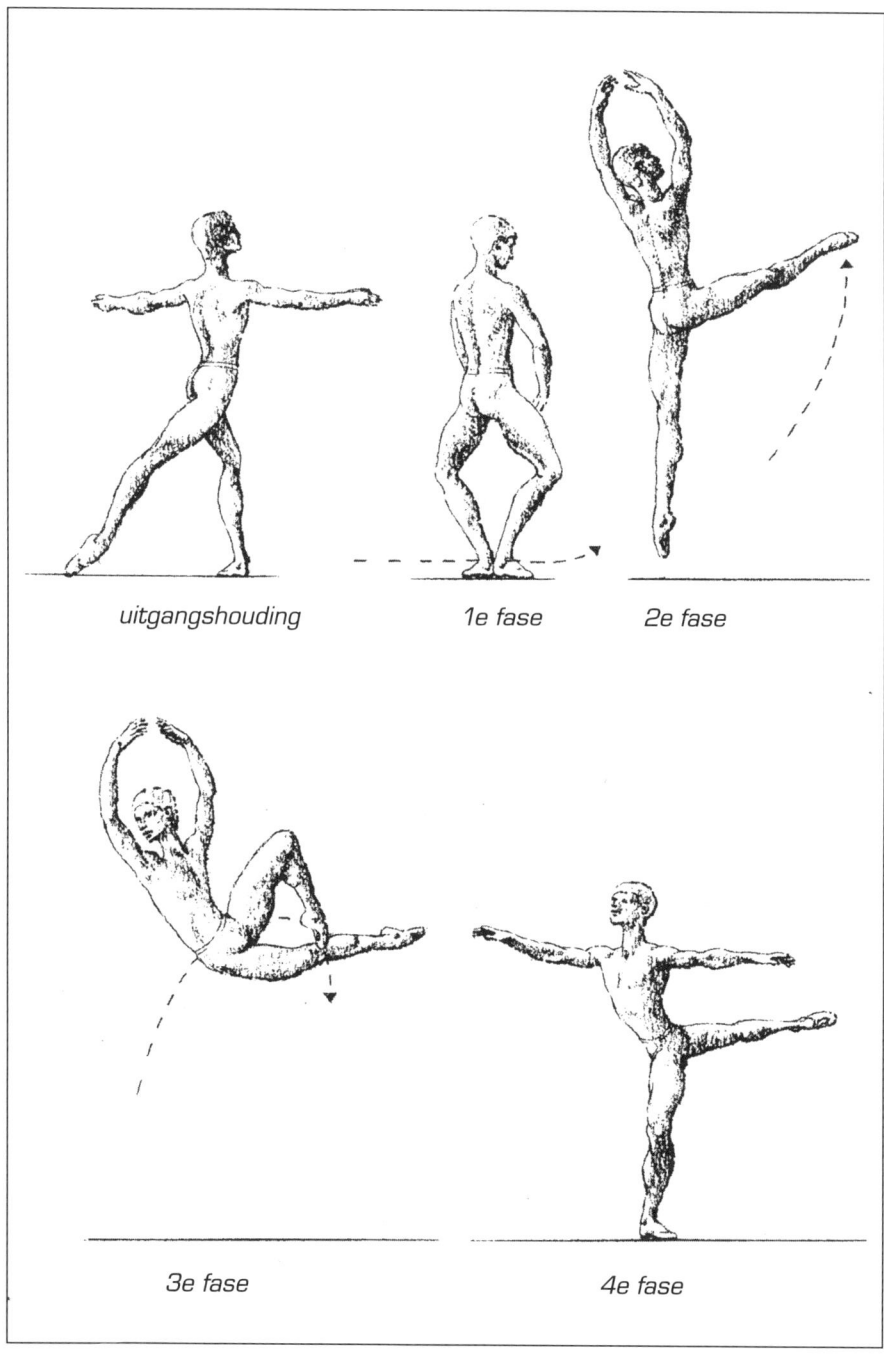

uitgangshouding   *1e fase*   *2e fase*

3e fase   *4e fase*

Rivoltade by Toer van Schaijk. From: René Vincent, *Klassieke Ballettechniek* (1982), p. 253. Courtesy of Walburg Pers. Reproduced with permission of the artist.

on assuming a direct connection between movement and feeling. His theory explains the impact of these dances as resulting from the effect of how movement seen on stage evokes feelings. These feelings are ones that Martin, rather problematically, understands to be universal.

Notwithstanding this problematic aspect of his theory, his approach remains interesting for its presentation of movement not only as a medium of expression but also as a medium of perception. Movement, according to Martin, is central to our way of responding to what we are confronted with, both in and outside the theatre. There is a close relationship between sense impression and movement response. With 'movement response' he refers to the (possible) actions undertaken by a body in response to the situation this body finds itself dealing with. This does not mean that the body will actually perform all these actions. Many motor responses are registered but not carried out. Yet, as motor impulse, they still play an important part in our experience of what we see. These motor responses connect what is seen to previous experiences and thus awaken earlier sense perceptions and the feelings, emotions, expectations, etc. related to current events. The result is that, when we are watching dance:

> We cease to be mere spectators and become participants in the movement that is presented to us, and though to all outward appearances we shall be sitting quietly in our chairs, we shall nevertheless be dancing synthetically with all our musculature. (Martin, 1965, p. 53)

And from this dancing along, our perception of the dance emerges.

Martin's theory aims at explaining modern dance from the standpoint of how our bodies are involved in seeing. Ironically, it is precisely in his account of seeing modern dance that his own bodily investment in what he sees – this central concern of his argument – is obscured. For when it comes to explaining how our bodies play their part in how we perceive dancing bodies onstage, Martin argues that our motor responses make us feel not our own feelings, associations, etc. connected to the movement, but those of the body seen. In the theatre, Martin feels not his own feelings but what the dancer feels, or at least that is how it feels for him, how he understands what he feels. Whereas his whole theory aims at explaining how our own bodies are involved in seeing other bodies (and actually presents a very useful theoretical approach to this question in many ways), it is precisely when he, finally, comes to the theatre that his own kinaesthetic involvement is obscured.

The theatre, so it seems, invites a conflation of his feelings with the feelings of the bodies seen on stage. The theatre thus mediates in a conflation similar to that of the Lacanian mirror stage identification – the conflation of a body felt over here and the image of a body seen over there – with the difference that Martin does not (mis)recognize the body seen as his own but rather the other way round. He mistakes his own feelings for the feelings of the body seen.

Martin's mirror stage moment, one might argue, demonstrates how the theatre mediates in bringing about a change in the cognitive perceptual practices constitutive of how the world, as an object of perception, appears to Martin. Crucial to these changes is a shift in kinaesthetic awareness. Instead of feeling his own movement/sensations, Martin now becomes aware of his movement/sensations as if they are housed in the body onstage. The theatre mediates in a 'bracketing out' of his movement/sensations, turning them from something constitutive of his perception of the world into something merely observed 'over there', something observed from a stable point of view.

Knowing Kung Fu

With his theory of movement response, Martin comes up with a theoretical explanation of looking that is unmistakably embodied, a way in which what is seen is the product of a body responding to what it experiences, which involves movement. More than that, his theory seems to move in the direction of an understanding of the body as the site of multi-sensual, perhaps synaesthetic, interpretative activities, where the border between perception and cognition fades in a process of embodied thinking, just like the 'activities' of the corpses in 'anatomy that is alive'. Martin himself would probably not have understood his theory of dance as a mode of embodied thinking. What I want to argue is that his theory seems to move in the direction of such a theory, or may be taken in this direction. This is especially true when we read his theory through the lens of what has happened during the now almost 70 years since he wrote his book. I will elaborate this potential through confronting Martin with Massumi, beginning with establishing a 'third term' as mediator. This 'third term' also starts with 'M': it is a scene from *The Matrix*.

Here we witness *The Matrix*'s hero, Neo, during his first combat training session. We see how Neo is plugged into a computer. On the little computer screen in front of him, we see a schematic image of a body in poses representing Kung Fu and other combat training, not unlike the images in the ballet book. But this is not what Neo sees. Neo does not learn Kung Fu from looking at images and mimicking the poses and positions represented with his own body. Instead, he lays back and closes his eyes and what happens inside him remains a mystery. And this mystery involves his body. For, to echo Martin, although to all outward appearances Neo may seem to be lying quietly in his chair, we are also given all kinds of signs that his body is actually very actively involved in something. Ten hours later, he opens his eyes again and says: 'I know Kung Fu.'

'I know Kung Fu,' says Neo. What does he know? How does he know it? What does it mean to know Kung Fu? To know Kung Fu in this film is to be able to move, respond, anticipate, and improvise in a Kung Fu-ean manner. It means to meet his master Morpheus's challenge and be able to respond to it. It remains unclear how exactly Neo learned to do so and what exactly happened to him while being plugged into the training program. Nevertheless, the result fulfils the purpose of movement sense as described by Martin, namely 'to pre-pare the body for appropriate movement with relation to the objects reported upon' (Martin, 1965, p. 42). Neo's training allows him to move along with his master's movements, to understand and interpret them and meet them with ad-equate action. Perhaps Martin's description of 'dancing along synthetically with all our musculature' is not exactly the right metaphor to describe his bodily in-volvement. A better image might be that of the 'thought-athlete' introduced by Deleuze and Guattari, in their *What is Philosophy?* (1994). Deleuze and Guat-tari propose an understanding of philosophy as a mode of thinking that takes the shape of a friendly contest between claimant and rival, in the context of a general athleticism.

In *The Matrix*, Neo's Kung Fu training is presented as a way to make him think, and a way to make him think differently. This training takes the form of a friendly contest. To know Kung Fu is to be changed by his own new ways of responding. This, explains Morpheus, is what it is all about. In *The Matrix*, learning to think differently is staged literally, as learning to move differently or by changing one's movement responses. The result is that Neo develops a different sense of reality, including a different sense of his own involvement in this reality.

In *The Matrix*, learning to think differently involves a change in the rela-tionship between movement and vision and how these are involved in the way we constitute the world as an object of perception. Learning to think through movement is staged as the change from what Massumi terms mirror vision to movement vision. In everyday life, Massumi argues, we form mental pictures of what it means to be who we are: parent or child, mother or father, boss or employee, cop or criminal. We embody these visualizations. We are involved in multiples of such mirror identifications. These identifications are connected by narrative lines, carrying us across a series of regulated thresholds. This is mirror vision. The term brings to mind Lacan and his account of mirror stage identification. Massumi, however, speaks of mirror vision, not of mirror stage identification. Mirror vision describes a way of imagining the self and the world that involves a separation of isolated moments from the multitude and blur of impressions, the flux of feelings and memories that are constantly folding into each other, resonating together in embodied perception. Mirror vision involves an act of bracketing that allows for stable cognitions that can then be connected by means of a narrative logic that explains the change from one into the other.

More than a way of perceiving, therefore, mirror vision describes a mode of understanding, of making sense, in which perception and cognition are inextricably intertwined.

Mirror vision, we might argue, constructs the world according to parameters that are in many ways similar to those of the ballet book. This involves a logic similar to the one implied within the Lacanian mirror stage essay, in which vision is opposed to the feelings of the body seeing, and where identification with the stable image of the body seen allows these feelings to be bracketed, in order to produce a more stable sense of self. But according to Massumi, this opposition of vision and the body felt is not a given, as is suggested by the Lacanian mirror stage. It is not a fact of life. Actually, it is the other way around. It is the effect of a particular mode of looking. Of mirror vision.

Mirror vision is distinguished from movement vision. In movement vision the imaginary distinction between vision and the feelings of the body seeing is lost. Entering the space of movement vision involves leaving behind the empirical world as we know it because movement vision undermines some of the basic presumptions concerning how we think we know the world, and what it means to know. Massumi describes this shift from mirror vision to movement vision in terms of 'entering the space of' movement vision. The shift from mirror vision to movement vision involves leaving the optical space of mirror vision.

> Movement vision is sight turned proprioceptive, the eyes reabsorbed into the flesh through a black hole in the geometry of empirical space and a gash in bodily form. Vision is a mixed mode of perception, registering both form and movement. For it to gain entry in the quasi corporeal, the realm of pure relationality, it must throw aside form in favour of unmediated participation in the flesh. Movement vision is retinal muscle, a visual strength flexed in the extremities of exhaustion. (Massumi, 2002, pp. 59-60)

This is almost literally what happens to Neo at the beginning of his combat training. Closing his eyes, he leaves empirical space. He is absorbed into the flesh through the black hole of the data plug in the back of his head. He turns away from the images in front of him, which are showing him Ju Jitsu and Kung Fu in visual form, to experience it through direct participation in the flesh. He enters this world with his eyes closed. Vision here is a matter of corporeal imagination, of movements that bring Neo, lying in his chair, to the extremities of exhaustion.

Unlike the case of John Martin watching Martha Graham, Neo's corporeal imagination is not stimulated by what he sees in front of him. Rather, what he sees is an imaginary world in which he participates through his corporeal imagination. This is also an important difference between the virtual reality of *The Matrix* and the kind of virtual reality presented by, for example, virtual reality goggles that produce virtual space in front of our eyes. The reality of *The Matrix*, its space, has no ocular existence. It is a world in which the characters participate only through the computer interface plugged directly into the black hole in the back of their heads. This world is radically relational in that it has no existence outside their imagination. Perceiving it is producing it in response to the electronic stimulation provided by the computer interface.

Although the world in which the characters in *The Matrix* participate has no ocular existence, we do see this world when watching the film. Large parts of *The Matrix* consist of visualizations of precisely this imaginary world. This is the irony of the film. An irony that is understandable from a commercial point of view. These visualizations are a way for us, the viewers of the film, to imagine what takes place within this non-ocular world. In order to do so, the makers of the film have to stage this world according to the logic of mirror vision, i.e. according to the type of vision for which theatre presents the model. These visualizations show the world of *The Matrix* as if it is a world that does exist independently from the corporeal investment of the ones participating in it.

This process of visualizing is thematized at several moments. One of these presents an interesting suggestion concerning the relationship between mirror vision and movement vision. It happens during Neo's fight with Morpheus. As viewers, we watch this scene as if it takes place in ocular, objectified space, while in fact, Neo and Morpheus are lying in their chairs and fighting each other in the non-ocular space of the corporeal imagination. In the next shot we see the other characters watching Neo and Morpheus fight. They are watching a little screen showing a visualization of the fight between the two men that are actually physically lying behind them. The little screen appears as a means to visualize what is not visible. At one point, one of the characters grabs the screen as if holding on to it; holding onto that which provides him with a visualization of what he cannot see. The next shot shows him mimicking (with his hands) the movements he sees Neo making during his fight, suggesting that this imagining of what happens to Neo involves a translation of what he sees into his bodily imagination, illustrating Martin's argument regarding bodily mimicking and movement response as a way of understanding what is seen.

Mirror vision and movement vision are discontinuous. There is no mediation between them. We cannot simply translate one into the other, because they are different ways of engaging with the world, different modes of cognitive perception or perceptual cognition. *The Matrix* suggests that we might think of them as two different ways of distributing the sensible, involving different realms of corporeal imagination. Crucial to their difference is a shift in attentional awareness concerning kinaesthetics. At this point, mirror vision as described by Massumi seems to function in ways similar to what Hubert Damisch

(1995) has described as the perspective paradigm. I am referring here to his *The Origin of Perspective*, in which Damisch argues that as long as we understand perspective merely as a mode of representing the world, we keep missing the point. Perspective is a way of understanding and imagining the world, a way of thinking the world, and this way it is deeply integrated in our perceptual encounters with the world. These perceptual encounters produce the world as a world of objects, an objective world in relation to a point, a subject, a 'person'. Perspective objectifies the world in a way similar to Martin's objectification of the dancing body seen on stage. This objectification involves a particular type of vision, a mode of looking in which visibility appears as a property of the world observed rather than the product of the encounter between the world and our perceptual systems (J.J. Gibson). In this situation, kinaesthetic awareness appears as tool for observing feelings and movement in other bodies in a world observed from a stable point of view.

Damisch's argument is historical, focusing on exposing elements of this paradigm at work, without addressing the question of the possibility of change. At this point, the distinction between mirror vision and movement vision allows for a different perspective. In movement vision the subject-object symmetry/duality of mirror vision is broken. Movement vision is 'a vision that passes into the body and through it to another space' (Massumi, 2002, p. 57). Conceptualizing the implications of movement vision requires a shift from movement/sensation understood as kinaesthetic awareness (i.e. the experience of a subject) towards movement/sensation as an aspect of the relationship from which self and world emerge, and into which both disappear. Here, kinaesthetics is not a matter of awareness (an awareness that allows for a decoding of aspects of a world out there) but of responsiveness. In movement vision, movement/sensation, rather than being the experience of an 'I', is itself constitutive of an 'I' emerging from the way our bodies hallucinate the world for us.

Maaike Bleeker is a Professor and the Chair of Theatre Studies at Utrecht University. Her current research project, for which she received a VENI grant from The Netherlands Society for Scientific Research (NWO) is provisionally titled *See Me, Feel Me, Think Me: The Body of Semiotics*. In addition to her academic career, she has worked for the last fifteen years as a dramaturge in theatre and dance. Her articles have appeared in *Performance Research, Theatre Research International, Maska, Women & Performance* (among others) as well as in various anthologies. She co-/edited several books, including *Body Check: Relocating the Body in Contemporary Performing Arts* (Amsterdam, Rodopi, 2002), and is author of *Visuality in the Theatre. The Locus of Looking* (Basingstoke, 2008).

References

Crary, J., *Suspensions of Perception. Attention, Spectacle and Modern Culture.* Cambridge and London, 1992.

Damisch, H., *The Origin of Perspective.* Cambridge and London, 1995.

Deleuze, G. and F. Guattari, *What is Philosophy?* New York, 1994.

Gibson, J.J., *The Senses Considered as Perceptual Systems.* London, 1966.

Grosz, E., *Volatile Bodies: Toward a Corporeal Feminism.* Bloomington and Indianapolis, 1994.

Lacan, J., *Ecrits: A Selection.* London, 1977.

Martin, J., *Introduction to the Dance.* New York, 1965 [1939].

Massumi, B., *Parables for the Virtual. Movement, Affect, Sensation.* Durham & London, 2002.

Vincent, R., *Klassieke Ballettechniek. De techniek en de terminologie van het akademische ballet.* Zutphen, 1982.

Wachovski, A. and L. Wachovski, *The Matrix.* Warner Bros., 1999.

Performance Documentation 5:

sensing presence no. 1: performing a hyperlink system

Isabelle Jenniches, Stefan Kunzmann and Renée Copraij presented a short performance in spring 2001, in the historical anatomical theatre in De Waag in Amsterdam. This was once the 'hometheatre' of anatomist Nicolaes Tulp, 'surgeon and representative of the civil authority, anatomist and frequent office holder in the bourgeois government,' to quote Francis Barker (1995, p. 103). Tulp is the man depicted by Rembrandt in his famous *The Anatomy Lesson of Dr Nicolaes Tulp*, which shows Tulp's magisterial dissection of the executed criminal Aris Kindt:

> at which Descartes was probably present; anatomist himself, philosopher and legislator of modern subjectivity, who, mediating by the stove, considering strangely whether his body exists, uses the wax that is to hand to prove that corporeal objects have no consistency or essentiality but extension in space. (Barker, 1995, p. 103)

Jenniches, Kunzmann and Copraij chose this theatre for a performance in which they engage with the Cartesian mind-body opposition, and the identification of mind with that which does the thinking.

One day prior to the performance, the audience received an e-mail with an invitation to visit the project website, http://www.9nerds.com/sk/waag/. Here, the audience encountered: a) a figure consisting of several lines and several small circles 'dancing' rhythmically up and down; and b) a discontinuous line, moving in the same rhythm. The visitor was given no clue as to the purpose or intention of this figure. The only way to try to understand it was to engage with it, and to engage with it meant to move through it. After clicking on the image, the visitor was able to move the discontinuous line through the figure. When this line hit one of the small circles, the appearance of a little hand sign invited the visitor to click again. As a result, a connection between two little circles was made, and the line in the diagram connecting these two little circles would become slightly thicker. After clicking, several of the circles would disappear and/or others appear, allowing for new connections to be made. Exploring the figure, the visitor marked the diagram with his or her movement through it, finally producing a figure dancing rhythmically up and down, as if floating on

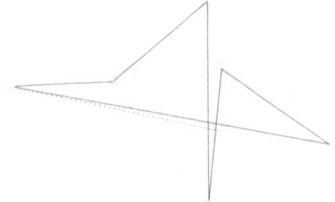

One of the patterns created by a visitor of the website of *sensing presence no. 1*. Courtesy of the artists.

top of the static line drawing. When the visitors decided to leave the page and close it, they would receive a message saying 'Thank you'. The pattern they had created would be added to the collection on the site.

During the performance, dancer Copraij was lying on the floor of the anatomical theatre space in a yoga position called the corpse position. The audience was seated in a semi-circle, very close to her, looking down at her. Lying on the floor, Copraij performed a series of movements, some of them so slow and so internal as to be almost unrecognizable for the audience. The only sound was that of Kunzmann, standing behind the rostrum, clicking a mouse. After a while, he started reading the names of body parts aloud: toe, knee, right hip, finger, right

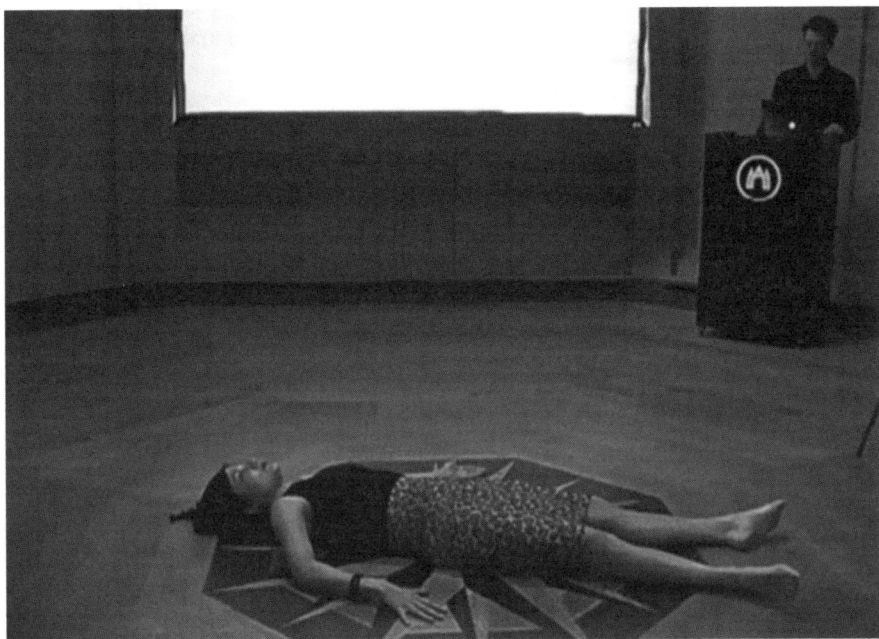

Renée Copraij and Stefan Kunzmann in *sensing presence no. 1*. Photo: Isabelle Jenniches. Courtesy of the artists.

shoulder, left shoulder, left hip, left foot, navel, heart. Now, it became possible to recognize Copraij's movements as attempts at connecting the parts of her body, named by Kunzmann, through internal body movements. These body parts, it appeared, corresponded to the points of intersection of the various lines in the diagram. Kunzmann thus 'read' the 'messages' left by the audience on the web-site. Copraij then would respond to these codes by making connections between corresponding points in her body. Instead of being a mute object subjected to the demonstration of the anatomist, inscribed by his superior knowledge, this body presented an interpretation directly through her body. She turned what she heard into a stream of energy (internal movements), thus translating the code into a neuromuscular experience. She literally incorporated the message.

Looking back at their performance, Jenniches, Kunzmann and Copraij ex-plained how it all started from the question of how to conceptualize a process of thinking through the body. If we consider the body to be a thinking entity, what then could thinking be, how does it take place? They decided to explore this through the analogy of the body and the computer. Computers are often used as a metaphor to imagine aspects of thinking. Yet, usually the computer is equated to the mind (or vice versa). Jenniches, Kunzmann and Copraij, on the other hand,

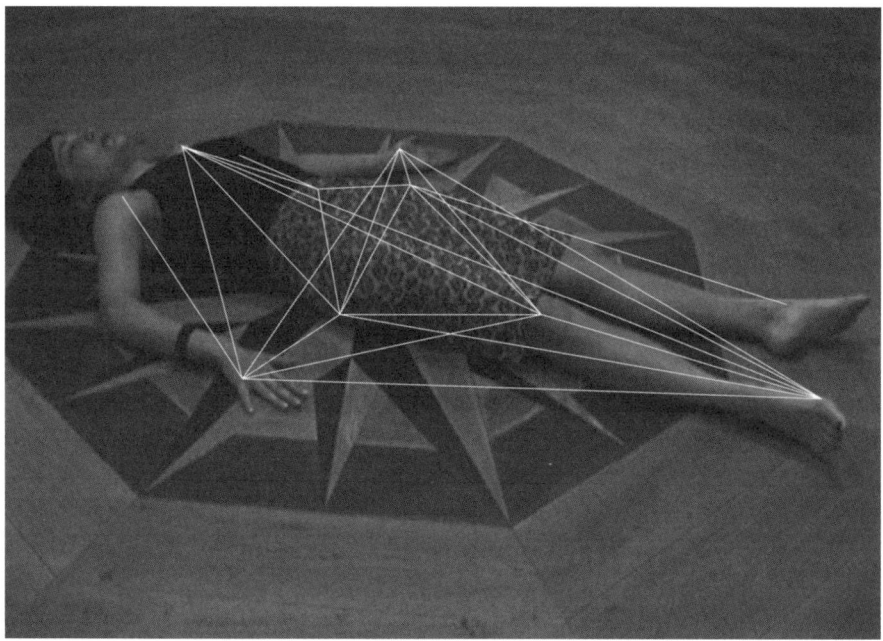

Renée Copraij with a projection of the figure on the website. Photo: Isabelle Jenniches. Courtesy of the artists.

proposed to explore the comparison of the computer with the body in order to come up with a Deleuzian-like conception of thinking in terms of movement. They showed the body, like the computer, to be a 'place' where links are being made as a result of which thought starts to move. Here, thinking does not proceed through mental representations or thought content somehow stored within the mind. Instead, thought is affected by the movement called thinking.

Text by *Maaike Bleeker*

Renée Copraij worked with Jan Fabre from 1987 to 2007. She spent twelve years as a performer, later working as his assistant for pieces such as *Parrots and Guinea Pigs*, *Swanlake* and *Tannhauser*. She did collaborations with Dennis O'Connor *(Interview)* and Martin Butler *(Protocol of Desire)*. Since 2004, she teaches regularly at the Amsterdam School of the Arts (SNDO/School for New Dance Development).

Isabelle Jenniches received her Master's degree in Scenography from the Academy of Applied Art in Vienna, Austria, and a postgraduate degree in Digital Media and the Arts from Media-GN in Groningen, the Netherlands. In performances and photographic series that seek out the intersections between physical and virtual space, she often draws upon such 'low tech' sources as the public or private webcam, and her ongoing compulsive collections of found footage from the Internet. Real-time collaborative creation plays an important role in connected performance events and her work with musicians and dancers. Having spent most of her life in major cities and travelling extensively, Isabelle is now in pursuit of a more sustainable life in the Santa Cruz Mountains in California.

Performance Data

Dialogue between Isabelle Jenniches, Renée Copraij and Stefan Kunzmann in the Theatrum Anatomicum in De Waag (Amsterdam). Saturday April 27 and Sunday 28, 2001. Special thanks to Andrea Leine, Harijono Roebana, Robert Steijn and Waag Society.

References

Barker, F., *The Tremulous Private Body: Essays on Subjection*. Ann Arbor, 1995.

'Where Are You Now?': Locating the Body in Contemporary Performance

Susan Leigh Foster

The Renaissance anatomy theatre, and the culture of dissection it represents, inaugurated new paradigms of subjectivity and corporeality. It helped to establish the body as a stable and consolidated entity capable of providing a singular perspective onto the world. The inert and mute body of the corpse came to vivify the body as machine, the body that transported a perceiving and thinking subject. As Maaike Bleeker has shown, this regimen of visuality, installed as part of the culture of dissection, began to consolidate a single and seemingly objective perspective from which to view the world (Bleeker, 2002). And, as Jonathan Sawday has observed, the adventure of discovering and charting the interior of the body coincided with and perhaps enabled the exploration of the foreign world (Sawday, 1995, pp. 22-32). Colonization of the body's matter took place using the same guiding principles as the colonization of foreign peoples and resources.

The invention of the anatomy theatre coincided with a new kinaesthetic awareness of one's positionality in the world. New cartographic technologies, such as Mercator's implementation of a horizontal and vertical grid to contain and locate the world's land masses, required a way of reading that privileged the single and stationary subject.[1] Just as the body in the anatomy theatre presented itself as a stationary object of study to be investigated by the anatomist, so too, the landscape that emerged with the latest cartographic innovations of the sixteenth and seventeenth centuries offered up a static territory for survey by a viewer who could see all from a singular, elevated position. Rather than the narrative approach to conveying directions, identified by Michel de Certeau as the 'tour', all those who would explore the world now relied upon the 'map' (De Certeau, 1984). They learned to place themselves within and upon this grid, an abstract horizontal plane that, as Paul Carter has shown, uprooted all living things from their local ecologies and placed them within the taxonomic rubric that measured difference in standardized terms as a product of degree (Carter, 1987).

Yet when anatomy theatres first came into use, the principle means of guiding transport across and around the world was a form of map that De Certeau never considered, one that required an entirely different corporeal intelligence. The Portolan chart, intended for use on shipping vessels, assumed its reader to be a body already in motion. Labelling towns or geographical features perpendicular to their location on the coastline, regardless of its curve or shape, the Portolan chart requires either the reader or the map to move continually. Rather than offering a bird's-eye view of the world as projected from a static viewing subject, the Portolan chart documents identity as a fluid collaboration between reader and landscape. Only in the late seventeenth century did the culture of dissection coalesce with regimes of bodily disciplining and cartographic technologies to yield a different orientation, one that presumed a static body that could view the world 'objectively'.

More than five hundred years later, a new system of orienting oneself in the world has emerged that, like the Portolan chart, helps to locate a map reader who is on the move. The Global Positioning System technology now being utilized in airplanes, automobiles, boats, and hand-held devices provides immediate topographical coordinates courtesy of multiple satellites circling the globe. Its companion technology, the cellphone, likewise hooks bodies up so that they can communicate while in motion. As a result, the map-reading skills that accompanied the culture of dissection are becoming obsolete. Like the new intelligent machines that diagnose bodily incapacity by scanning and anatomizing physical substances, the GPS creates a prosthetic interface between bodies that assists them in knowing where they are.

What do these changes in cartographic technologies tell us about the daily experience of the body? What do they predict about the body's role in performance? What do they intimate about the structuring of power in and on the global stage? What kinds of bodies are able to resist the regimes of surveillance implanted in these technologies? In what follows, I will focus on the ways that bodies discerned their locatedness in the world prior to the establishment of the anatomical subject, and compare that worldview with current trends in mapping and orienting. By examining what came just before the anatomy theatre alongside what is happening now in contemporary performance, I hope to contribute to our understanding of corpo-realities and corpo-politics.

Berlin, May 2005, 17:00: I've reserved at the Hebbel Theater am Ufer (HAU) to participate in their production *Call Cutta*, a new experience in theatre. The production was conceived and organized by a collaborative group of artists known as Rimini Protokoll. The group consists of artists Helgard Haug, Daniel Wetzel, and Stefan Kaegi.[2] I'm handed a cellphone and told to wait outside. After thirty seconds, the phone rings and a voice greets me by name, then introduces herself as Aisha from Calcutta. She asks me to cross the street and then turn right towards the glass doors of a seemingly abandoned building. Not at all abandoned, she explains, I am headed towards one of the main office centres for telecommunications in the city of Berlin. Aisha explains that hundreds of workers in small cubicles on the many floors above are busy processing data, much as she is doing in her home city, the difference being that she is working for Citibank, a transnational finance corporation whereas the Berliners are working for their city and country.

She directs me through the building, across an adjacent parking lot, and into a wooded vacant lot. Here, she points out a group of pictures attached to a tree. As I examine them she explains that her great uncle came from India to Berlin to seek Hitler's assistance in his campaign against Gandhi. Nearby, she points out the remnants of train tracks and a loading dock where armaments were shipped to the various war fronts. Obscured by weeds and small trees, these archaeological remains of a not very distant past seem all the more startling because they are unveiled by a voice from so far away. Her geographical remove combines with the intimacy of her voice and her uncanny connection to Hitler to create a new cybernetic world, one that requires new kinds of skills to navigate.

Indeed, as she directs me for over an hour to move through housing projects, across a bridge, into a shopping mall, and finally out onto the street again, I have lost all sense of orientation. I have been too engrossed in her stories and *her* observations about things *I* am looking at to keep track of my progress through space. Unable to determine the direction from which I came, I am rescued by the theatre's bus, which ferries the 'audience members' of this performance back to their point of origin.

Call Cutta, with its many starts and stops, its requests to focus near and far, is unusually disorienting. Casting the city and its inhabitants as stage set and performers, it invites audience members to become immersed in the action. As a result, participants would seldom be able to draw a map of their path, or to return directly to the starting point, without retracing many of the loops and detours they had taken. Having been asked to scan the entire city from a bridge, then to gaze at a tree trunk, and to look under a stairwell, the audience member loses any standard frame of reference, such as the proscenium provides, for calculating one's relationship to events being represented.

Call Cutta was created, in part, to advertise the working conditions of South Asian labourers who man banks of phones daily to answer questions concerning financial and commercial transactions of multinational corporations.[3] These corporations have outsourced voice communication with their customers to highly articulate and well-mannered assistants who will work for a fraction of the salary required in the First World. The work is quite hard on the body, and it also produces a distinctive anxiety, in that the assistant must pass as a member of the economy s/he is serving while remaining solicitous of all the customer's needs. Typically, this involves soothing, pacifying, and jollying the customer while following the rules of corporate exchange. Neither party ever witnesses the other or enjoys the opportunity to get to know them. The system offers no way to acquire a history of familiarity, reliability, or favour, since each phone call routes to a different worker. These workers are interchangeable and completely anonymous within the social economy.

The woman who is my guide is well aware of all this. Her joking, alluring confidence asserts an ironic distance from the labour that she and her co-workers typically perform. Satirizing her role as the agent who can sell you anything and make you feel good about the transaction, she instigates a series of questions about my love life, foregrounding the possibility for a long-distance romance. 'Do I have a boyfriend? Have I ever had phone sex?' This line of questioning backfires when she finds out I'm a lesbian in a long-term relationship. Her disingenuous efforts to switch sexual orientation and claim a flirtatious interest in me cause some awkward silences between us. Yet, we move past the topic, hurried on by the new landscape I am encountering – the backyard of a shabby housing project. Some of the inhabitants, Turkish, judging by their dress, are having a picnic. I feel strange, intruding on their semi-public leisure, since my actions, probably privileged and even voyeuristic from their point of view, are not entirely in my control.

I feel more at ease once we enter a shopping mall where many anonymous shoppers stroll, with or without purpose. But now I've lost the 'audience member' who had been ahead of me for most of the 'performance'. Although he has evidently been asked to attend to slightly different details, his general trajectory has matched mine, and I have found his presence reassuring, even though it breaks the illusion of my special relationship with Aisha. But Aisha is now urging me to find a camera store where, she announces proudly, we will meet. Suddenly I see a young South Asian woman waving glibly in the screen at the front of the store. She urges me to take a picture of myself with my cellphone, so that she can see me as well, and then she entreats me to 'stay in touch'. I can write to her any time at the e-mail address specified in my program.[4]

Why don't I feel like contacting her again? We've spent an hour and a half together, improvising a conversation, while at the same time completing a score that she knew well and that I could only suspect. Yet she set each new segment of our journey as a task for me to complete, always praising me when I had arrived at the specified location. Asking for reports about what I could see at a given moment, she responded only by confirming my descriptions. Thus, even though we conspired together to create a piece of 'theatre', I felt more like another of the many customers she would service in a day at her 'real' job.

The artists who conceptualized *Call Cutta* privileged the improvised structure of the piece so as to make possible a more lived and enduring connection between Aisha and myself. Rather than actually implement a GPS navigational system so that the caller could constantly track the audience member, they intended for the duo to develop a sense of mutual trust with each member contributing equally to the fulfilment of the score.[5] However, Aisha's role as a worker at the call centre conflicted with this dialogic goal. In order to perform the worker, she had to appear to know where I was at each moment, simulating a GPS system that was not actually in use. She could never appear in need of assistance or lacking in information. And this contradiction reverberated throughout the piece, most especially when I was walking through Turkish tenements as though they were just another feature in a neutral landscape. As a result, the performance evoked more than it critiqued the culture of digital surveillance in which we live today.

Still, *Call Cutta* problematizes in intriguing ways the theatre itself, the performer, and the audience. It partakes in a topos quite distinct from the perspectival and volumetric prescriptions for representation inaugurated by the proscenium theatre and the culture of dissection of which it was a part. In order to further interrogate *Call Cutta's* effects as well as the anatomy theatre from which it emerged, I want now to jump back in time to the early Renaissance courts and look closely at how they crafted self-presentation in the semi-theatrical occasion of an evening's dancing. At these balls, many of the same features are strikingly present: improvisation, an assessment of economic gain or loss, credibility, and most importantly a particular kinaesthetic sense of one's own orientation.

Taking place in a single room rather than outdoors, the balls nonetheless presented all performers and viewers with a socialscape that was constantly changing. Certain fixed features, such as a throne, stabilized and demarcated power, yet the perambulation of bodies throughout the space constituted a flux that required constant scrutiny and response. Renaissance courtiers were asked to calculate their distances from one another - to track all bodies and to keep track of their relative motions. Each body performed for every other body, although those with higher vantage points clearly saw more.

As they jockeyed to maintain or enhance their respective positions, courtiers drew on skills that are well documented in the courtesy and dance manuals beginning with Domenico da Piacenza's *De arte saltandi et choreas ducendi*, c. 1416, and continuing through Thoinot Arbeau's *Orchesography* from 1589.[6] In these texts major pedagogical emphasis is placed on learning to compose the body according to the principle of moderation, so that no movement is too large or too small; responding sensitively to the music's metre; remembering the sequence of steps; and, most crucially, adjusting this sequence to the size of the room in which the dance is being performed. Whether a slow bassadanza, or a livelier balli, all dances involve a presentation, a scrutiny, and an intermingling of performers. Reigning the body in and then calibrating its position and distance in relation to others, each dancer should evidence the ability continually to readjust one's location in relation to all the other bodies moving through the space. As Jennifer Neville has demonstrated in her analysis of fifteenth-century courtesy and dance literature, the distance among bodies is key to relative nobility (Neville, 2004). Courtiers continually deciphered the proximity between bodies, how close someone was sitting or standing to someone else, as a sign of their relative status.

In this continual flux of bodies mutually readjusting and reassessing their relationships to one another based on each body's most recent movements, pathways through the space were not defined against a stable, constant, and eternal plane. Instead, the room itself had to be read and re-read based on the ongoing progress of each dancer. Only through this ability to self-accommodate to a changing spatial fluidity could dancers participate effectively in the civil intercourse of dancing.

Mark Franko, along with Neville, notes that the Renaissance dancing body strives to become a rhetorically eloquent body, one that converses effectively and graciously with other dancing bodies and with viewers who witness the dancing as a form of conversation (Franko, 1986). Dancing Master Thoinot Arbeau describes dance as a form of mute rhetoric that enables dancers to persuade viewers of their nobility, spiritedness, modesty, and grace. Far from being ornamental, their decorousness offers proof of morality. In this way, dancing seamlessly attaches to quotidian interaction as an extension of the ongoing project of fashioning oneself in manner and measure, while at the same time, one scans others for any lapses or ruptures in their composure.

Franko argues that in its eloquence, the dancing body serves as a means of acquiring social and political capital. Citing the 1586 courtesy manual of Stefano Guazzo, Franko notes that social intercourse is dominated by the desire to conserve and increase one's means.[7] Income is acquired through the practice of silent and sympathetic attention in which 'one avoids a harsh expression in the eyes, twisting the body, a frowning seriousness, looking around (...)' (Franko, 1986, p. 74). Yet speaking can also be used to acquire wealth. Guazzo notes: '(...) well-received words bring profit to the listener and honour to the speaker. And just as different sorts of money come out of a purse, some gold, some silver and some copper, so sentences issue from the mouth and other words of more or less value' (Franko, 1986, p. 75). As all bodies continually decipher their manner and measure in response to one another, they build up a framework of mutual indebtedness. Needing both to profit and to please, they perform the proof of goodness that yields the profit of power over others.[8] And this ongoing indebtedness augments with each successive movement performed.

Perhaps this is the kind of mutual reliance that the authors of *Call Cutta* intended to evoke. Perhaps they aspired to knit back together, one call at a time, the social fabric torn asunder by the workings of transnational capital. Yet, according to the Renaissance model, several skills would be necessary, including an ability to note one's own placement in space in relation to others and an ability to respond appropriately to the flux of all bodies' changing positions.

Cellphone technology, however, discourages an awareness of other bodies in the space. It isolates the individual within his or her surround and creates a new privileged contact with another body across an unspecified distance. As a result, the single most asked question on both ends of the receiver is 'Where are you now?' And as they ask this question, cellphone users exhibit a notorious disregard for the loudness of their voices and the space they are occupying. They slow down unpredictably, stumble into other people or objects, and seldom assist in sustaining the modulated flow of bodies moving through public space. For them, profit results not from performing well in front of each body with whom they come into contact but from multi-tasking so as to accomplish more contacts in a shorter length of time. These bodies, equally comfortable in stillness or motion, transporting themselves or being transported, have learned that the body's motion alone is no longer responsible for the changes in volume or vision that they experience. These bodies rely on an apparatus to modulate physical changes such that they no longer correlate directly with sensory experience.

If cellphone users are no longer required to track their progress in space and to correlate physical motion with a changing sensorium, how do they know where they are? They are able to rely on the Global Positioning System to provide them with exact coordinates for their longitude, latitude, and vertical height. Developed by the US Department of Defense, the GPS consists of twenty-four satellites, four in each of six orbital planes, that emit signals designed to be decoded by a receiver to compute the receiver's position, velocity, and time (Dana, 1999). Four satellites are required for each reckoning, usually provided in less than a tenth of a second, with an accuracy of 1-10 metres. The computation can be displayed as a set of numbers indicating longitude and latitude, or it can be reconciled with a map that locates the receiver, in motion, with respect to various features of the landscape, such as roads or buildings. This map continues to unfold on the screen, locating and tracking the receiver as it moves.

In many respects, the GPS bears a strong resemblance to the Portolan charts used by the earliest Renaissance explorers. Detailing trade routes across and around the Mediterranean, these charts were constructed from a network of intersecting lines, or rhumb lines, originating from sixteen equidistant points spread about the circumference of a 'hidden' circle. Like the twenty-four satellites, these points gave mapmakers the stable reference with which to calculate star positions and ground locations. This information was translated on to a chart with towns and other geographical features labelled so as to be read when one is navigating along the water route at that place (Goss, 1993, p. 41).

Both chart and GPS project each body's motion onto a two-dimensional map, and both assume that the map-reader is on the move. Each also relies on an omniscient apparatus, either the sixteen points and their rhumb lines or the twenty-four satellites in the orbital planes, to compute locale. Prior to the culture of dissection that installed omniscience in the singular viewing subject who surveyed the world, Portolan charts allocated all-knowingness to the arbitrary yet evenly-spaced points that connect the rhumb lines. Now, in a post-anatomy theatre world, GPS similarly relieves the individual body of omniscience and instead specifies the computational system, the equations that reconcile data concerning five distinct points in space, as the sovereign source of knowledge about one's location.

Cellphones and the GPS work synergistically to inform users of their location. The cellphone de-activates the awareness of how one's motion alters the sensorium as measured in terms of the formal geometry of the grid-like map. The GPS then moves into the space of needing to know one's location with its ever-accessible screenic rendition. Where the anatomy theatre constructed a sturdy body, one that could carry the subject from place to place and track the results of that portage through a comparison of motion with sensory change, the new cellphone and GPS systems construct a prostheticized body that relies on digitized input to determine its whereabouts. Where the anatomy theatre's subject could claim, 'I have travelled this far, past these things, and I can locate that passage symbolically on this sheet of paper that projects my surround onto a two-dimensional geometric plane,' today's bodies instantly track their progress on a screenic version of the two-dimensional map.[9] No longer required to judge their whereabouts relationally or to continually reassess the relative motions of all relevant bodies, today's bodies are perpetually in touch with those they need to connect with. Today's bodies navigate a new transnational space by relying not on kinaesthetic sensibilities, but on redial, call waiting, and directories of contacts. Within this transnational space, theatre is no longer cordoned off and separated from daily life so as to confer and confirm its specialness. Now, as *Call Cutta* has demonstrated, theatre is all around us.

So, what did it mean that Aisha and I, physically distant by 6,000 miles, were talking together on cellphones in order to create a piece of theatre? How might the technology be subverted so as to provide a non-disembodied period of contact between the two of us? I think that one tactic of resistance would involve acknowledging that bodies moving through space do not experience all points in space as equal or equivalent. Each place supports an ecology and contains histories that are highly distinctive. That is why *Call Cutta* began so promising-ly as an inquiry into an extraordinarily local set of events – the uncle, the war, the almost absurdist connections between India and Germany. But these events became interchangeable with the Turkish tenements, the mall, and workers ev-erywhere. Even though each point in space contained its specific story, all sto-ries were rendered equivalent through the persona of the call worker and the standard amount of time spent at each location. In this sense, *Call Cutta* suc-cumbed to the culture of surveillance rather than resisting it.

But I can imagine a version that would not render all experience equivalent. Nor would it project all events onto the horizontal geometry of the Mercator-inspired map, as the culture of dissection did. Rather than substitute any point for any other, or fix them in hierarchized chains of relative meaning, *Call Cutta* might construct a variegated terrain, dense with memories and associations in some areas, and more sparse in others. But in order to do this, Aisha and I would have to practise improvising together. We would have to learn to depend on one another and to solicit candid responses from each other in order to mutually ex-plore the locality of our shared experience. With practice at being spontaneous, and a shared score for our actions, we could use disorientation to reaffirm and even enhance public protocols of comportment through which individuals rely on and sustain one another. And we could celebrate the fact, always a delight to rediscover, that theatre is all around us.

Susan Leigh Foster, choreographer and scholar, is Professor in the Depart-ment of World Arts and Cultures at UCLA. She is the author of *Reading Danc-ing: Bodies and Subjects in Contemporary American Dance* (University of Cali-fornia Press, 1986); *Choreography and Narrative: Ballet's Staging of Story and Desire* (Indiana University Press, 1996); and *Dances that Describe Themselves: The Improvised Choreography of Richard Bull* (Wesleyan University Press, 2002). She is also the editor of two anthologies: *Choreographing History* (University of Indiana Press, 1995) and *Corporealities* (Routledge, 1996) and co-editor of the journal *Discourses in Dance*.

Notes

1   Gerardus Mercator (1512-1594) was a Flemish cartographer and geographer who is best known for the mapping technique that became known as the 'Mercator projec-tion'.
2   *Call Cutta* grew out of a Goethe Institute-sponsored trip to the city of Calcutta, where the artists viewed a call centre first hand and began to speculate about how they could interact with it.

3   In an interview with Florian Malzacher, the artists comment: '(...) Yes, two complete-ly different markets are connected over the phone. And through employees who are constantly acting as though they were part of the Western market but are actually part of the Indian market.' Florian Malzacher, 'Do You Find That Interesting Too?' March 2005, Goethe-Institut, www.goethe.de/kue/the/prj/cak/int/enindex.htm. Last accessed December 28, 2006.

4   The program handed out along with the cellphone identifies e-mail addresses for each of the ten callers participating in the event.

5   [Florian Malzacher] Are your scripts for the performers in the call centre entirely written out?
[Helgard Haug and Daniel Wetzel] There'll be plenty of room for improv. But also, of course, a fairly clear-cut text, a sort of descriptive roadmap. Like a GPS – though with information about the things you're seeing and not just: 'Turn left.' It's about lots of minute visual details – and the call centre people have to keep track of the callers' exact whereabouts at all times.
[FM] Well, why don't you actually use GPS at the call centres?
[HH/DW] It's important to us for the two parties to really do the rounds together. That serves as the basis of an interchange based on mutual trust. What's more, groping their way forwards together will provide a source of stories and questions. Malzacher, www. goethe.de/kue/the/prj/cak/int/enindex.htm. All spelling in context.

6   These include: Antonio Cornazano *Libro dell'arte del danzare*, 1455; Guglielmo Ebreo da Pesaro *Trattato dell'arte del Ballo*, 1455; Giovanni Ambrosio n.d. Fabritio Caroso *Il Ballarino*, 1581; and Cesare Negri *Le Gratie d'Amore*, 1602.

7   See Franko, 1986, p. 72. As justification, Franko points to Guazzo's observation: 'As a wise man was asked why nature has given us two ears and only one tongue he replied because we should hear more than we speak. That answer gave me reason to attribute income to the ears and expenditure to the tongue.' Quoted in Franko, p. 73. Silence, and by extension, stillness prompt the accumulation of income because they please others and dispose others favourably toward the listener. See Franko, pp. 73-75.

8   According to Franko, movement performs the proof of goodness which both dissimulates the clandestine appeal to the emotions of the first proof and yields the 'profit' of power over others: glory (Franko, 1986, pp. 76-77).

9   A second type of map, the route survey, documents a similar mobility on the part of its maker. Using a perambulator that endeavours to measure distances, but is always inaccurate because of twists and turns, potholes, etc., the mapmaker moves forward from one major geographical feature to the next in sight, notating relevant data on either side, so as to draft a regularly unfolding narrow band of landscape. Each segment comes to an end, and the next starts based upon the surveyor's sense of direction and the views onto the path ahead afforded by a rise in elevation. See Matthew Edney, 1990, pp. 94-5.

References

Bleeker, M., 'Locus of Looking. Dissecting Visuality in the Theatre.' Ph. D. dissertation. Amsterdam, 2002. Published as *Visuality in the Theatre: The Locus of Looking*. Basingstoke, 2008.

Carter, P., *The Road to Botany Bay: An Essay in Spatial History*. London, 1987.

Certeau, M. de, *The Practice of Everyday Life*. Berkeley and Los Angeles, 1984.

Dana, P.H., *The Geographer's Craft Project*. Boulder, 1999.

Edney, M., *Mapping an Empire: The Geographical Construction of British India, 1765-1843*. Chicago, 1990.

Franko, M., *The Dancing Body in Renaissance Choreography*. Birmingham, Ala., 1986.

Goss, J., *The Mapmaker's Art*. New York, 1993.

Neville, J., *The Eloquent Body: Dance and Humanist Culture in Fifteenth-Century Italy*. Bloomington, 2004.

Sawday, J., *The Body Emblazoned: Dissection and the Human Body in Renaissance Culture*. London and New York, 1995.

Performance Documentation 6:
Under My Skin

In Ivana Müller's *Under My Skin*, a group (maximum 20) is invited to 'step inside' Müller's own body to participate in an intimate guided tour through its interior. Ivana's 'body' consists of a maze of wood-framed, variously sized rooms, separated by red curtains. Each room contains different body processes, accomplished by the body's inhabitants. Tour guides explain the phenomena encountered by the spectators. For instance, the guides point out how body tissue can be repaired (by seamstresses, in the Mending Room) and how accelerated heart beats, which are produced by amplifying the sound of a fly swatter, are pre-recorded in the Sound Studio. In this bodily maze, the guides try to orientate the spectator by means of a map of the different rooms, and how they are connected. The body is a maze, and also a theatre, most specifically backstage. Entering this theatrical body, the audience literally is offered a look behind its curtains.

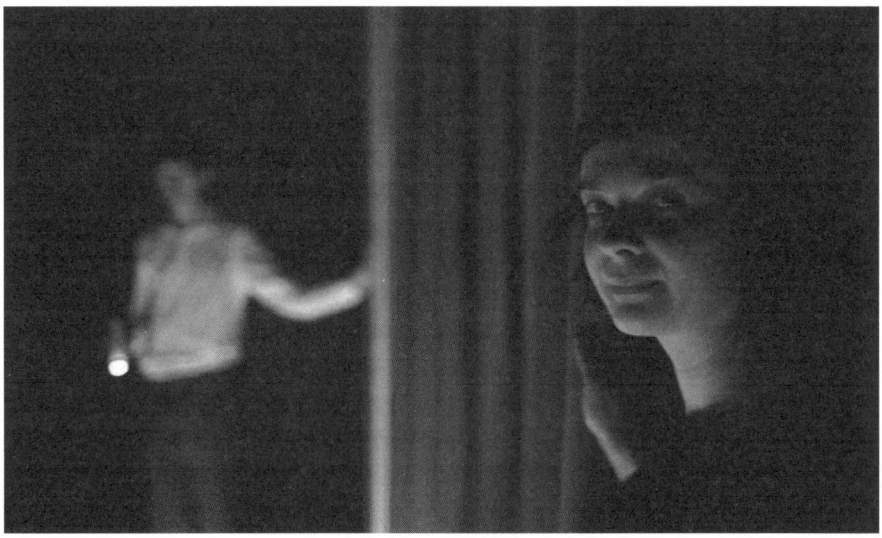

Under My Skin by Ivana Müller (2005). Photo: Anja Beutler. Reproduced with permission of the photographer.

Under My Skin can be regarded as the second part of a performance diptych in which Ivana Müller explores her imagining of the relationship between body and mind. In the first part of the diptych, *How Heavy Are My Thoughts*, Müller asked: 'If my thoughts are heavier than usual, is my head heavier than usual too?'[1] She then proceeded to subject this essentially metaphorical question to a series of empirical experiments, presented on stage in the form of a scientific lecture. Engaging in *Under My Skin* with themes similar to those in *How Heavy Are My Thoughts* — such as the comparison of scientific and artistic research, the identity and presence of the performer, and the reflection on 'non-theatrical' modes of representation — Müller continues to explore the relationship between body and mind, but now with a focus on the body. In the performance announcement, she provides an explanation for her fascination with her body interior: '[T]he most physical part of me is the most difficult to imagine, and once I do it becomes an invented fictional place.'[2] *Under My Skin* is a theatre performance that explores the metaphorical concepts and ideas we use to think and fantasize about our bodies. By employing the formal conventions of a guided tour, it evokes questions about the representation of the body as a space that can be explored and mapped.

After the first tour guide has introduced himself to the audience, he opens a curtain covering a screen on which a picture of Ivana Müller, standing on a sidewalk, is projected: 'This is an external view of the body we are all standing in. It is, as you can all see, a female body. She is known by the name of Ivana Müller.'[3] The image zooms in on Ivana's head, the screen fades white, and then zooms out again, now showing a heavily schematized image of Müller's body. The 'inhabitants' of the body and their different rooms can now be seen. In the middle of the screen a red circle starts to blink, marked with the words 'you are here'.

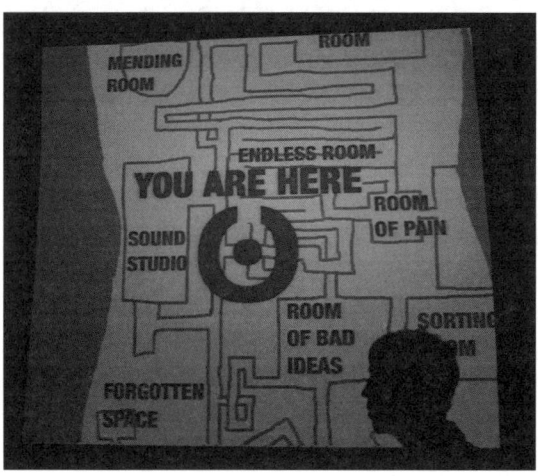

Under My Skin by Ivana Müller (2005). Photo: Anja Beutler. Reproduced with permission of the photographer.

The spectators are invited to look at this abstract overview as a ground plan of the body they are in, which they are about to discover in a guided tour. The schematized representation of Ivana's body inevitably evokes associations with anatomical imagery. The image, with pathways connecting the rooms, is reminiscent of depictions of the network of blood vessels that links the organs in a human body. The 'you are here' sign emphasizes the function of the representation as a means to orientate the spectators, and invites them to consider the bodily space that is surrounding them as a topographical terrain.

The representation of Ivana's body as a space that can be explored and mapped is directly reminiscent of the features of anatomical imagery in the early modern period. The visualization of the body in the 'anatomical atlases' of that time was based on a similar metaphor.[4] Jonathan Sawday has argued that the journeys of discovery in the sixteenth century were not accidentally coincident with the emergence of these first modern scientific works on human anatomy (Sawday, 1995, p. 23). Sawday observes that the way the geographic discoverers were mapping the world influenced the conception of the body as an 'undiscovered country', an alien, unknown place that was yet to be explored. The anatomical atlases presented the positivist promise that, just like the most remote areas in the world, the body was a space that could be colonized and charted through the efforts of the anatomists.

The relationship between visualization, knowledge and control of the body that Sawday refers to is also one of the leading themes of *Under My Skin*. The tour guides are clearly concerned with showing the audience that they (the guides) 'master' their surroundings. Their intention is to present the body as a comprehensibly structured system. Yet, they have a lot of trouble with trying to maintain their authoritarian status when, time and again, they are confronted with various bodily phenomena they cannot explain nor control.

Soon after their entrance, the visitors are informed that 70% of the body will be left out of the tour 'due to safety reasons'. The tour guide explains that two Japanese tourists recently got lost and still have not been found. Despite these precautionary measures, at the beginning of the tour black creatures are already invading the room, crawling over the floor and harassing the audience. As the creatures return throughout the tour, the spectators are encouraged by the guides to stamp their feet at the floor next to them, to chase them away. Despite this, it is clear that the guides cannot control the creatures' behavior, and that they are unnerved by these recurrent appearances. The mysterious black creatures also appear on the screens of the 'monitoring system', which shows the images of cameras that are supposedly set up all through the body. According to the guides, this surveillance system was installed to prevent disturbances and irregularities in the interior.

The monitory system in *Under My Skin* presents a view of the body as a repressive political system in which alien or dangerous elements, like the black creatures, are to be kept under surveillance to prevent any possible revolts that could threaten the existing establishment. This system illustrates the endeavours of the guides to exercise power over the body by means of visualization. Moreover, a successful demonstration of the body as a fully intelligible system contributes to their authoritarian status.

Just like modern anatomists, the guides set out to show that every phenomenon encountered has its own function, one that fits logically within the functioning of the body as a whole. They present the body as an anatomical body, which is visually represented in a way in which it can be known and, hence, can be controlled. Near the end of the tour, the keeper of the Forgotten Space confronts both guide and audience with this (their) view of Ivana's body as an anatomical body: 'I suppose you want to see all the exciting and more glamorous places... but there is more to this place than meets the eye,' he tells the audience. 'The body has its mystery things that it doesn't know what to do with.' In this way, the keeper challenges the ability of using either functionality or spectacle, which are both features typical of the anatomical body, as a means to understand the body.

At the end of the tour, the body map of Ivana Müller returns. The guide uses it to retrace the route that the group has just followed. A red dot appears on the screen and starts to move, following the quirky turns of the schematized paths that connect the rooms on the map. Although the audience members can recognize the names of the rooms they just passed through, the weird twists and turns of the connecting paths hardly correspond with their experience of the tour. The tour guide confirms this observation: 'I suppose this schematic diagram is not so much like your experience of being here inside the body, is it?'

Once again, a specific feature of the visualization of the anatomical body is brought to the fore. Proceeding from Sawday's remarks on the anatomical atlas, the sociologist Catherine Waldby, who has specialized in the social aspects of biotechnologies and the body, has observed that anatomical representation relies on a spatialization of the body in order to create a communicable knowledge (Waldby, 2000). Waldby argues that the form of the atlas 'suggests both a spatiality and a temporality, insofar as one reads and turns its pages in a sequence [and hence] lends itself to a spatialized narrative about the body's constitution' (Waldby, 2000, p. 94). The body in *Under My Skin* is similar to the body as it is represented in the anatomical atlas because in both cases it is impossible to perceive an overview of the whole body at once. Just like different pages in an anatomical atlas, every room in the tour through Ivana's body represents a different bodily function or process. The guided tour in *Under My Skin* can also be regarded as a spatialized narration of 'the body as a sequence of systems' (Waldby, 2000, p. 94).

The representation of the body as a theatre in *Under My Skin* draws attention to the metaphorical nature of our conceptualization of the body interior. Müller presents the body as a dramatic world, a fictional place that we can only enter through our imagination. Whether we consider the body as a scientific object or as a fantastic space that can be explored, our understanding of the body is constructed by the way it is visualized and narrated in representations. The inability of the tour guides to explain and control the body reiterates the fascination, the wonder, but also the fear that characterized some of the main questions of the sixteenth-century natural philosophers' main questions about the body: Will the soul be able to control the body? How do the soul and the body relate to each other? *Under My Skin* playfully engages with these questions, bringing up issues about the relationship between visualization and knowledge that have all but lost their relevance. 'We've spent an hour discovering the inside of the body,' the tour guide concludes the tour, 'and we have only seen a glimpse of the body at work. Which is not surprising because the body is as infinite as the imagination.'

Text by *Laura Karreman*

Ivana Müller is a performance artist/choreographer/theatre director. She studied literature in Zagreb, dance and choreography in Amsterdam, and fine arts in Berlin. In her artistic work she develops defined performative concepts that use twists in perception or logic as a starting point, creating pieces that are poetic and scientific, philosophical and humorous, intimate and political at the same time. In her recent work she has explored the notions of self-invention and story telling, often working on the borders between fiction and reality. Most of her work is made for theatres, although she also creates installations for galleries and museums and publishes texts. Ivana Müller is founding member of LISA. She lives and works in Amsterdam and Paris.[5]

Laura Karreman is currently finishing her RMA in Art Studies with a major in Theatre Studies at the University of Amsterdam.

Performance Data

Performed by: Bill Aitchison, Andrea Bozic and Ivana Müller
Text: Ivana Müller in collaboration with Bill Aitchison and Andrea Bozic
Video: Nils de Coster

Sound and technique: Xavier van Wersch
Set design: Ivana Müller, Nils de Coster and Bill Aitchison
Set advice: Nuno Almeida
Thanks to: Bojana Kunst and Maaike Bleeker

Under My Skin is a LISA production. It was co-produced by Productiehuis Rotterdam (Rotterdamse Schouwburg); Stuk, Leuven; and Monty, Antwerpen. It premiered in Monty, Antwerp on April 28th, 2005.

Notes

1   *How Heavy Are My Thoughts* was made by Ivana Müller, in collaboration with Bill Aitchison and Nils de Coster. It is a LISA production and was co-produced by Mousonturm, Frankfurt, and Gasthuis Theater, Amsterdam. It premiered at the Plateaux Festival, October 24, 2003.
2   Association LISA has its website at: www.associationlisa.com.
3   All quotes from the performance are my transcriptions from the DVD registration of *Under My Skin.*
4   The Flemish physician and anatomist Andreas Vesalius is generally regarded to be one of the first medical scientists to create an 'anatomical atlas'. His work *De humani corporis fabrica libri septem* ('Seven Books on the Working of the Human Body') was published in 1543.
5   This biography was quoted from the LISA website. More information and texts on this and other performances by Ivana Müller can also be found on this site.

References

LISA. www.associationlisa.com.
Sawday, J., *The Body Emblazoned: Dissection and the Human Body in Renaissance Culture.* London and New York, 1995.
Waldby, C., 'Virtual Anatomy: From the Body in the Text to the Body on the Screen.' In: *Journal of Medical Humanities,* 21, pp. 85-107, 2000.

Anatomies of Live Art

Sally Jane Norman

Our constant invention of machines and interactive processes to multiply and extend bodily relations to the world is mirrored in the transformations of theatre, its physical organization being tightly intertwined with its dramatic contents. In the past, the shaping and experiencing of theatre have been hugely modified by advances related to mechanics and electricity. Information and communications and biotechnologies are in turn prompting new means to expose live art, and new conceptions of the performing body. Yet all these technological forces continue to animate a theatrical corpus, which is as ancient as it is metamorphic. This text cuts across history to reveal some of the ways in which anatomies of contemporary live art seem to perpetuate the primitive vitality of theatre.

Theatre Architectures as Social Anatomies

The structural characteristics of theatre architectures reflect the anatomy of the body politic that they convene and contain. The principles of social organisation are written into theatrical venues ranging from early open air settings for processions and site-specific action, through to dedicated, sealed architectures which have marked theatre history since the Renaissance. Like the anatomical theatre, these architectures have been shaped by multiple, mutually determinant forces and goals. Vectors of perception (sightlines, acoustics) and social mores dictating public rank and station are instrumental in 'exogenous' concrete design questions like choices of scale and materials, to be compared with simultaneously active 'endogenous' questions proper to the poetics of theatre, attempts to engage, enthral or alienate an audience being as bound up in dramaturgical processes as in physical construction.

The endo/exogenous distinction is however largely formal, in that social and physical architectures are inextricably and vitally interwoven in the staging of live art; indissociable links between dramaturgical and architectural languages are evident throughout theatre history. Staged space literally offered readings to French court ballet spectators: social status and correlative physical positioning of royal gallery viewers allowed them to decipher symbols in choreographic floor patterns. Three concentric circles represented Perfect Truth, two equilateral triangles within a circle represented Supreme Power, etc., in addition to imposed values such as the sovereign's monogram (McGowan, 1963). Early modern English theatre architecture and spectator experience were likewise tightly coupled, as shown by Martin White's research involving simultaneously filmed viewpoints of historical reconstructions of several Jacobean plays, aligned in accordance with distinct seating emplacements whence very different light – literally and figuratively – is shed on the staged action.[1] White shows how the viewer's social status as borne out by the seating confirms tight links between whence and where you see (therefore where you are seen, i.e. who you are socially) and what you see, audience experience being patently conditioned by inter-determinant relations between dialogue, stage directions, lighting and physical architecture. Because spectators at the ground level and those placed in galleries are very differently caught up in viewpoints and exchanges between the protagonists, they experience distinctive interpretations of the work. Relations like these entangle writings, buildings and audiences throughout theatre history.

To set theatre anatomies shaped by high-tech prostheses in a historical context, it is worth emphasizing the spatial and temporal flexibility that empowers ostensibly non-technological theatrical forms to outstrip apparent physical boundaries or frames. Through imaginative investment in theatre for two and a half thousand years, we have prepared ourselves for the miracles whereby space and time are seemingly infinitely reshaped by contemporary technics. The Greek amphitheatre spawned novel physical/dramaturgical forces by multiplying places that could be imaginatively embraced by the actors' and spectators' sweeping gaze, as indicated by the opening lines of Sophocles's *Electra* where the Paedagogus addresses Orestes as follows:

> Son of him who led our hosts at Troy of old, son of Agamemnon! (...) There is the ancient Argos of thy yearning,- that hallowed scene whence the gad-fly drove the daughter of Inachus; and there, Orestes, is the Lycean Agora, named from the wolf-slaying god; there, on the left, Hera's famous temple; and in this place to which we have come, deem that thou seest Mycenae rich in gold, with the house of the Pelopidae there, so often stained with bloodshed (...).[2]

Identification of five near and far landmarks in a single glancing sentence and gesture might be read as an early form of distributed, networked spaces, causally meshed by past and future events. Just as imagination gave us wings and supernatural human sight long before we invented aircraft and satellites, we seem to have readily shared our dreams about conflated and dovetailed spaces thousands of years before inventing the technical means to instantiate them.

In parallel to its concentration and concatenation of spaces, theatre has evolved architecturally to offer an arena for recreating temporal structures: its containment within premises freed from nycthemeral cycles has spurred techniques to command day and night at will. Abstraction from the constraints of natural space and time prefigures today's distributed performances, interwoven by virtue of data transmission rates rather than physical proximity. Integrating the technical characteristics of networked platforms is core to online performance works, as in the first *Ballettikka Internettikka* creation by Igor Stromajer and Brane Zorn, which foregrounded differential bandwidths and data packet delivery rates.[3] The piece was choreographed to be seen as a webcammed, webcast work for 20-second low- or high-bandwidth uploads, breaks in transmission being considered by the artists to mirror the aesthetics of human computer interaction. Discontinuities in space and time were integral to the communication experience, the viewers being free to imagine whatever happened between uploaded 20-second intervals.

Whereas previous theatre forms tended to draw geographically unified groups around obvious temporal markers and physical boundaries, activities bundled under the term 'locative media' (media that are grounded, so to speak, in mobile technologies based on location awareness) encompass participants and forge identities at levels ranging from the most intimate to the most distant: singular located occurrences bleed into distributed events, which in turn colour local experience. Our sense of rhythmic constructs underlying live art, traditionally imbued with the visceral metrics of bodies in a shared physical locus, is being extended to embrace geographically remote spaces, spectators and actors. Like the subtle flow regulation gestures that modulate our face-to-face communication, new means of scansion and meta-synchronization are emerging to tune the social exchange in distributed, hybrid, multi-agent systems. Such evolutions resonate with Victor Turner's reflections on the cultural roles of the communitas, interaction and synchronicity.[4] Rather than staging the gestures of individual human protagonists as in traditional theatres, the networked anatomies of nascent theatres are relaying gestures and patterns of encounter that are at once multiple, collective and complex,[5] bearing out Turner's suggestion that new communications technologies may enable unprecedented genres of cultural performance, and thereby new modes of self-understanding.[6]

Life Support Systems and Skenabiotopes

Technologies that foster spatial and temporal coincidence, linking previously isolated moments and places, alter our sense of presence and embodiment essential to the live art of theatre. Moreover, the vivacity characteristic of interactive art through its more-or-less programmatic staging of spectator behaviours depends on uncannily hybridized relations between human and electro-mechanical and informational resources. Artefacts belonging to this body of work might be described as life support systems, analogous to the medical apparatus which upholds vital functions. Life support systems in the context of theatre's willfully mixed realities and blasphemous trafficking in life-likeness designate an array of dynamically open, evolving processes that endow all manner of living and pseudo-living entities with autonomy.

A conceptual framework for these systems is offered by the *skenabiotope*. Coined by artist Louis Bec, the skenabiotope derives from the *skena* or stage and the biotope, and is defined as

> an artificial space specially constructed to enhance the spectacular activities of certain organisms and/or models. It is a 'dispositif', a system whose parameters can be manipulated, provoking programmed or random behaviours. One might say that it is constructed quite precisely to study and amplify certain types of theatricalising or theatricalised behaviours in artificial organisms. (Bec, 1992, p. 116)

The *agon* or contest that has whetted the performing arts ever since opposition between the chorus/soloist or actor/spectator engendered the first proto-agonist subtends skenabiotopes in which disparate species vie for survival and supremacy. Places of primitive physical spectacle ostensibly devoid of discursive elements, including the Coliseum and the more generic cockpit and bearpit, constitute strong precursors for the anatomical theatre.[7] The tenuous border separating man and beast stands as an ancient and lasting locus for the performing arts: for thousands of years, parades and circuses (then rodeos, agricultural fairs, dog and cat shows, etc.) have celebrated humankind's ability to capture, tame, train and 'civilize' wildlife. Skenabiotopes for these celebrations feature devices which focus attention on the mongrel entities formed by animals and their masters: cages, pools, nets, ramps, harnesses and leashes, sticks and whips, obstacles and podiums highlight demonstrations of conquest, complicity, shared intelligence and cunning. These props reinforce what might be called the crossing of the inter-species barrier ('artistes', entertainers who showcase physical virtuosity, often share the bills and sawdust of the arena with other trained animals). Human-animal partnerships as deranging vectors of cross-species communications have long enthralled semi-clandestine halls of miracles and road-shows, alongside teratological freaks and other quasi-human, quasi-living apparitions.

This tradition is perpetuated in skenabiotopes that today celebrate species engendered by unholy marriages of bodies and machines, software and wet-ware, from popular culture's 'robot wars' to more subtle hybrids fashioned by eclectic arts and sciences. Anatomies of live art refer not just to linkages of physically distant entities, but also to linkages of phyletically distant entities to create startling new chimeras. SymbioticA, the Art and Science interdisci-plinary group based at the Science Collaborative Research Laboratory in the School of Anatomy and Human Biology, University of Western Australia, tack-les this question with its 'TC&A' – Tissue Culture & Art Project – research.[8] Oron Catts and Ionat Zurr have developed semi-living sculptures for over a decade by growing cell cultures on scaffolds made of biocompatible substrates in sterile, homeostatic environments. This technique of three-dimensional tis-sue engineering has produced emblematic works like *Pig Wings*, a set of wing-shaped skin growths cultivated from scavenged porcine tissues, and *The Pro-cess of Giving Birth to Semi-Living Worry Dolls*. The latter work translates into bio-art the Guatemalan Indian tradition of giving worry dolls to children; at night, the children can take one doll at a time from its bedside box and share their worry with it, confident that their problem will be solved by the morning. TC&A hand-crafted seven dolls from polymers and surgical sutures, sterilized and seeded with endothelial, muscle, and osteoblast cells grown over the poly-mers which degraded as the tissue grew, bringing the dolls to life. The chamber in which the live cell cultures were maintained was accessible via video images taken at regular intervals and uploaded to a website; viewers could enlarge and modify resolution of the images to follow the growth process (a whimsical take on controversy surrounding zealous echographic monitoring of human foetus-es in utero). Announced doll-feeding times were an exhibition artifice, since nutrient supply was necessarily permanent.

MEART (Multi-Electrode Array Art), a SymbioticA Research Group work created in collaboration with the Department of Biomedical Engineering at the Georgia Institute of Technology (Atlanta), consists of a brain comprised of nerve cells (embryonic rat cortex grown over a multi-electrode array) cultured in the Atlanta neuro-engineering lab, and of a robotic drawing arm functioning as its remote body.[9] Brain and body communicate via software and the internet to produce unique, non-reproducible artworks for *MEART* exhibitions, raising questions about the nature and systems which allow creation to be sustained. Catts and Zurr feel that the bioreactor core of their works 'should be treated as an art object and not a mere tool. Conceptually a bioreactor (in conjunction with the semi-living sculptures growing inside it) represents an artificial "life-giving" and maintaining force.'[10] As a skenabiotope, 'constructed to study and amplify certain types of theatricalizing or theatricalized behaviours in artificial organisms' (Bec), the bioreactor and its contents pose questions analogous to those posed more generally by the pseudo-lives integral to theatre: what existence and significance might they enjoy beyond the artificial and artefactual worlds which guarantee their survival?

Distributed theatre anatomies formed by networked bodies stand for an interesting conundrum in the domain of conjoined biotechnological and artistic activity. Because they involve living systems, biotechnological developments including those modelled by highly abstract means are too hastily seen as directly espousing the real-life world they are designed to engage with. This results in tendencies to ascribe the robustness of real-world phenomena to hyper-regulated in vitro and in silico phenomena, despite discontinuities between their respective underlying processes of raw emergence and idealized modelling (however much stochastic grit is integrated by the latter). Artists working with biotechnologies are pushing for acknowledgement of this hiatus and recognition of the determinant role played by scientific artefacts, albeit and especially in the vital domain of living systems.[11] Instantiation of these imperatives traces new links between art and life, and between art and science, and reinforces our need for the skenabiotope as a place designed to creatively explore the particular liminality represented by radically artificial organisms. The strength of groups like SymbioticA lies in their ability to create unique sites of public engagement with biotechnologies through creations that elude the positivistic confines of scientific explanation, standing as wilfully poetic feats and triggers of the imagination.

Because the essence of theatre resides in its interlacing and weaving of chimeras and flesh, humans and machines, it offers ideal ground for exploring fringe zones between the natural and the artificial, between living and inanimate phenomena, between humans and other autonomous evolving creatures. The meltdown of registers of presence and modes of communication brought about by biotechnologies, and the correlative emergence of search patterns through live information spaces, demand platforms to reconcile bodies and spectres, life-lines and codes, signals and signs, anticipating and projecting new languages. Skenabiotopes are a theatrical manifestation of such platforms, which integrate and model physical life processes and behaviours, and vampirize attributes from the human world with which they interact. They serve as protected zones or cyberzoos for evolving species which cannot be attached to the wall or floor like traditional artistic creations, and which are generally durably neotenic: even when fed with appropriate energisers (current, bandwidth, software updates, etc.), they show a propensity to misbehave, break down, lose their code, and run unpredictably amok. Today's skenabiotope inhabitants must be turned on and off, networked, rebooted, rewired, updated – in short, looked after like rare living specimens.

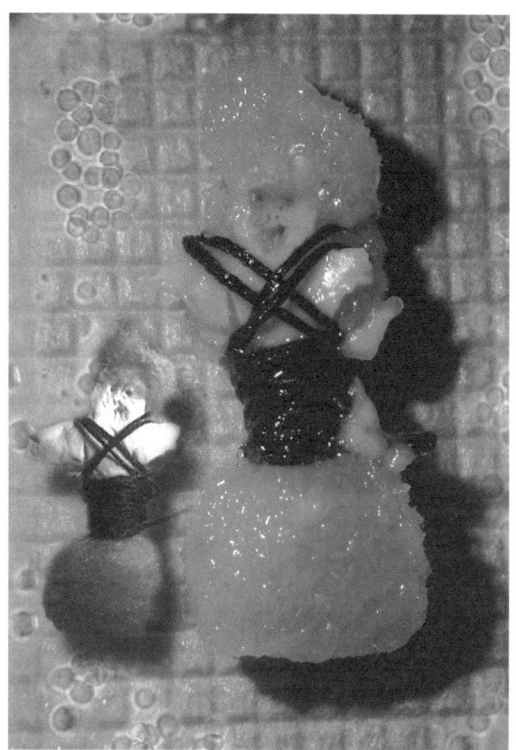

Left: A Semi-Living Worry Doll by
The Tissue Culture & Art. Medium:
McCoy Cell line, Biodegradable/
bioabsorbable Polymers and Surgical
Sutures. From *The Tissue Culture &
Art(ificial) Wombs Installation*, Ars
Electronica 2000. Photo Axel Heise.
Reproduced with the permission of
Oron Catts.

Below: Semi-Living Worry Dolls
Display by the Tissue Culture & Art.
Photo Axel Heise. Reproduced with
the permission of Oron Catts.

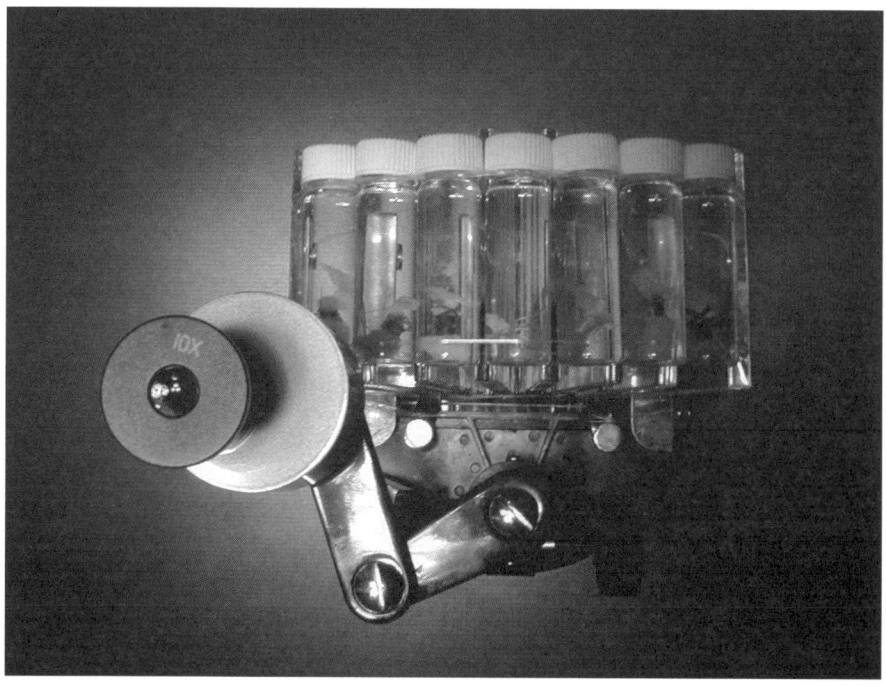

Theatres of Life and Death

Skenabiotopes challenge our sense of what it is to be alive and what it is to be human. Rituals associated with hosted living processes (breeding, feeding, grooming), including their demise and death, might represent as much aesthetic interest as their birth. Framed as instants of a new kind of theatre, such rituals could provide exciting, creative insights into the hybrid anatomies peopling our increasingly humachine world. Funerals for the semi-living Pig Wings and Worry Dolls might be as culturally valuable as exhibition openings, emphasizing their peculiar states and categories of aliveness. This would challenge obsessive desires to preserve life and traces of human endeavour, which tend to overlook or underestimate the poetics of absence, loss, and ephemerality. Who gets to switch off hybrid life forms, how, when and why, and what does this signify in ethical and aesthetic terms? Is the inert or empty bioreactor a stage or is it a mausoleum, a site of rituals to do with homage and mourning?

Symbolic 'transitional objects'[12] frequently underlie our attempts to reconcile the cycles of life and death, creating linkages between different categories of matter, effigies, and the afterlife. Many masks exemplify the recognition of the liminal qualities of living and non-living matter by integrating bodily relics: artefacts incorporating human bones, teeth, hair, and skin have been central to ritual performances all over the planet, and the corpse is borne to its grave as a highly animated figure in numerous cultures. Western vestiges of such traditions can be seen in relics, death masks and memento mori. In Ancient Rome, funeral processions starred professional players called arch-mimes masked to resemble the deceased, whose gestures and voice they cunningly imitated and thus rendered acutely present for the mourners.[13] Similarly, in traditional Yoruba death ceremonies, a member of the tribe donned a specially sculpted wooden mask and the shroud of the deceased, considered as being invested by his/her life, in order to convey the spirit of the lamented person. Congo chiefs' dead bodies were traditionally dried then wrapped in layers of fabric to form an imposing effigy, laid on a litter energetically displaced to make the figure dance and leap to its burial. In funeral rituals in Gabon, the corpse was borne by a porter made 'invisible' thanks to a palm-leaf disguise, by whose intermediary the deceased could 'walk' and 'speak'. The Mofu-Gudur in the Cameroons would break the bones of the deceased person, who would dance to the tomb in a final public appearance of superhuman grace. The Slavic tradition of placing the deceased upright in the coffin for a final round of visitors went as far as animating the corpse with string devices in the Ukraine. These traditions verge on the art of puppetry, which mocks human mortality, reproducing life by imitation and artifices that violate purportedly natural laws of reproduction (Darkowska-Nidzgorski and Nidzgorski, 1998). Tadeusz Kantor's creations

constitute a powerful theatrical legacy in this ambivalent realm, where the obscure, seditious aspects of human activity are spectacularly staged in blasphemous recreations of life.[14] Kantor's *Theatre of Death* with its incessant traffic of
dehumanized actors and replicas, and its maniacal mechanisms of repetition
and reproduction, appears as a quintessential form of black art and of durably
disturbing live art.[15]

If we were unable to freely anthropomorphize and see objects outside of our
own organisms as capable of bearing or deploying vital functionalities, in other
words, as entities to which we can delegate activities that we would otherwise
have to perform ourselves, we would probably not have been able to imagine,
let alone fabricate, the vast majority of artefacts that have transformed our civilization. It is by virtue of this same ability that ostensibly simple narratives
that play with the boundaries of living and non-living phenomena can be oddly
spine-chilling. One such story is Steve Tillis's account of puppeteer Bart Roccoberton Junior's visit to the home of a famous American puppet artist, where
his viewing of a puppet collection was to be followed by dinner. The artist's
best-known puppet greeted Roccoberton and presented the collection, while
the artist, in his own voice, made just a few comments. Towards dinnertime, an
argument broke out between the artist and the puppet: the former suggested
a drink and dinner, while the puppet, complaining of fatigue, insisted that the
wearisome visitor should leave. The artist ended up reluctantly agreeing with
the puppet, and Roccoberton was shown to the door, his host apologizing for
the puppet's behaviour (Tillis, 1992, p. 33). The story 'works' because we recognize how readily we operate irrational affective transfers, emotionally investing
in ostensibly banal objects. To write this off as superstition or naivety is to miss
the point. Far from betraying juvenile weakness, our capacity to invest in transitional phenomena to create complex symbolic systems is a vital determinant
of the imaginative agility we must collectively develop in order to face a largely
unknown and unknowable future.

Skenabiotopes devoted to the survival of existing life forms are a cultural
counterweight to bioreactors and arenas for emerging life forms. Throughout
history, the ownership and display of rare species have served to affirm wealth
and social prestige, entertain the masses and, more recently, educate the wider
public about our planet's rapidly declining biodiversity. Illegal traffic of live
flora and fauna has today reached unprecedented levels, to rival transactional
values of weapon and drug commerce in a doubtless irreversible development
foreseen by authors like Philip K. Dick, whose characters in *Do Androids Dream
of Electric Sheep?* (1968) highly esteem authentic living animals that are mas-
sively outnumbered by their artificial surrogates. From the 'vasculum' or tin
carrier case of the eighteenth-century botanical collector to entire territories
delimited to protect our dwindling ecosystems, a diverse array of techniques to

frame 'natural' life contrasts with containment systems specifically devised for hybrid and artificial entities. Comparison of these different kinds of skenabiotopes can shed light on our visions and redefinitions of life.[16]

Questions of survival, extinction and evolution have haunted networked creations since the earliest experiments in artificial life and ecosystem modelling, epitomized by Tom Ray's milestone Tierra software project.[17] Bearing in mind the risk of blithely mapping ideally wrought phenomena to real-world settings, computer-generated, networked dealings with life forms like Ray's elucidate emergent and evolutionary processes in ways that enhance our sense of life. An ironically overt link between real and virtual worlds is manifest in artist collective Transnational Temps' *Novus Extinctus* (2001), a web-based work building edgy tension between abstract, highly individuated entities that make up domain names on the internet, and formidably real, frighteningly irreplaceable entities on lists of endangered flora and fauna.[18] The economy of rarity encountered in the frenetic appropriation of internet property or domain names is compared with the economy – or lack of – that characterizes human management of the biotope: while thousands of domain names are registered annually for new websites, thousands of species are becoming extinct. In this work combining online creativity and offline ecology, the website offers as 'free' the Latin names of recently extinct species, emphasizing the momentous die-off that is making the names 'available'. The work was inspired by the realization that images of endangered animals online often outnumber the animals themselves in the wild, hence that the disappearance of real living species that formerly occupied taxonomists is perversely offset by growing populations of data miners hunting down available names with which to label the infinitude of new phenomena being created in cyberspace.

A human twist on the issue of survival and extinction in dataspace is presented by Rob Lycett's *Portable Memorial Meme Pool [Interval]*, which he describes as a book of souls for the internet age.[19] The book lists the 209,444 lapsed domain names for the period 16 May 2000 to 8 May 2001, and visitors to the exhibition where it is displayed are encouraged to highlight individual names as an act of remembrance. Another poignant project designed to offer a public setting for mourning and remembrance that can resonate in our context of globalized and secularized lifestyles is Ulrike Wachtmeister's *Transitions*.[20] The artist proposes to create a physical, networked installation on the artificial island of Pepperholm, a road and rail transportation link between Malmo Island in Sweden and the nearby Danish mainland. The installation consists of a field of solar-driven light poles stretching from the land into the water on the thinnest part of the island, visible from the train and road. By visiting websites built as virtual repositories for their lost ones, internauts trigger the pole-mounted physical lights connected to these sites, creating an uncanny glimmer of pooled recollections watched by travellers who may be the internauts themselves, using hand-held devices, or desk-bound website visitors. Lycett's and Wachtmeister's works raise questions about rituals and shareable affect in the heterotopic networks of increasingly fused 'natural'/virtual worlds, and about processes whereby the experience of communitas might become the memory of communitas, serving as a means of social scansion and structure (Turner, 1982, p. 47).

Bodies Without Organs

Live performance and the skenabiotopes that house it are a key component of the means we humans have built to evolve and survive, proposing models of existence in barely conceivable spaces. Because of its dual anchorage, in the flesh of the human actor and in what Artaud referred to as the virtual reality of theatre,[21] performance shapes and stretches the collective imagination, and the fact that the public shares this experience is crucial: the mass of spectators is enlightened and welded by its collective revelation. By offering life models, the skenabiotope feeds the hoard of possible models that we hang onto jealously like a mental spare wheel, as a means to fire visions of our future evolution. Both dreams and art reactivate our memorized stock of locomotor schemes by incarnating and conveying 'impossible' acts. But whereas dreams remain individual, theatre as a socially networked art offers shareable visions and possibilities for 'intersubjective illumination' (Turner, 1982, p. 27).

There are kinds of live performance that move us by reactivating the buried phylogenetic memory we possess as an evolving species. Acrobats propose projections of living bodies that defy the rules of locomotion that govern the rest of us, heavy earthlings as we are. Their kinetic performance transcends the laborious conquest of our fragile biped status, to remind us of the wings, scales, gills, and other appendices that endowed our evolutionary forebears with very different behaviours. Beyond the staging of forgotten and premonitory biomechanics, the human being's triumph over the constraints of normal existence is vivaciously manifest in the art of jugglers and tumblers, who present in vivo proof of impossible relations to other bodies, conjuring up spectacular instants of space and time where objects display unthinkable behaviours and deride known physical laws. The impossible bodies and gestures of certain species of performers gnawingly reveal strangely déjà vu ways of being. Perhaps this sensation is bound up with our enchanted recognition of the feasibility of acts we had ruled out as impossible yet continue, irresistibly, to dream of, like a haunting kinaesthetic memory.

When you will have made him a body without organs,
then you will have delivered him from all his automatic reactions
and restored him to his true freedom.
Then you will teach him again to dance wrong side out
as in the frenzy of dance halls
and this wrong side out will be his real place. (Artaud, 2004, p. 1654)[22]

The body without organs that spectacularly concludes Artaud's *To Have Done with the Judgement of God* (1948) is without weight and direction, freed from the reflex reactions and spatial references that govern our organ-packed bodies. In its effort to learn to dance anew, this body evokes those of extraterrestrial pioneers, anticipating needs to reinvent expressive gesture in corporeally estranged situations. According to 'sentics' research founded by Manfred Clynes (who with Nathan Kline coined the word 'cyborg' in 1960),[23] centred on emotional communication and gesture, humans deprived of normal means of embodied expression — for example when subjected to long periods of microgravity where the weight of grief, the density of anger or the lightness of elation are no longer felt — experience major shifts in terms of affect and identity. Existential questions abound: is one simply the inhabitant of one's known body, albeit hard to recognize under unfamiliar conditions, or rather of a foreign body, to be invested and appropriated anew? Can recognizable reincarnation be attained through unfamiliar sensory structures? Under such circumstances, can we still be characterized as human? Like Artaud's body without organs, we must learn to dance anew, wrong side out and upside down, to create a new place and identity.[24]

Slovenian director Dragan Zivadinov has launched a theatre project whereby he will 'become empty-bodied'.[25] His *Noordung Prayer Machine* is a fifty-year epic production whose cast of mortals will be progressively replaced by robots, launched in 1995 and scheduled to take place at ten-year intervals until Zivadinov's own death at the final performance in 2045. In 1999, in conjunction with Marko Peljhan's Project Atol Institute,[26] Zivadinov created the *Noordung Zero Gravity Biomechanical Theater*, a performance staged in an Ilyushin-76 MAK aircraft used to train cosmonauts. Six actors before an audience of eight, their costumes and biomechanics choreography inspired by Meyerhold's constructivist works, offset by cabin decorations also reminiscent of constructivism, performed eight 30-second zero-gravity sequences. These were followed by the audience's release from passive observer status to join in the gravity-free action for three further parabolas, creating an experience described by film-maker participant Michael Benson: 'When I flew up to join the spinning, kinetic, angelic cloud of turning, shifting people, there was no question of difference; it was pure shared experience.'[27] Interacting individuals in this spon-

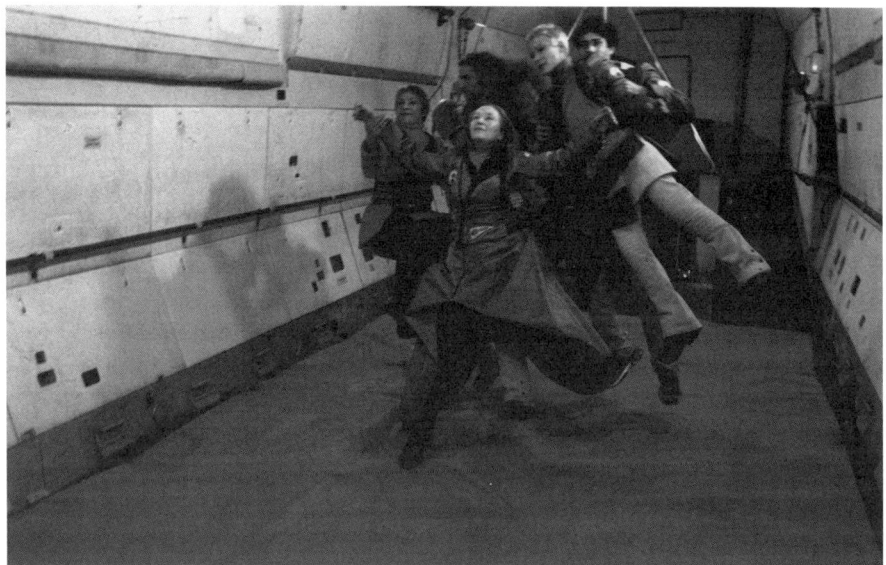

Biomechanics NOORDUNG, Star City, Russia, 1999, attractor Dragan Zivadinov. Reproduced with the permission of Dragan Zivadinov and Dunja Zupančič.

taneous communitas were thus 'totally absorbed into a single synchronised, fluid event' (Turner, supra, n. 4). Despite our having to experience this work by proxy, its traces are brought home to us with epiphanic force, fulfilling one of theatre's essential functions by acting as a mutagen for the collective imagination.

Theatre as an inherently shared form of live art is a unique vector for communicating creative visions of living beings and experiences. The anatomical theatre was a collective viewing place designed to allow biological cut-ups (*ana* – up – *tomia* – cutting) to disclose the mysteries of the human body. By contrast, emerging twenty-first century theatres are spatially and/or temporally bounded venues for staging the peculiar splicings of space, time and personae afforded by hybridized, networked, distributed environments. Like their historical forebears, they offer powerful means for us to reckon and resonate with our new corpora, to map their and our vital signs.

Sally Jane Norman is a cultural theorist/practitioner working on live art and technology; her publications include texts for the French Centre National de la Recherche Scientifique (Laboratoire des arts du spectacle), Ministry of Culture and UNESCO. Docteur d'état (Institut d'études théâtrales, Paris III), co-/organizer of workshops, performances, and seminars exploring human interactions in digital environments at the International Institute of Puppetry (Charleville-Mézières), ZKM (Karlsruhe), STEIM (Amsterdam), Phénix Théâtre (Valenci-ennes), École supérieure de l'image (Angoulême/ Poitiers), IRCAM (Paris); founding member of Telefonica's VIDA Art & Artificial Life competition. Since 2004, she has been director of Culture Lab, an interdisciplinary research labo-ratory at Newcastle University, UK. http://www.ncl.ac.uk/culturelab/people/profile/s.j.norman.

Notes

1   Martin White's research is conducted with a group of professional actors using a full-scale, candle-lit reconstruction of a Jacobean playhouse in Bristol's Wickham The-atre, based on plans by Inigo Jones and realized by stage designer Jennie Norman. Recordings employ high-definition cameras that can operate in very low light levels, for transfer to an interactive, multi-perspective DVD publication. The project is led by Bristol University in collaboration with Ignition Films and Shakespeare's Globe in London. Authored by Caroline Rye, the DVD will include a virtual reality model of the original playhouse, created by a specialist team at the University of Warwick. www.bris.ac.uk/drama/staff_research/martin_white/; www.dartington.ac.uk/drha06/pa-pers/abstract.asp?uid=109.

2   Sophocles, mid-410s BC. *Electra* (Translated by R. C. Jebb), The Internet Classics Archive. Available from: classics.mit.edu/Sophocles/electra.html.

3   Projects by Stromajer and Zorn are documented at www.intima.org/. For *Ballettikka Internettikka 1*, see www.intima.org/bi/bi1/netballet.html.

4   'Individuals who interact with one another in the mode of spontaneous communitas be-come totally absorbed into a single synchronized, fluid event. Their "gut" understanding of synchronicity in these situations opens them to the understanding of such cultural forms (...) as Eucharistic union and the I Ching, which stresses the mutual mystical par-ticipation (...) of all contemporary events (...), if one only had a mechanism to lay hold of the "meaning" underlying their "coincidence"' (Turner, 1982, p. 48).

5   'Patterns of encounter' is an expression borrowed from mediaevalist Tom Pettitt, whose analysis of the dynamics of boundary crossings in social groupings was used by the author in a study of locative media as the site of emergence of new forms of theatre. See Pettitt (2001), and Norman (2006).

6   'New communicative techniques and media may make possible wholly unprecedent-ed genres of cultural performance, making possible new modes of self-understanding' (Turner, 1982, p. 79).

7   Circus-derived features characteristic of such places of spectacle are interlaced with subsequent theatre architectures, as evidenced by the 'Cockpit-in-Court' that graced Whitehall Palace in seventeenth-century England, and was apparently a multiple-use sport and performance facility until James I ordered its conversion from cock fighting to theatre. See Izenour (1977, p. 268).

8   See Catts and Zurr (2002, 2006).

9   *MEART*, documented at www.fishandchips.uwa.edu.au/project/collaborators.html, was partly inspired by chimera-based prosthetics research by Sandro Mussa-Ivaldi's Robotics Lab at the Sensory Motor Performance Programme, Northwestern Uni-

versity, Chicago, which in 2000 built a cyborg by connecting a lamprey's brain and part of its spinal cord to robot-mounted light sensors driving the disembodied brain's vestibular system, electrical impulses that would normally move along nerves to the lamprey's muscles being sent instead along a second set of wires to the robot's wheels. (sulu.smpp.northwestern.edu/robotlab/). Mussa-Ivaldi's work in turn recalls K.W. Jeters's novel *Noir* (1998), whose protagonist McNihil enforces intellectual property rights in a future where capital punishment is an insufficient deterrent for intellectual property theft which is a capital crime. In retaliation, enforcers capture culprits and extract their living brain and nervous system, which they embed into life-support systems, packaged as self-aware, natural intelligence components in everyday consumer items offered to slighted authors. Thieves who forfeit their intellect and suffer eternal hell as unspeaking wires thus form an odd science fiction parallel with anatomical theatre criminals subjected to twofold punishment, by execution and by subsequent dissection. Bojana Kunst usefully flagged this novel through work made generously available on the Internet.

10   'In the context of our project, the bioreactor should be treated as an art object and not a mere tool. Conceptually a bioreactor (in conjunction with the semi-living sculptures growing inside it) represents an artificial 'life-giving' and maintaining force' (Catts and Zurr, 2001, p. 369).

11   Workshops organized by SymbioticA, Critical Art Ensemble (www.critical-art.net/biotech/index.html), and Natalie Jeremijienko (visarts.ucsd.edu/node/view/491/31) provide contexts where lay persons can experience vitally hands-on, phenomenological rather than purely conceptual engagement with biotechnologies, obtaining the deeper understanding that is a prerequisite to broader, better informed social and ethical debate about these determinant new forces. The fact that such awareness-raising efforts are politically controversial is highlighted by the court case brought to bear against Critical Art Ensemble member Steve Kurtz, arrested by the FBI for conducting college-level type biotechnology experiments (www.caedefensefund.org/).

12   Introduced in *Playing and Reality* (1971), Winnicott's concept designates objects that polarize high levels of affective engagement and play a major role in infant development (blanket, teddy bear, etc.), symbolizing and facilitating the child's gradual distinction of the 'me' from the 'not-me' and thereby easing inevitable separation from the mother. The term is more loosely used here to designate the similarly intermediate status of phenomena that are life-like and/or invested with relics of living beings, which exude a powerful affective sway over their audiences in many ritual/theatre contexts.

13   Relations between these roles and the emergence of avatars in cyberspace are discussed in Norman (1996, 1995).

14   Kantor's *Theatre of Death* manifesto, first published in Poland in 1975, features in numerous publications and languages including Huxley and Witts (1996).

15   For a study of Kantor's repetitive structures and their theatrical effects, see Norman (1993).

16   Skenabiotopes include an array of performance arenas that favour the emergence of new protagonists and particularly of hybrid species: race courses where machines ride animals (e.g. robot jockeys now used to replace children in camel races in the Middle East), and extreme sports stadiums where humans ride and pilot machines (e.g. all terrain motorbike and heavy vehicle trials) are examples firmly entrenched in the public imagination, which are giving rise to new notions of humachine partnerships and experiences. Other kinds of skenabiotopes, including zoos, aquariums

and herbariums of various kinds, stage natural phenomena in ways that highlight their singularity. Artist Phil Ross designs and constructs controlled environmental spaces in which he transforms and refines sculptural artifacts as one might train the growth of Bonsai trees, or frames what he labels 'natural readymades'. See www.phil-ross.org.

17 Because evolution may occur in media other than our 'natural' environment, Ray's Tierra C source code was created to build a virtual computer and Darwinian operating system, which ensures that executable machine codes are evolvable. The system provides control for factors that affect the course of evolution (mutation rates, disturbances, allocation of CPU time to each creature, size of the soup, etc.), and an observational system to record births and deaths, sequence each creature's code, and maintain a gene bank of successful genomes. The operating system also allows recording of the kinds of interactions taking place between creatures. Communities that have emerged from this system have been used to experimentally examine ecological and evolutionary processes. See www.his.atr.jp/~ray/tierra/.

18 The website on which this project was located has (appropriately?) disappeared from the internet; a description by the 2001 Vida Art & Artificial Life Competition jury, which included the author, can be found at www.fundacion.telefonica.com/at/vida/paginas/v4/enovus.html. Ongoing projects by the collective can be consulted at www.transnationaltemps.net/.

19 See www.re-draw.org/-/artworks.html.

20 For a full description, see www.fusedspace.org/.

21 'All true alchemists know that the alchemical symbol is a mirage just as theatre is a mirage. And this perpetual allusion to the things and principle of theatre found in almost all alchemical books must be understood as the sense (of which alchemists were extremely aware) of identity between the plane on which evolve characters, objects, images, and more generally speaking all that constitutes the virtual reality of theatre, and the purely supposed and illusory plane on which the symbols of alchemy evolve.' Artaud (1964), p.75 (Artaud's emphasis).

22 The quoted version is Helen Weaver's excellent translation published in Artaud (1988), which however cannot render the spatial ambivalence conveyed by the French original. In the French text, reproduced below, the expression 'à l'envers' translates equally as wrong side out, wrong way round, backwards or back to front, or upside down; 'véritable endroit' plays on the term 'à l'endroit', meaning right way up or right way round.
Lorsque vous lui aurez fait un corps sans organes,
alors vous l'aurez délivré de tous ses automatismes et rendu à sa véritable liberté
Alors vous lui réapprendrez à danser à l'envers
Comme dans le délire des bals musette
Et cet envers sera son véritable endroit

23 See Clynes and Kline (1960).

24 Corporeal exploration of unusual physical spaces through acrobatics and microgravity experiments is set in the context of cyborg conceptualization in Norman (2002).

25 D. Zivadinov (not dated). The artist's activities are set in context as developments of the Slovenian artists' collective 'Neue Slowenische Kunst' (NSK) by Arns (1996). The participant and filmmaker Michael Benson provides an account of the zero gravity performance (1999).

26 For a discussion of links between Zivadinov's and Peljhan's works, see Brian Holmes (2006).

27 Benson (1999). The shared euphoria experienced in zero gravity is increasingly related by a community that is steadily widening beyond initially exclusively military and scientific participants in zero-gravity flights. Yet unlike such artists as Zivadinov, Peljhan and French pioneer Kitsou Dubois, whose forays have contributed inspiring legacies to the broader community, many cultural actors recently engaged on parabolic flights seem sadly unable to significantly translate their experience for non-initiates.

References

Arns, I., 'Mobile States| Shifting Borders | Moving Entities: The Slovenian Artists' Collective Neue Slowenische Kunst (NSK)', 1996. www.projects.v2.nl/~arns/Texts/NSK/finale.htm.

Artaud, A., *Le théâtre et son double*. Paris, 1964.

Artaud, A., *Selected Writings*. (Edited and with an introduction by Susan Sontag, translated from the French by Helen Weaver.) Berkeley and Los Angeles, 1988.

Artaud, A., *Oeuvres*. Paris, 2004.

Bec, L., 'Skénabiotope. Etude des comportements modélisés et pamphlétaires d'organismes artificiels'. In: Arnaud Labelle-Rojoux (ed.), *L'Art en scènes*. pp. 115-126. Bois-le-Roi, 1992.

Benson, M., 'Noordung Zero Gravity Biomechanical Theatre'. 1999. www.nsk-state.com/noordung/noordung-benson.php.

Catts, O. and I. Zurr, 'Growing Semi-Living Sculptures: The Tissue Culture & Art Project'. In: *Leonardo*, 35, pp. 365-370. 2002. www.leonardo.info/isast/articles/catts.zurr.pdf.

Catts, O. and I. Zurr, 'Towards a New Class of Being: the Extended Body'. In: P. Lichty (ed.), *Intelligent Agent*, Vol. 6, No. 2 (2006). New York. www.intelligentagent.com.

Clynes, M. and N. Kline, 'Cyborgs and Space'. Reprinted in C. Gray (ed.), 1995. *The Cyborg Handbook*, pp. 29-34. New York, 1960.

Darkowska-Nidzgorski, O. and D. Nidzgorski, *Marionnettes et masques au cœur du théâtre africain*. Saint-Maur, 1998.

Holmes, B., 'Coded Utopia'. In: *Mute*, www.metamute.org/en/node/7069. 2006.

Huxley, M. and J. Witts (eds), *The Twentieth Century Performance Reader*. London, 1996.

Izenour, G., *Theater Design*. New York, 1977.

Jeter, K.W., *Noir*. New York, 1998.

Kantor, T., 'Théâtre de la mort'. In: T. Kantor, *Le théâtre de la mort*. Texts grouped and presented by D. Bablet, pp. 215-224. Lausanne, 1977.

Kantor, T., 'The Theatre of Death'. In: T. Kantor, No. 2, *Cricot 2 and The Theatre of Death*, Exeter Digital Archives of performance practice, Theatre Papers

Archive (TAP). 1979-80. See www.spa.ex.ac.uk/drama/research/exeter-digitalarchives/tpcatalogue.html.

McGowan, M., *L'Art du ballet de cour en France (1581-1643)*. Paris, 1963.

Norman, S.J., 'Rondes et parades. Répliques et répétitions'. In: D. Bablet (ed.), *T. Kantor (2)*, pp. 224-237. Paris, 1993.

Norman, S.J., 'L'Art des marionnettes/ The Art of Puppets'. In: *Actes d'IMAGINA*, Bry-sur-Marne, 1995.

Norman, S.J., 'Dramatis Personae'. In: *Fifth International Conference on Cyberspace*, Telefonica Foundation. Madrid, 1996. Available at www.fundacion.telefonica.com/at/enorman.html.

Norman, S.J., 'Leap of Faith'. In: D. Canogar, *Zero Gravity*. Barcelona, 2002.

Norman, S.J., 'Locative Media and Instantiations of Theatrical Boundaries.' In: *Leonardo Electronic Almanach* 14, 2006. www.leoalmanac.org/journal/vol_14/lea_v14_no3-04/sjnorman.asp.

Pettitt, T., 'The Morphology of the Parade', paper delivered to the 10th Triennial Colloquium of the Société internationale pour l'étude du théâtre médiéval, 2001. Available from www.let.rug.nl/~sitm/pettitt.htm.

Sophocles, *Electra* (Translated by R. C. Jebb.), mid 410s BC. Available from The Internet Classics Archive: classics.mit.edu/Sophocles/electra.html.

Tillis, S., *Towards an Aesthetics of the Puppet: Puppetry as a Theatrical Art*. Westport, 1992.

Turner, V., *From Ritual to Theatre. The Human Seriousness of Play*. New York, 1982.

Winnicott, D.W., *Playing and Reality*. London, 1971.

Zivadinov, D. 'Das Problem der Befahrung des Weltraums. Empty-Bodied Directing'. (not dated) www.nskstate.com/noordung/dragan-empty.php.

Zivadinov, D. 'Zero Gravity Biomechanical Theater'. 1999. www.orbit.zkm.de/?q=node/271.

Performance Documentation 7:
Crash

In anticipation of *Crash*, performed by the Belgium group CREW, I am sitting in the foyer of the Rotterdamse Schouwburg. I am being welcomed, along with three other visitors – each *Crash* performance is for a maximum of four visitors – and my personal *Crash* buddy leads me to an individual 'cell'. She starts to dress me up, putting a helmet-like construction with video goggles and headphones on my head and hanging a bag in front of my belly. Then she buckles me onto an upright table, all the while giving me instructions. Attached to countless cables, I am completely wired.

CREW makes use of new technologies, like virtual reality. In *Crash* the visitor is immersed in another world through a VR-helmet. The performance is

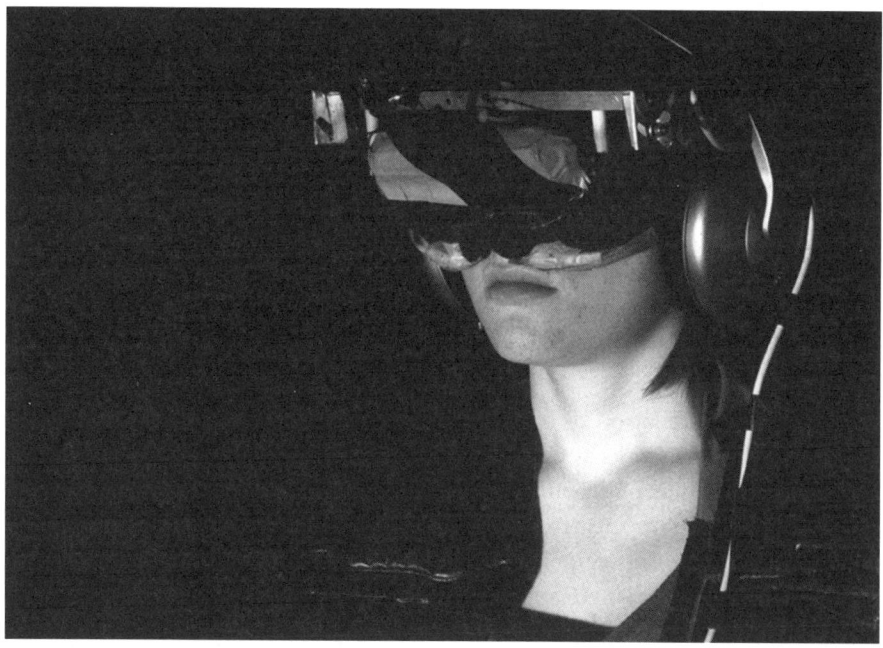

Immersant with video goggles and headphones. Reproduced with permission of Eric Joris.

not something happening in front of him/her, instead, s/he is invited to imagine a world created through projections onto the goggles, and through texts, sounds, and tactile experiences. The images s/he perceives are a combination of prerecorded and live images. The visitor is immersed in VR, and sees his/her own body as well. The live, real-time images are recorded by five tiny cameras attached to the visitor's helmet, and are then mixed with the prerecorded material, and transmitted to the goggles. Fiction and reality merge into an imaginary theatrical universe, and it is no longer possible to distinguish between VR and the actual world. The visitor is temporarily deprived not only of his/her usual sight, but of his/her sense of hearing as well. Through headphones, music and sounds penetrate the visitor's ears, acoustically disconnecting him/her from the here and now. As a consequence, the visitor feels completely isolated from the real world, and reality is replaced by the world evoked by CREW.

In this imaginary world I see projections of myself being driven around, and simultaneously the buddy moves the table I lean against. I *feel* that I am actually moving, while in fact I stay immobile. Because different senses are being addressed simultaneously, I get a remarkably realistic, almost uncanny, experience. The effect is amazing and disturbing at the same time – I find myself in constant sensory confusion, and I lose every sense of where I actually am. At a certain point in the performance, my buddy lowers the table, bringing my body into a horizontal position. The jolting table suggests a wheeled or hospital bed. I enter a room where someone is laid on an operating table. I am being pushed forward to the scene and forced to look at the naked, seemingly dead body. To my dismay, I see myself approaching the operating table, until my body coincides with the body laid on it. Through the mixing of live images of myself and prerecorded material, I become the body on the operating table. A finger is picking the abdominal wall, the skin comes off, and something – possibly an organ – is removed. After this dissection, my journey through the imaginary building continues. Finally, there is an open window, bright light radiating from it. I am pushed out of it and swung back into reality.

CREW is a constellation of artists and scientists within which Eric Joris is a key figure. CREW works at the intersection of live art and technology. Exploring the relationships between reality and fiction, man and technology, and the role of technology in theatre, their artistic outcomes often question and undermine seemingly self-evident assumptions about performance: 'CREW uses technology not only as an inventive scenography but as a main theme and starting point. High-tech theatre, not as shallow entertainment, but as a reflexive strategy' (CREW website).

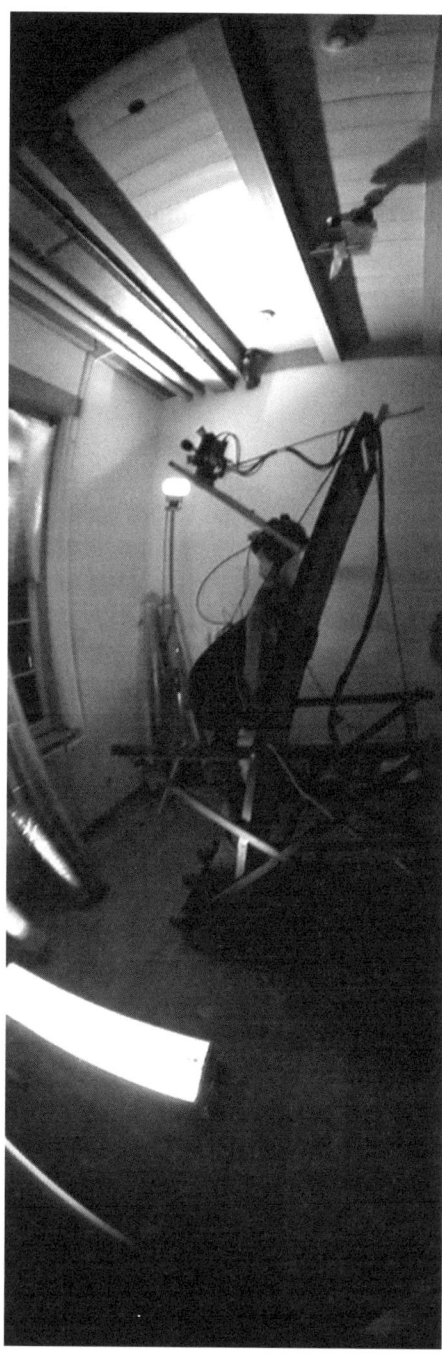

Immersant buckled onto an upright table that can be lowered. Reproduced with permission of Eric Joris.

In *Crash* the use of newly developed technologies leads to a redefinition of the theatrical situation. The performance is not a spectacle with a spectator, sitting safely in the dark, watching people perform for him/her. Rather, *Crash* is about an individual experience realized in the visitor's imagination and body. To quote Joris:

> The intention with *Crash* is to position people in another body (...) by working with new technologies. Usually, a theatre performance is a spectacle at which the spectator watches. We try to fulfil the idea of theatre in one's head: we want theatre happening in the spectators' heads. (Joris quoted in Rummens, my translation)

Crash draws attention to the historical anatomical theatre in several ways. Very explicitly, the dissecting scene revives the theatre wherein dead bodies were cut open in order to investigate the human physical interior. It also functions as a reference to famous representations of such sites and scenes. The finger picking the abdominal wall of a body stretched on an operating or dissecting table, with a few onlookers on the side, brings to mind Rembrandt's *The Anatomy Lesson of Dr Nicolaes Tulp*. More importantly, the theatre of CREW can be considered a return to the anatomical theatre – a place for artists and scientists to collaborate, and a theatrical space where (living) bodies look at (dead) bodies. However, whereas in the Renaissance anatomical theatre the watching itself was the case, *Crash* problematizes the distinction between the body seeing and bodies being seen. It is impossible to distinguish between them, because the visitor is at once spectator and performer. CREW evokes an experience in the visitor through a combination of visual, acoustic and tactile stimuli. Instead of looking at a body being dissected on stage, the visitor is brought into the position of that body him/herself. This transition occurs literally when the visitor in the imaginary world becomes the body on the operating table. *Crash* is an anatomical theatre without spectators. CREW creates an anatomical theatre of experience, CREW's collaborators being the anatomists subjecting the body to all kinds of sensory experiences. Just as anatomical dissection dismembers a body in order to produce a 'body of knowledge' (which replaces the original body), *Crash* frays sensory experience, utilizing its various sensory strands to create a world of experience within the visitor.

Text by *Fleur Bokhoven*

Fleur Bokhoven is currently finishing her RMA in Art Studies with a major in Theatre Studies at the University of Amsterdam.

Performance Data

Crash is a co-production of CREW vzw, Het Toneelhuis and Productiehuis Rotterdam (Rotterdamse Schouwburg). *Crash* premiered in 2004 in Het Toneelhuis in Antwerp, Belgium.
With: Kevin Janssens, Bert Haelvoet and Kristien de Proost
Buddies: Ellen Bernaerts, Celia Bogaert, Kristof Coenen, Uwamungu Cornelis, Bert Geets, Ellen Schoeters, Michel van Looveren, Karl van Welden, Ronald Verhaegen and Tinne Verhaert
Text: Peter Verhelst
Direction: Eric Joris
Concept: Eric Joris in collaboration with Peter Verhelst
Conceptual advice: Kurt Vanhoutte
Scenography: Martin Baarda
Dramaturgy: Griet op de Beeck in collaboration with David Cornille
Sound design: Christoph de Boeck
Technological research and development: Philippe Bekaert in collaboration with Tom de Weyer, Erik Hubo, Tom Mertens and Frank van Reeth

References

Rummens, T., 'Crash. Eric Joris en Peter Verhelst, achter je netvlies'. In: Syllabus compiled by CREW, unpublished.

CREW, www.crewonline.org. Accessed on September 2, 2007.

Restaging the Monstrous

Bojana Kunst

Introduction

The introductory story is old, it belongs to the turn of the sixteenth into the seventeenth century, with two anatomists as its protagonists. Both had an object of anatomical interest: hermaphrodites, wondrous beings combining two sexes in one body, often depicted in popular imagination as hairy masculine women or male warriors with satin skin. Both lived in France. The first was Realdo Colombo (writing c. 1550), anatomy practitioner and doctor; the other, also a (highly acclaimed) doctor, named Jean Riolan (writing c. 1614). Colombo described hermaphrodites as the most miraculous of human anatomical specimens because they combined the feminine and the masculine in a single body. He praised their complexity and originality, their ontological exclusiveness, and saw them as examples of nature's creativity. According to him, the excessive originality of their monstrous appearance demonstrated the wondrous creative side of nature. Jean Riolan, on the other hand, half a century later was highly critical towards such descriptions and cynical regarding the scientific authority of Colombo. Riolan found hermaphrodites to be not only disgusting, but unworthy of serious scientific attention: they should be forbidden as objects of research.[1]

Both authors are academic anatomists, writing in similar traditions of natural philosophy. Yet their quarrel is not simply a disagreement about scientific accuracy. Riolan thought hermaphrodites should be forbidden objects of scientific research because of their transgressive nature. In his view the coexistence of both sexes in one body is not possible. Hermaphrodites, he argues, are nothing but deformed women, who can, should they ever 'take advantage of their sex', be accused of 'scandalous crimes'. Monsters of all kinds are nothing but 'a perversion of the order of natural things, people's health and King's authority' (Daston and Park, 1998, p. 203). The problem, therefore, is not simply that Colombo's scientific conclusions are wrong but that he was already mistaken in what he chose to research. Whereas Colombo's observations on hermaphrodites — praising their ontological complexity — imply an understanding of the monstrous as primarily a sign of the originality and creativity of nature (disclosing the generative excess of nature in the given order of the macrocosm), Riolan excludes the monstrous from the possibility of being a proper object of scientific observation. Their existence has no ontological basis. The monstrous thus becomes a kind of *quasi object* — an object pretending to be something it is not, requiring scientific observation to put it in its proper place, regulating it by pointing out that it is not what it seems.

On a micro-scale, this story reveals the status of the monstrous in early modern science. Riolan, accusing the hermaphrodite of 'scandalous crimes', turns the monstrous into a perversion of the natural order of things, as well as a perversion of authority. In his vision, the monstrous represents a site of potential disruption of the political order of society. From having been an object of scientific attention, the monstrous (pretending to be something it is not and with its excessive presence disturbing the given order of things) now becomes a player on the political stage.

I would like to uncover the consequences of this change in the status of the monstrous and connect those consequences to the present situation. I am particularly interested in the moment of the temporary visibility of the monstrous during the Baroque era, when the foundation is laid for the ways in which the monstrous will be regulated in early modern science and politics. In the Baroque, the monstrous (exhibited during that period in many museums of curiosities, private collections, etc.) was not only a kind of 'entertainment' for the sceptical mind, but also a topos for the temporary visibility of connections between man and animal, human and non-human, natural and artificial. Following Bruno Latour's arguments, I will show how this visibility of connections quickly became subject to different regimes of representation. To be more precise, I will argue that it is exactly the regulation of the monstrous — the attempt to make the monstrous invisible — which enabled the continuous production of hybridity in the scientific 'black box' as well as in political procedures. The appearance and disappearance of the monstrous, therefore, are somehow two sides of the same coin: the monstrous *theatrum mundi* was a kind of spectacular prelude to early modern science and politics. I am interested in the staging of such connections: how disclosing fluid connections between what is (supposedly) divided also allows irregularities and connections to be regulated, making possible the division between human and non-human. Today, confronted with hybrid connections between nature and culture, it is interesting to observe how the connections are once again becoming visible, and to question what are the similarities and differences from the Baroque disclosure of the monstrous. Following Agamben's analysis of the anthropological machine, I would like to show that despite the omnipresent visibility of connections, we are still not done with the mystery of separation. Today, the potentiality of the generative potential of the monstrous is at the core of such a separation, or to put it differently: the generative potential of the monstrous is being subjected to contemporary economic and political power.

Domestication

With the objective and rational approach towards nature, with the 'sweeping of the irregular under rules' (Canguilhem, 2004) during modernity, everything monstrous is not only excluded from positive scientific observation of the physical world, but also put on the stage (anatomical, political, scientific). The significance of the monstrous is no longer a matter of metaphysics, with its cause connected to the irregularities of creation, to the accidents of nature that are always in complex relation to the work of the Creator. Instead, the significance of the monstrous shifts to a different territory, and represents a threat to authority and to the natural order of things. Its pretentious, tricky nature needs to be emphasized to an audience eagerly searching for new ways of defining the political order of living beings and things.

The Baroque, then, was the era grounding this shift, the period when the monstrous was visible everywhere (in cabinets of curiosities, gardens, anatomical theatres, private collections). Its visibility was brief, the monstrous was common only for a moment. At the end of the seventeenth century, monstrous imagination was already becoming generally ridiculed and despised.[2] The monstrous was a kind of a public thing in the Baroque era, because revealing the monstrosity endemic to the field of the in-between (between man and animal, natural and artificial, man and woman, etc.) enabled early modern procedures of establishing humanness. It was a kind of spectacular entertainment, through which the procedures of recognizing what is human were disclosed, and the divisions between different regimes of representation were established. Within the temporary visibility of the monstrous, we can observe a change in its understanding, moving in two directions. On the one hand, the monstrous is becoming instrumental and invisible (in the sense that it becomes an object in a laboratory): a functional object of science. On the other hand, the monstrous is restaged on the political stage: due to its tricky and pretentious nature, it is endangering a political order. As a result, all future explanations of its nature will lead to attempted domestication.

This restaging of the fundamental nature of the monstrous occurs in the middle of the processes establishing the modern regimes of representation; the processes that install the division between different territories of knowledge and power, where the division between science and politics has a decisive role.[3]

The monstrous becomes a public object because it has a special function in the sphere of politics: its role is connected to establishing the political division between the human and non-human, where domestication, civilization and culturalization of the monstrous will play a decisive role. As Park and Daston said, 'monsters interested the anatomists not because of their rarity or singularity and the concomitant wonder evoked by nature's sports, but because they revealed still more encompassing and rigid regularities' (Daston and Park, 1998, p. 205).

Staging the monstrous coincides with the ways in which in our modern world 'the representation of things through the intermediary of the laboratory is forever dissociated from the representation of citizens through the intermediary of the social contract' (Daston and Park, 1998, p. 27). These divided regimes of representations are, as Latour writes, in a very special relationship throughout the modern era: 'the more we forbid ourselves to conceive of hybrids, the more possible their interbreeding becomes' (Daston and Park, 1998, p. 12). Or, to rephrase: precisely at the moment when the monstrous appeared and disclosed the complexity of the connections between man and animal, men and women, artificial and natural, it was also emptied of its transgressive content. Monsters not only lost their metaphysical function and purpose, they became *instrumental*. When shown in public, when visible, the monstrous body becomes a theatrical one, associated with make-believe, imitation, transgression as its main (anatomical) characteristics: an obscene trick. Politically, monstrous bodies serve the purpose of demonstrating what is and is not 'human'.

In his book *The Open: Man and Animal* (2004), Agamben writes that the privileged position of the human has always been strategically produced and ensured by the 'anthropological machine' of Western thought. 'Homo sapiens, then, is neither a clearly defined species nor a substance, it is, rather, a machine or device for producing the recognition of the human' (Agamben, 2004, p. 26). The monstrous can therefore be understood to be a consequence of a political/ontological apparatus of separation which may disclose to us the difference between human and non-human. In the Baroque the prime example of such a mechanism is an optical machine, constructed of a series of mirrors in which man, looking at himself, sees his own image already deformed. The images could resemble the features of an ape, black Ethiopian, or some other 'monstrous' being.[4] It is not enough to understand these machines as only triggering perception and playfully blurring the line between human and non-human. The huge popularity of such museums can be also linked to their specific function in the understanding of the human (which in this case meant white and western human beings). They were mechanisms for recognition: only when the spectator can see himself as (for example) an animal, he can really define what he is. He has to include what is outside, see himself with an animal face. As Agamben said: 'he has to recognize himself in a non-man in order to be human' (Agamben, 2004, p. 27).

The monstrous becomes the 'ever present possibility to destroy the natural order of authority'[5] not because it is some externalized other which has to be swept into the arms of regulating order, but because it is a constant production of the otherness in the very *human* being, so that the human can recognize and define itself. There is no nature proper to Homo, writes Agamben, thus, 'he is being always less or more than himself' (Agamben, 2004, p. 29). Such recognition can be found as early as the humanist discovery of man. Agamben is quoting humanist philosopher Pico della Mirandola, who wrote that the human being was created without any definite model, without even having a face of his own. The paradox here is that Homo, says Agamben, 'is constitutively nonhuman; he can receive all natures and all faces' (Agamben, 2004, p. 30). Monsters therefore remind us of the fact that the lines of separation have always been inside the human being, that instead of the mystery of conjunction we have to 'deal with the practical and political mystery of separation' (Agamben, 2004, p. 26). Exactly this practical and political mystery of separation is at work in the early modernity, grounding the staging of the monstrous in the political field. The assumed pretension and the tricky nature of the monstrous being are threatening because they point to the instability of the process of separation inside the human being. The caesura inside the human turns out to be visible. The monstrous shows us that the caesura is not between the human and the outside, but it is always internal and shifting: human is constitutively unhuman.

It is no wonder that the main modern political occupation with the monstrous became its domestication and cultivation, evidence of which can be found in the ways in which the other (animal, slave, machine, woman, etc.) is continuously humanized to reflect back the face of 'our' (white, western, and male) own humanity. The main strategy of dealing with the monstrous becomes that of a paternal patronage where the monstrous appears from time to time as an excessive rebellion (the untamed son), an image that still strongly inspires popular and artistic imagination. Moreover, the modern artist himself often took the role of the non-domesticated son, showing artistic imagination to be a safe ground for challenging the fragile borders of humanity via aesthetic means.

After the domestication?

The monstrous, with its hybrid nature and ontological instability, is a recurring topos in postmodern cultural theory. In many cultural and philosophical observations from the 1980s and 1990s (Baudrillard, Kroker, Gibson, Haraway, etc.) dealing with the development of technology, biology and cyberspace, the topos of the monstrous marks the transgressive moment where previously invisible connections between nature and culture become visible and force us to rethink what is human. For it seems that our contemporary experiences are constituted more and more through a subtle matrix of connections, not only those between bodies, but between everything from the non-physical to the most material. The process of domestication of the monstrous seems to be finished. We are living in a time when, to quote Latour, 'heads of state, chemists, biologists, desperate patients and industrialists caught themselves in a single uncertain story mixing biology and society' (Latour, 1993, p. 2). Hybridization between natural and artificial, woman and man, nature and culture seems to have become part of everyday life. It even looks like the appearance of monstrous connections is again opening up the question of the division of territories (politics, science, technology). During the past decades, many distinctions have been reconsidered, and this is surely also one of the characteristics of contemporary artistic projects. Instead of the mystery of separation, it seems we have to deal today with the mystery of conjunction, which has often been praised in postmodern cultural theory.

Hybrid connections between nature and culture force us to rethink the borders between different regimes of representation (like science, politics and art). Contemporary culture is obsessed with connections, that is true. Nevertheless, one might wonder, are we really done with the mystery of separation, when our understanding of humanness is at stake? How then to understand our inability to keep pace with the speed of contemporary production, celebrating the mystery of conjunction with an excessive and hegemonic production of hybrids and monstrous objects? Hybrids may be literally pouring out of the laboratories, but at the same time, it seems, they have even stronger tendencies to divide and separate when it comes to ownership and power over natural and artificial entities. Take, for example, genetically modified corn seed, which pours into the neighbour's field, blown by the wind. Natural causes at work or not, the neighbour will be sued for illegal use of the crops.

Hardt and Negri observe that:

> Today when the social horizon is defined in biopolitical terms, we should not forget those early modern stories of monsters. The monster effect has only multiplied. Teleology now can only be called ignorance and superstition. Scientific method is defined increasingly in the realm of the in-determination and every real entity is produced in an aleatory and singular way, a sudden emergence of the new. Frankenstein is now a member of the family. In this situation then, the discourse of living beings must become a theory of their construction and the possible futures that await them. Immersed in this unstable reality, confronted by the increasing artificiality of the biosphere and the institutionalisation of the social, we have to expect monsters to appear at any moment. (Hardt and Negri, 2004, p. 196)

After the domestication of the monstrous, it is important to know 'how to love some monsters and combat the others' (Hardt and Negri, 2004, p. 196). What kind of 'show' is at work here in this division, in this caesura within the monstrous? When Agamben describes the anthropological machine defining the human (and dividing it from animal), he notices two variants of this machine at work in our culture, two variants which are the two sides of the same performance of division. One side of separation can be described as the inclusion of the outside, the humanizing of the animal, wherein the human recognizes itself in the human. As observed above, its consequence is domestication and cultivation of the monstrous. The anthropological machine is today performing the other side of the performance of division. It doesn't perform separation through the *inclusion of the outside*, where non-man is defined by the humanization of the other (animal, slave, savage being, etc.), but via opposite means. The other side of the machine performs through the *exclusion of the inside*: through isolating the non-human within the human, the non-man is produced inside man, like the contemporary neo-mort or comatose person, that is, the distinction between human and non-human happens within the human body.[6] The contemporary appearance of the monstrous can then be understood as the operation of this other side of the performance of the anthropological machine. It is not the consequence of fluidity and visibility of conjunctions or — if we are talking about the language of disciplines — of crossing, interplaying and disappearance of borders. It is the consequence of isolation of the monstrous inside the human being deeply affecting our understanding of what is a human being today.

Today this type of separation takes the shape of the total management of biological life, the very animality of man, where, writes Agamben, 'genome, global economy and humanitarian ideology are the three united faces of this process' (Agamben, 2004, p. 77). What is at stake is a face without the body, a life that is excluded from life. The early modern monsters reminded us of the empty spot of humanity. The similarities between human beings and monsters were grounded in early modern divisions, placing the human being in the centre of the world. Today monsters remind us of the exclusion of the human from life, of life that is more and more being divided from humanity; of the ways in which 'total humanization of the animal coincides with a total animalization of a man' (Agamben, 2004, p. 77).

Agamben is reflecting on the anthropological machine because he wants to challenge the apparatus established in early modern politics for the recognition of the human, which is also deeply embedded in our contemporary political and human disasters. With the speed and efficiency of contemporary separation, the non-human isolated inside the human is increasingly abandoning the human outside the human. 'And faced with this extreme figure of the human and the inhuman, it is not so much a matter of asking which of the two machines (or the two variants of the same machine) is better or more effective, or rather less lethal or bloody, as it is understanding how they work so that we might eventually be able to stop them' (Agamben, 2004, p. 38).

Potentialities of non-domestication

One of the consequences of this two-sided separation is fear of 'monstrous' deeds of non-domesticated entities, which, paradoxically, strengthens the very process of separation that produces the fear in the first place. We are living in the world where there is no real outside. The monstrous lost its 'location' from whence it could look back at us, restaging our intimate, social and political understanding. 'Today we are confronted with a situation, where, strictly speaking, there is no instance in which the monstrous could have the role of "constitutive outside".'[7] There are no others who could enable the construction of us, because as us, they too are already included (Agamben, 2004, p. 61). One way to describe our contemporary humanized and globalized world is that there is no exclusion. Moreover, exclusion itself has been already excluded, which is not at all to say that exclusion has disappeared.

When thinking about bringing together nature and culture, we have to be very critical towards the operation of separation at work within the production of omnipresent hybridity. We are living in a hybrid world, but nevertheless power is today strongly grounded within, and maintained through, processes of separation. Many zones of exception exist in the present world, like the socially and politically outcast territories and masses of people who are not allowed to move freely in the 'connected' world. Such exclusions are basic to contemporary global political and economic power, based as they are on the endless production/reproduction of the caesurae between life and non-life. Or, take the example of the privatization of natural resources, where the potential for hybridity is issued with a patent belonging to international corporations and secured with the permanent war state. Another example comes from the contemporary media, where imagination and liberating processes are not only fictionalized and transformed into the surplus value of the product, but their ownership is simultaneously increasingly concentrated in big corporations. Or take a case from the more intimate, micro-level, for instance life and death decisions about prolonging the existence of persons in severe comas that are being more and more left to politics. Another example comes from the management of our biological life, which is becoming a transparent imprint for identification and surveillance purposes. In all these cases, we can observe operations of separation in which life is somehow excluded from itself.

Contemporary power structures strongly regulate the generative potential of the monstrous, its enormous creative potential, its potentiality to reproduce and mutate, to create different forms of life, different perceptions and understandings of life. This generative potential is currently at the centre of the scientific, economic and military interests. On one side it is separated from life itself and given to the laboratories. On the other it is separated from life itself and given market value. What made this taking over of the generative potential of the monstrous possible is the operation of excluding the inside. The double-sided machine of separation functions by establishing a zone of indifference at its centre, which, as Agamben says, is 'perfectly empty and the truly human being who should occur there is only the place of a ceaselessly updated decision in which the caesurae and their re-articulation are always dislocated and updated anew' (Agamben, 2004, p. 38). With this operation, more and more zones of exception are produced, enabling continuous shifting between life and death according to the pragmatic needs of capital in the production of contemporary hybrids. How then would it be possible to conceive of the monstrous outside the operation of separation, and what would be the stage whereon the new processes could be heard and seen?

If we understand the monstrous as a primary topos of hybridity, we can conclude that there is a certain tension at work today among the omnipresent production of hybridity and the very productiveness (the generative potential) of hybridity. We are living in a hybrid world, but at the same time the generative potential of hybridity is regulated all the time, separated out, subject to surveillance, and controlled. In a world where imagination, processes of liberation and thinking about the future are already fictionalized and transformed into the surplus value of spectacle, it is hard to generate processes, things, relationships, emotions, hopes, imaginations and desires differently. In such a world, it is difficult to think outside the anthropological machine precisely because the very productivity of hybridity, the generative potential of the monstrous, is so ruthlessly exploited and separated from the world. In this situation of radical contingency, where the generative powers of language and imagination of the future no longer belong to us, it has become even more difficult to ask the question about potentiality. How to act once again in the open, how to provide our actions, work and generative thinking once again with the potentiality of the monstrous future?

Hardt and Negri find the answer to this question in the 'monstrous expressions of the multitude to challenge the mutations of the artificial life transformed into the commodities, the capitalist power to put up for sale the metamorphoses of nature, the new eugenic that support the ruling power' (Hardt and Negri, 2004, p. 196). They understand the multitude as a kind of generative force, materializing the very potential of hybridity to open up possibilities for a different world, where humans belong without any representable condition of co-belonging. Monstrous expression would be in this sense the possibility of that which Agamben describes as what is most threatening for the state, a 'whatever without an identity' (Agamben, 2001, p. 86). Latour also tries to rethink hybridity, arguing for a return to things. 'Are we then going to slow down, reorient, and regulate the proliferation of monsters by representing their existence officially? Will a different democracy become necessary? A democracy extended to things?' (Latour, 1993, p. 12). The monstrous is here being restaged in the sense that it is provided (again?) with generative potential; it gets a language to speak, a possibility to be represented.

What is interesting from the perspective of our question — how the monstrous is being restaged today — is the way in which processes of change are described: what exactly are the material qualities of these processes? In Hardt and Negri we are dealing with the murmur of swarms, with the innumerable qualities that we cannot rely on counting any more. These are the processes of bubbling, growing and intensifying, whose power is similar to the tension of bending the law. It is a potentiality of different sensory orientations and qualities, of hearing and seeing, of languages, which can disclose a life without any representable condition of belonging. Latour, on the other hand, writes about representation through slowing down and reorienting, about the processes of waiting, about decelerating. In both cases generative processes of monstrosity open up the potential for conjunction, which is not so much about new beings and things, as about beings without origins. Their descriptions demand that we take into account the processes of life. The topos of the monstrous points to the ways in which we sense and experience the process of life: in life itself there is a potentiality, a generative potentiality that opens towards the future.

Then there is the question regarding how theatre might contribute to disclosing the generative potentiality of the monstrous while at the same time avoiding becoming an empty spectacle. It is true that the linguistic nature of contemporary spectacle is somehow taking language away from us, but it is also true, to quote Agamben, that in 'the spectacle our own linguistic nature comes back to us inverted. (...) This is why the violence of spectacle is so destructive; but for the same reason the spectacle retains something like a positive possibility that can be used against it' (Agamben, 2001, p. 80). What needs to be stressed is that, unfortunately, questions about life and death are today being uttered on a different (closed) stage, which has no visibility and where unfortunately there is no space for representation. The divisions between life and death, human and non-human are being produced by expelling the human outside of the human and leaving the inert life to the mercy of the contemporary flaws of political and corporative ownership. Here, there are no cognitive and aesthetical relationships between stage and audience at work, there is no (public) place offered for the observer, no possibility to return the gaze, and no possibility of being heard in many directions. To restage the monstrous today therefore means resistance to such operations of separation and closure. There is a strong need at this moment for a place to show the monstrous, for a place to open up the material qualities of the monstrous and disclose it in public. The processes of conjunction have to be brought to light with all their potentiality. The conjunctions and hybridity have to be brought to visibility and representation to resist separation and exclusion, and to disclose the mechanisms of contemporary understanding of human. In this way the positive possibility of anatomical spectacle is used against its own spectacular nature, and the dense fluidity and inventive time of life can begin to act.

Bojana Kunst is a philosopher and performance theorist working at the University of Ljubljana, Faculty of the Arts – Department of Sociology. She is a member of the editorial board of Maska. Her articles have appeared in numerous journals, and she has taught and lectured extensively in Europe. She has published three books, among which are *Impossible Body* (Ljubljana, 1999) and *Dangerous Connections* (Ljubljana, 2004). She is also a dramaturge and leads the International Seminar for Performing Arts in Ljubljana.

Notes

1   The story is taken from Daston and Park, 1998.
2   In England there was a strong resistance to the poetry of John Donne due to its unusual analogies. French Enlightenment thinkers like Jean-Francois Marmontel or Chevalier de Jaucourt were also condemning the strange similarities and monstrous images in art as a sign of disturbed artistic imagination. See Coleman, 1971.
3   The discussion between Robert Boyle and Thomas Hobbes in the middle of the seventeenth century is a clear example of that division. The main hero of the discussion is an air pump. Even if Boyle and Hobbes agree with basic political principles – they both want a king, a Parliament and unified Church– their opinions diverge as to what can be expected from experimentation and scientific reasoning. As Bruno Latour writes, Boyle is not simply creating a scientific discourse while Hobbes is doing the same thing for politics. 'Boyle is creating a political discourse from which politics is to be excluded, while Hobbes is imagining a scientific politics from which experimental science has to be excluded' (Latour, 1993, p. 27).
4   Many of these optical machines can be found in one of the most popular seventeenth-century museums, *Musaeum Kircherianum*, founded by Athanasius Kircher (1602-80). In the catalogue of that museum, published in 1678 by its secretary, we can find several optical machines that were changing the spectators into monsters and animals. In another popular museum from that time, owned by Manfredo Settala, we can find a

mirror in which the spectator could see himself with the black skin of the Ethiopian. Many such examples can be found in Hanafi, 2000.

5   Riolan, quoted in Daston and Park, 1998, p. 203.

6   This is the concept of homo alalus, the ape-man, a concept that was formed by Ernest Haeckel in 1899. 'And it is enough to move our field of research ahead a few decades, and instead of this innocuous paleontological find we will have the Jew, the non-man produced inside the man, the neomort and overcomatose person, that is the animal separated within the human body itself' (Agamben, 2004, p. 37).

7   Šumič-Riha, J., 'Kako drugačen je drugi v politiki?' ('How other is the Other in politics?'). In: *Problemi*, 35, no. 1-2, pp. 61-80, 1999.

References

Agamben, G., *The Open: Man and Animal*. Stanford, 2004.

Agamben, G., *The Coming Community*. Minneapolis, 2001.

Canguilhem, G., 'Monstruosity and the Monstrous'. In: M. Fraser and M. Greco (eds), *The Body: A Reader*. New York and London, 2004.

Coleman, F. J., *The Aesthetic Thought of the French Enlightenment*. Pittsburgh, 1971.

Daston, L. and K. Park, *Wonders and the Order of Nature, 1150 – 1750*. New York, 1998.

Hanafi, Z., *The Monster in the Machine, Magic, Medicine, and the Marvellous in the Time of the Scientific Revolution*. Durkham and London, 2000.

Hardt, M. and A. Negri, *Multitude: War and Democracy in the Age of Empire*. New York, 2004.

Latour, B., *We Have Never Been Modern*. Cambridge, Massachusetts, 1993.

Šumič-Riha, J., 'Kako drugačen je drugi v politiki?' ('How other is the Other in politics?'). In: *Problemi*, 35, no. 1-2, pp. 61-80, 1999.

Delirium of the Flesh: 'All the Dead Voices' in the Space of the Now

Michal Kobialka

> Estragon: All the dead voices.
> Vladimir: They make a noise like wings.
> Estragon: Like leaves.
> Vladimir: Like sand.
> Estragon: Like leaves.
>   (Silence)
> Vladimir: They all speak at once.
> Estragon: Each one to itself.
>   (Silence)
> Vladimir: Rather they whisper.
> Estragon: They rustle.
> Vladimir: They murmur.
> Estragon: They rustle.
>   (Silence)
> Vladimir: What do they say?
> Estragon: They talk about their lives.
> Vladimir: To have lived is not enough for them.
> Estragon: They have to talk about it.
> Vladimir: To be dead is not enough for them.
> Estragon: It is not sufficient.
>   (Silence)
> Vladimir: They make a noise like feathers.
> Estragon: Like leaves.
> Vladimir: Like ashes.
> Estragon: Like leaves.
> (Beckett, *Waiting for Godot*, 1954, p. 40)

In the celebrated *The Body Emblazoned* (1995), Jonathan Sawday places the dead body at the centre of enquiry into the Renaissance culture of dissection. The abstract idea of theological knowledge about the body (*Hoc est corpus meum*), which had been given visibility by the dogma of transubstantiation in 1215,[1] was now under a knife, which cut through a corpse. That which was revealed was assigned a non-theological status as well as a rational, not to say empirical, function. From now on, it will be possible to arrange and rearrange the elements constituting the bodily knowledge, displayed both as a corpse and as a *nomos* on a dissecting table.

Sawday's argument, however, not only draws attention to how what was seen on the table of the Renaissance culture of dissection was constructed rationally and discursively, but also, how the Renaissance culture of dissection divided the bodies (or their parts) into those that mattered or did not matter. At the same time, Sawday's *The Body Emblazoned* marks a shift in the field of Renaissance studies from logocentric towards corporeal investigations. A multitude of volumes and conferences that followed and whose subject-matter is bodies tremulous, bodies single-sexed, bodies enclosed, bodies intestinal, bodies consumed, bodies carnivalized, bodies effeminized, bodies embarrassed, bodies sodomized, bodies castrated, or approximate bodies is an example par excellence of this shift.[2] And there will be many more volumes, since gazing at the images of oneself, plunging our hands into the body or the corpse, or of fondling body parts or the entrails of the dead, manifests the quest for a body whose intelligibility will and can only be established in the process of representing that which can be seen or understood about it.

If a body is a complete and rational object delimited by a particular political and social coding, corporeal investigations, as well as complex ideological structures, what happens when its very materiality — the fidgety 'liveness' of the flesh — or the lack thereof 'disrupts' this coding and its critical prose? What becomes visible or thinkable through the body's being unhoused in being, that is, once it has been freed from concrete knowledge and the nature of the object? What are the consequences of such a shift in the perception of a body for modes of perception as well as for bio-politics, theatre historiography, gender/ethnic identity formation?

This essay is an attempt at addressing some of these issues by thinking about the body and theatre using Tadeusz Kantor's *The Dead Class* and the Old People inhabiting a space which could not be appropriated by the gaze of the spectators; a performance and the dancing body of Marta Becket at the Amargosa Opera House in Death Valley Junction, California; and Samuel Beckett's prematurely old woman with unkempt grey hair moving to and fro accompanied by the mortal silence of her words and the noise of a rocking chair in *Rockaby*.

Let me start with the body emblazoned in the anatomy theatre designed by Inigo Jones in 1636 for the Barber-Surgeons at their premises in Monkwell Street in London. The surviving plans of the theatre show an elliptical structure with a table in the middle surrounded by four concentric elliptical rows. A note, published in 1708, describes the interior of Jones's anatomy theatre in the following manner:

> [the theatre was] fitted up with four degrees of seats of cedar wood, and adorned with the figures of the seven liberal sciences, and the twelve signs of the zodiac. Also containing the skeleton of an ostrich, put up by Dr. Hobbs, 1682, with a bust of King Charles I. Two humane skins on the wood frames, of a man and a woman, an imitation of Adam and Eve, put up in 1645. A mummy skull (...). The skeleton of Atherton with copper joints (...). The figure of a man flead (flayed), where all the muscles appear in due place and proportion, done after the life. The skeleton of Canberry Bess and Country Tom (as they then call them); and three other skeletons of humane bodies. (Quoted in Sawday, 1995, p. 76)

The figures of the seven liberal sciences, twelve signs of the zodiac, the skeleton of an ostrich, the image of Charles I, two human skins on the wooden frames, skeletons of notorious criminals, and a figure of a flayed man remind me of a passage in *The Analytical Language of John Wilkins*, an essay on the seventeenth-century English mathematician and philosopher, in which Jorge Luis Borges refers to a 'certain Chinese encyclopedia' to demonstrate a different system of thought for organizing knowledge about 'animals': animals belonging to the Emperor, embalmed, tame, sucking pigs, sirens, fabulous, innumerable, having just broken the water pitcher, etc. (Borges, 1964). Here, too, Jones's anatomical theatre, designed according to architectural specifications for perspectival viewing (Alberti, 1435), is filled with objects breaking up that ordered and normative social structure in order to remind the viewers about the principle of death — natural, juridical, and biblical demise — even when the table in the middle of the room stood empty.

Sometimes, however, that table was not empty. When Samuel Pepys visited Jones's anatomical theatre in 1662, he witnessed an anatomy demonstration on the kidneys. The body displayed on the table was that of a seaman who was hanged for robbery. After the dissection by Dr. Tearne, 'a fine dinner was served' in the Hall. After the dinner, Pepys returned to the anatomy theatre in the company of Dr. Scarborough 'to see the body alone.' There, he stretched out his hand and 'touched the dead body with (his) bare hand: it felt cold, but, methought, it was a very unpleasant sight' (quoted in Sawday, 1995, pp. 77-78).

Discomfort, and I may add, pain, death, social or religious prohibitions separate us from our bodily interiors. But the gazing at these interiors, touching the dead body with bare hands, or finding oneself in the presence of Gunther von Hagens's collection of anatomical specimens, produced and preserved with the process called plastination, is that which leads us back to what is known and familiar (see Von Hagens, 2001).

The culture of dissection not only provided us with the voyeuristic opportunity to see the body interior; with the impossible knowledge of ourselves by mapping it out or subjecting it to a new regime of language of property and appropriation; with the representation of the body-exterior as surfaces, but also, as Sir Francis Bacon observed in *Novum Organum* (1620), it made us see the body not as mysterious, but rather as a system, a design, a structure, whose rules of operation, though complex, can be comprehended with the help of reason or a microscope (technology) — the famous 'artificial Eys' (quoted in Sawday, 2005, p. 32).

Cartesian rationalism, English empiricism, and everything else from the classical age via the Enlightenment to the postmodern condition cut into the body to facilitate the confrontation as well as adequation between pedagogy, medicine, economics, politics, and representational practices. Julien Offray de La Mettrie's *Machine Man* (1747), a materialist reduction of the soul and the denial of Leibniz's balance between the mechanistic world and a theological concept of God;[3] a discussion in England about a woman's place determined by her body and sexual desire;[4] a distinct desire to create a new personality type defining the 'living body' and placing it under the surveillance of a new economic mechanism;[5] the Enlightenment discourse of Kant's empirico-transcendental doublet; Comte's positive philosophy; Marx's defence of the mechanized human being; or Freud's explorations of death and pleasure drives, etc., constitute multiple inscriptions of social, economic, and ideological meanings in their specificity, which are visible all over the body.

It is not therefore surprising that, for writers as diverse as Judith Butler, Jean-François Lyotard, Luce Irigaray, Gilles Deleuze, Jacques Derrida, and Michel Foucault (and those who followed their theoretical investigations), the body is conceived as a fundamentally historical and political object. Indeed, for many it is the central object over and through which relations of power and resistance are played out. Each is anxious to challenge the ways in which the body has been relegated to a subordinate or secondary position relative to the primacy of the mind, consciousness, or reason. Each is committed to non-reductive materialism. Each convincingly argues that the subject is produced by social and institutional practices or techniques, by the inscriptions of social meanings, and by the assigning of psychical or indexical significance to body parts and organs.

Making these bodies visible or readable on the level of a diagram or a sentence is to gloss over that moment when something happens which cannot be fully folded into the known — a process of syncopation (see Clément, 1994). A white sheet covering the dead body of a boy was, for Roland Barthes, such a moment, which he called a punctum. A punctum is that split second when something 'rises from the scene, shoots out of it like an arrow', and rips across a cultural field of critical thought or across a communicable experience of it (Barthes, 1981, p. 26). A punctum is that split second that activates the aporia between the living or dead body and logos. A punctum is that split second that gives voice to a thought freed from critical language now ripped open. That human body, formed, and yet not reducible to the historical or theoretical determinations that its presence contests (as recent political events in Europe, the Middle East, and Africa make painfully obvious), is a tear in the studium; that human body — that body defined in the anatomy theatre — is unhoused in being in the space of the now.

The presence of that body covered by a white sheet reminds us that a punctum is a shared and constant 'now' between the dead body visible on a photograph and us voluntarily or involuntarily staring at it. This shared and constant now expresses itself on the historical plane which, as Juan Goytisolo poignantly argued in *State of Siege*, is ontological and cannot be glossed over by the narrative of the 'there-and-then' and the 'here-and-now', or the silences that enveloped everything having to do with the siege in Sarajevo, or in his imaginary Paris, which should never have taken place (Goytisolo, 2002).

The condition of a human unhoused in being in the space of the now discreetly dissects the pretty anatomy of thought and practice, producing gender, ethnic and sexual identities on stage, where all the gazes are supposed to see the same body. The condition of a human unhoused in being haunts the space of the now by giving visibility to that which fulfils itself in the anguish of verbal hallucinations:

> The human being can survive the human being, the human being is what remains after the destruction of the human being, not because somewhere there is a human essence to be destroyed or saved, but because the place of the human is divided, because the human being exists in the fracture between the living being and the speaking being, the inhuman and the human. (Agamben, 1999, pp. 134-5)

If the human being exists in the missing articulation between the living being and logos, in being unhoused in being, what happens to the body which can no longer find itself along the narrative itinerary prompted by the perspectival vision experienced by Pepys (and the scores of others after him) seated in one of the elliptical rows of Inigo Jones's theatre? What happens if a voyeuristic experience of a morgue no longer enables the body to be seen as a readable and teachable sign to all? What happens if that human body cannot be reinscribed into politics, ideology, and epistemology/philosophy that its living existence contests? What happens if the fidgety liveness of the flesh disrupts critical cod-

ing and its critical prose? What happens to the body when it refuses the consolation of correct forms, the consensus of taste permitting a common experience
of nostalgia for the voyeuristic experience of ourselves, and rearticulates itself in
the non-place — in a different kind of theatre.[6]

That theatre which materializes as 'an activity that occurs when life is pushed
to its final limits, where all categories and concepts lose their meaning and right
to exist; where madness, fever, hysteria, and hallucinations are the last barri-
cades of life before approaching TROUPES OF DEATH and death's GRAND
THEATRE' — as Tadeusz Kantor says (Kantor, *The Infamous Transition from the
World of the Dead into the World of the Living*, 1993, p. 149).

Indeed, what happens when the body refuses the consolation of correct
forms, the consensus of taste permitting a common experience of nostalgia for
the voyeuristic experience of ourselves...?

Kantor was on stage staring intensely at the audience as they entered the space
where *The Dead Class* was to be performed.[7] Whether it was a live performance
or a video recording of one, in one corner, rather than in the centre, four rows
of old school desks, pulled as if from the memory of the immemorial past, stood
facing the audience.

The audience entered the performance space expecting, with narcissistic
pleasure, to be projected onto the inaccessible performance surface. This narcissistic pleasure of thought was foiled by a rope and school desks populated by
the Old People in black exactly in front of the audience. It was as if an impassable barrier had been raised, rupturing the perspectival order which had, for
centuries, constituted the metaphysical and political program organizing the
visual and the social as well as modern notion of culture (Lyotard, 1991, pp.
119-20). It was always there in subsequent stagings or incarnations of *The Dead
Class* — the space with the audience, trying to see its reflection in the representations on stage, and the space where Kantor moved among the school desks
occupied by the actors, the Old People, staring silently and motionlessly, like
wax figures, at the entering audience.

The silhouettes of the Old People were enveloped in a bright and misty light.
Caught by this brightness, the spectator's gaze encountered the motionless
gaze. Their eyes expressed an infinite emptiness. Unlike Diego Velázquez's *Las
Meninas*, the emptiness of *The Dead Class* can never be filled by the image of
Philip IV, and his wife Mariana, arrested in the silver surface of a mirror in the
back of the painting; that King who was called upon to cruelly restore 'what is
lacking in every gaze: in the painter's, the model, which his represented double
is duplicating over there in the picture; in the king's, his portrait, which is being finished off on the slope of the canvas that he cannot perceive from where
he stands; in that of the spectator, the real centre of the scene, whose place he

himself has taken as though by usurpation' (Foucault, 1973, p. 15). In *The Dead Class*, emptiness remained in the centre of an anguished perception. In the language of mirrors, reflections, doubles, transferences, and transformations, one heard a distant, murmured, anxious question: 'who is there?' (Shakespeare, *Hamlet*, I.1). Like Clove in Beckett's *Endgame*, the viewers were however forced to see their light dying (Beckett, *Endgame*, 1981, p. 929):

> In the school desks,
> the actors — the Old People,
> are sitting or standing,
> staring directly at the crowd entering the space,
> motionless,
> like WAX FIGURES,
> masterfully resembling the living (...)
> They are exhibited shamefully,
> like the condemned at a public execution,
> more than that: as if they were DEAD.
> From the moment the audience enters,
> a separation should be felt —
> simultaneously, they should feel repulsed by and attracted to this horrible inhuman condition.
> Like the dead!
> 'On the other side!'
> School desks like catafalques.
> (Kantor, *Umarla klasa — Partytura*, p. 3)

On the other hand, there was the inhuman condition of the actors, drastically repositioning traditional relationships between spectators and actors in the theatre: FOREIGNESS. From *The Theatre of Death* manifesto: 'it is necessary to reestablish the essential meaning of the relationship: spectator and actor. It is necessary to recover the primeval force of the shock taking place at the moment when, opposite a human (a spectator), there stood for the first time a human (an actor), deceptively similar to us, yet at the same time infinitely foreign, beyond the impassable barrier.'

> Foreign ... the impassable barrier ... and deceptively similar to us, the spectators.
> One day, or one night, I found a model for the actor which would ideally fit into these conditions: the dead — I felt afraid and ashamed. (...) The DEAD and the ACTOR, these two notions started to overlap in my thoughts. (Kantor, *Umarla klasa — Partytura*, p. 1)

Kantor achieved this foreignness by placing the school benches and the Old People on the side of the performance space, in a corner of the room, beyond the organizing gaze of the spectator. 'WAX FIGURES', 'infinitely DISTANT, shockingly FOREIGN as if DEAD'. This idea seemed to him inexhaustible and, as the production made clear, he could never exploit it enough, as if, liberated from the constraints of linear time and from standards of visibility, Kantor had located his theatre in 'the silence at the eye of the scream', where death and his actors escaped the voice of banality (Beckett, *Ill Seen Ill Said*, 1982, p. 29). The school desks, like catafalques, 'infinitely DISTANT, shockingly FOREIGN', were like a punctum, a hallucinatory rip, a fissure, cut, hole, or tear, an eruptive detail in the studium of forgotten or repressed school days.

Suddenly, the immobilized wax figures at the school desks started to move, as if life had been injected into them. Their returning to life was marked by slow and minute movements of the bodies denatured by time and reduced to nothing more than the mannequins, whose stone-frozen faces expressed an infinite emptiness. The torsos were upright, the hands on the desks, the faces looked forward, ready to embark on an unknown journey. Silence. 'Grace to breathe that void' (Beckett, *Ill Seen Ill Said*, 1982, p. 59). After a split second, one of the Old People raised her hand, as if asking for permission to leave. She was joined by other Old People. 'Something is taking its course' (Beckett, *Endgame*, 1981, p. 935). The hands were in the air, the request to leave becoming more and

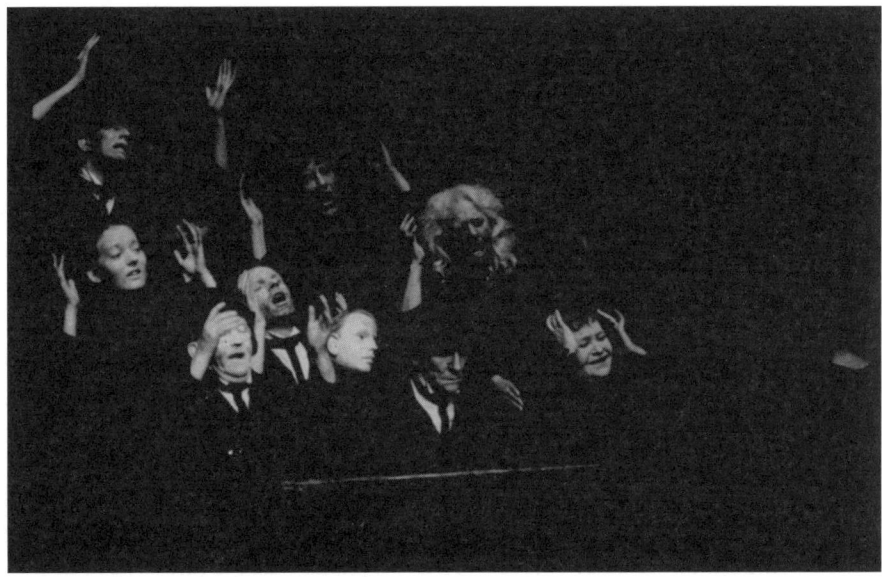

Tadeusz Kantor. *The Dead Class* (1975). Reproduced with permission of Jacquie Bablet.

more pressing. 'The meaning of this sign is slowly changing. THE OLD PEO-
PLE ARE ASKING NOW FOR SOMETHING . . . SOMETHING FINITE'
(Kantor, *Umarla klasa — Partytura*, p. 4). As always, in Kantor's theatre, mun-
dane matters were mixed with everlasting concerns — here, the irrepressible
need to go to the toilet was mixed with the desire for eternity. Eschatology and
sacrum; there was no escape from that something which tore the fabric of the
studium. The Old People, one by one, disappeared into the opening, the black
hole, the open grave at the back. The school desks were empty. Emptiness and
silence provided a momentary relief from the unexpected and sombre image.
What was going to happen next? 'Birth was the death of him. (...) Words are
few' (Beckett, *A Piece of Monologue*, 1984, p. 265). Kantor's characters were
being born and dying into the thought of a theatre materializing 'on the other
side', where 'life is pushed to its final limits, where all categories and concepts
lose their meaning and right to exist' (Kantor, *The Infamous Transition from the
World of the Dead into the World of the Living*, 1993, p. 149).

The Old People reappeared in the black hole of the opening. Their grand
entrance was accompanied by the nostalgic sounds of a waltz, whose opening
tune brought back the memory of its title, 'If only once again the past could return...'[8] But it was not only the past that returned with a melancholy regression
into a bygone area. The dreams, desires, hopes, and memories of failure did
return, too. The Old People circled the school benches. Their awakening to the
dreams and nightmares of history, this Grand Parade of the Circus of Death, as
Kantor called it, would have been incomplete without that which testified and
bore witness to their dying light. The Old People carried with them the wax
figures of children — of their own childhood:

> the dead children hang over (the Old People), cling to their bodies with
> strength; others are pulled as if they were a heavy weight, a heavy remorse
> of the soul, a burden; others 'crept around' the bodies of the ones who
> grew old, and who killed this childhood with their adulthood in a sanc-
> tioned and 'socially acceptable' manner. (Kantor, *Umarla klasa — Par-
> tytura*, p. 5)

The Old People carried with them the tumours of childhood. 'The eye will
return to the scene of its betrayals' (Beckett, *Ill Seen Ill Said*, 1982, p. 27). These
tumours, like a painful image in the service of violent and bloodied thought
brought forth the possibility that

> the memory of their childhood had became a poor and forgotten storage-
> room where dried up and forgotten people, faces, objects, pieces of clo-
> thing, adventures, emotions, images are stored...

> ... The desire to bring them back to life is not a sentimental symptom of old
> age.
> It is a condition of TOTAL life,
> which cannot be limited to a narrow passage in the present moment. (Kantor, *Umarla klasa — Partytura*, p. 6)

Unlike the Maeterlinckian or Symbolist ambition to present a *Gesamtkunstwerk* of evocative images of life before and after the present moment, Kantor's Old People walked onto the stage with the dead bodies of their childhood. Like runaways trying to escape the soul's remorse, they were excited by the possibility of living their past again, to the tune of a familiar waltz, to prove that they were still alive — more, as if to prove that their light reflected the impossible thought of 'total, undialectical death.'[9]

The idea of undialectical death marked the moment of revelation to the audience, 'on the other side', of the meaning of the word 'defunctus' (Beckett, *Proust*, 1931, p. 72). 'The place was crawling with them! Use your head, can't you, use your head, you're on earth, there's no cure for that,' says Hamm in *Endgame* (Beckett, *Endgame*, 1981, p. 941). Indeed, the place was crawling with them, until they returned to the school desks where they sat down together, with the wax figures of their childhood — another frozen moment, during which the audience had a chance to face the 'DISTANT, shockingly FOREIGN' possibility that there is no cure for a past which is discharged and finished (*defunctus*), yet not dead (defunct). It is an undialectical death that grows in the mind, through Kantor's images and scenes, 'grain upon grain, one by one' (Beckett, *Endgame*, 1981, p. 926).

Kantor's opening vision of an infinite emptiness was filled with the Old People regressing into the past in their present moment. They could never be dead, for, though deceased, the dead live in our memory of them. The audience could have no memories of these dead, for the Old People were subject to Kantor's desire to make them be what he or his autobiography wanted them to be. Thus, the audience 'remembered' only what filled their sight by force.

It was not enough for Kantor to bring memory back to the present moment and make it visible through art. He needed to separate it from the audience with a rope, so that the process of exploration became the process of recovering from the shock 'taking place at the moment when opposite a human (a spectator) there stood for the first time a human (an actor) deceptively similar to us, yet at the same time infinitely foreign, beyond the impassable barrier' (Kantor, *The Theatre of Death*, 1993, p. 114). Kantor faced the mirror of memory — the school benches and the people sitting in them. It is a mode of thinking which begins with something existing outside, but then it surpasses the dialectics of the visible by folding back upon itself in order to disrupt its own history and shape. Kantor's solitary figure activated the mirror, turning a flat, fetishized memory into a multidimensional spatial fold on 'the other side'. In the performance space, where linear time ceases to function, this fold perpetually breaks up, and forms itself anew.

Across the space and across the time, there is the Amargosa Opera House in the Death Valley Junction. A set of buildings — now a motel, private apartments, and a theatre — is marked by time, which peeled the paint from the walls to the shriek of the peacock and the wind moving in and out of the empty blue windows. A peacock — a bird of death; a wind — a howl in the desert, in the void. The long corridor is empty; there is only a set of doors and a sign in a broken window — 'Not Responsible for Accidents.' A perfect set up for Anselm Kiefer, whose works — *Isis und Osiris* (1987), *Sulamith* (1990), *Lilith* (1990) or *Liliths Töchter* (1990) — one by one cut through the remnants of metaphysics which have inhabited our thought since the Enlightenment. Marta Becket, a ballerina who, as an apocryphal story goes, stopped in this now defunct town erected by the Pacific Coast Borax Company in 1907 on her way to Las Vegas, because her car had a flat tyre:

> It was as if suddenly I found myself in a place where time stopped. An invisible wall seemed to surround this place — impenetrable, creating a retreat from today. My eyes then wandered down to the colonnade to where it turned a corner. Small buildings with gates leading to possible courtyards continued and suddenly my eyes fell on the largest structure in the row. It was a theatre. (Quoted in Wolska, np)

The phantasmagoric life of the theatre ended at that very moment. After laborious renovations, the theatre opened to the audience who would come from the desert towns nearby to see this strange woman/ballerina perform on stage. When I saw the performance, *The Masquerade*, in April 2005, Death Valley Junction was in bloom. We were supposed to gather at 7:45 PM at the doors of a building marked the Amargosa Opera House. The doors were locked, and nobody was allowed to enter. The music of Puccini and Verdi came from the sound speakers and filled the space around us. We waited outside, until given a sign to enter the theatre by an MC, an eccentric handyman and a clown/performer on Saturdays and Mondays — the show days. The theatre was brightly lit and ... already full. Above the doors, in the box painted on the walls, there were the King and Queen of Spain richly dressed in seventeenth-century costumes, painted too. They were surrounded by their courtiers and servants, monks and nuns, musicians and vagabonds, gypsies and prostitutes, painted in bright colours, seated in the gilded balconies all around the auditorium. They were talking; someone was pouring a glass of wine; someone else was playing

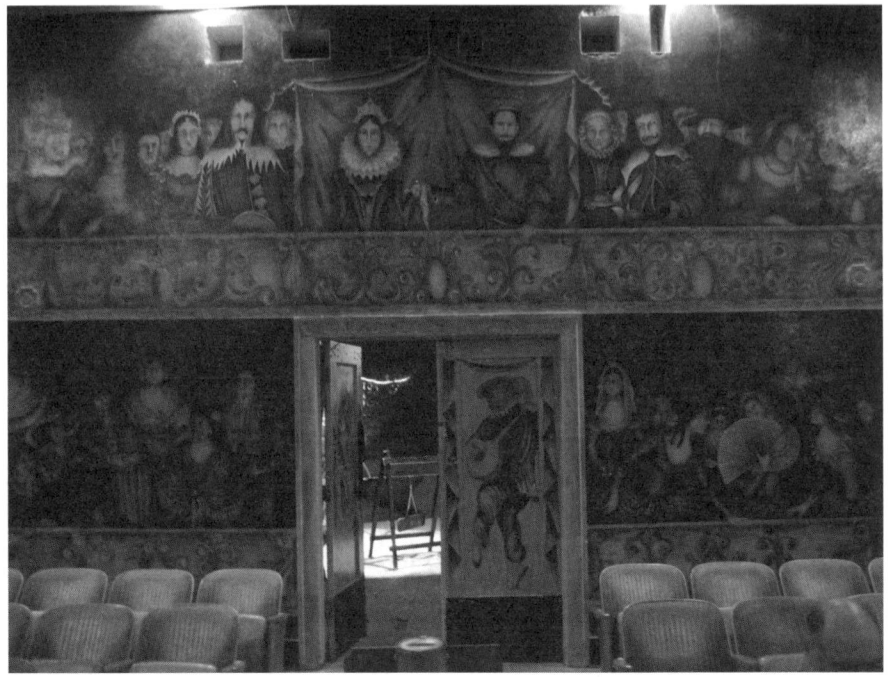

Amargosa Opera House (interior); Death Valley Junction, CA. Photo by Michal Kobialka. Reproduced with his permission.

a harmonica; still someone else was gossiping while covering her face with a fan. Native Americans entertained the spectators gathered around. The royal court of the Spanish Golden Age and the bodies transported from the New World stared at each other and at the audience filling the seats; and, if no one comes, they stare at Marta Becket dance onstage transversally moving between the past, the present, and the future. The movement of her body fills their sight by force. The movement of their eyes fills her body with presence by force...

When she finally appears on stage, wearing a black cape covering her body and a bright red lipstick, this 81-year-old diva startles us and the courtiers, for different reasons, of course, with her incorrigible desire to conquer time and dominate the space. The cape is removed, and the body is revealed. Wearing a black ballet dress and a high-cut top, she moves across the stage marking her position with a blue fan. Becket seems to cut through the pressures and the demands of the real — the real world. At 81, in the dance she performs in front of the painted spectators, she lifts her leg to the impossible height, pirouettes on point, and allows the fan to reveal her face, which seems to escape the ravages of vulgar time. In the lights of the ramp, the theatre in the desert — in the void — marked by history and theory cutting into the body or into the space now divided into the stage and the auditorium, is perhaps only a fantasy of the brain or the void it has peopled. *The Masquerade*, a homage to the impossible, is a fantasy in which a pauper becomes a prince, a ladies man a movie producer, and a secretary an Esmeralda. Their stories are told with a wink and an occasional kick until that final scene veiled in the blue hues of the inevitable loss — at midnight, everything stops, and the everyday, marked by that 'poisonous ingenuity of Time'[10], claims the movement and the body. The audience leaves marked by the loss which can only be reclaimed by the uncanny or the ritornello hummed by the memories of the performance in the service of thought, commerce, or signed memorabilia. 'There, he stretched out his hand and touched the (...) body with (his) bare hand: it felt cold' (quoted in Sawday, 1995, pp. 77-78).

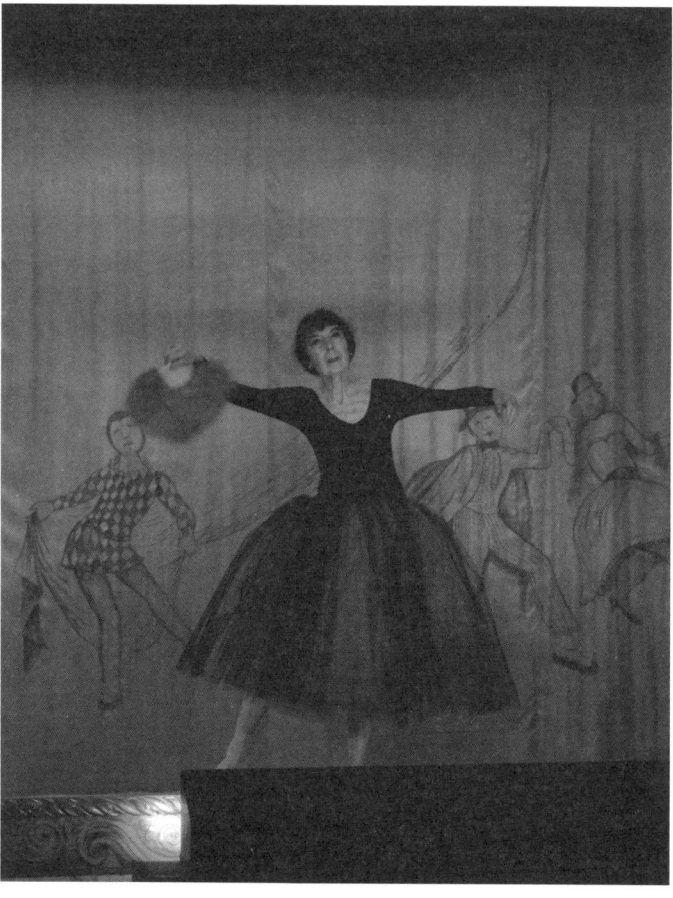

Marta Becket in *The Masquerade* (April 2005). Photo by Michal Kobialka.
Reproduced with his permission.

Marta Becket remains outside of this touch. Despite the loss of her acting partner, Tom Willett, who died last year and can only join us in our memory of him, she continues to perform every Saturday and Monday, dancing her own body with the memories of Esmeralda and in memory of a performer who, with every movement, must understand the notion of time embodied. But to embody time means to allow time to cut through the body and mark the singularity of this movement with a scratch and a noise like wings, like leaves, like sand, like desert:

> Nagg: Could you give me a scratch before your go?
> Nell: No.
> (Pause)
> Nagg: In the back.
> Nell: No.
> (Pause)
>   Rub yourself against the rim.
> Nagg: It is lower down. In the hollow.
> Nell: What hollow?
> Nagg: The hollow!
> (Beckett, *Endgame*, 1981, p. 863)

The hollow — 'the silence at the eye of the scream', where Becket escaped the voice of banality. Amargosa, emptied of the material bodies, which will inevitably end up on the dissecting tables, is the void peopled by her. Thus, it is the Spanish courtier in a white wig who continues to look at her through his spectacles — 'You are one in your memory. You are another in the time you cannot remember' (Fuentes, 1976, p. 445). He will never stop. The painted spectators, 'infinitely DISTANT, shockingly FOREIGN', are like a punctum, a hallucinatory rip, a fissure, cut, hole, or tear, an eruptive detail in the studium of forgotten or repressed days. Rub yourself against the rim of the Spirit of Illusion, also played by Becket in the closing moments of *The Masquerade*, and maybe you will be able to observe what you can think. Dare to think — sapere aude — but do not think about the mechanized body, but about that body that, while moving through this three-dimensional theatrical space, forces us to acknowledge our own constructedness, which remains on this side together with the memory of her materializing the fictions of its many bodies. The dance of seven veils. Rub yourself against the rim and think about Maurice Merleau-Ponty's flesh of the world — 'my body is made of the same flesh as the world (it is perceived), and moreover, this flesh of my body is shared by the world, the world reflects it, encroaches upon it and it encroaches upon the world. They are in a relation of transgression and of overlapping' (Merleau-Ponty, 1968, p. 248).

A body unhoused in being, existing in the missing, articulating between the living being and logos. A theatre in the Death Valley Junction, a vortex, where absolute time collides with immaterial time defined. It cancels, even if temporarily, the condition by which to live; and finds its voice and destiny in the anguish of verbal hallucinations.

The anguish of verbal hallucinations in the space of the now. That space and that now through which all the voices, blasted out of the continuum of history or being, might enter:

> From the dim recesses,
> as if from the abyss of Hell,
> there started to emerge
> people, who had died a long time ago,
> and memories of events,
> which, as in a dream,
> had no explanation,
> no beginning, no end,
> no cause, or effect.
> (Kantor, *Silent Night*, 1993 p. 182)

'Little is left to tell' (Beckett, *Ohio Impromptu*, 1984, p. 285). Except maybe that all the voices make a noise like wings, like feathers, like ashes, like leaves. They all whisper at once: 'to see/be seen' (Beckett, *Rockaby*, 1984, p. 279). To be is to be heard in this vulgar conception of time and space as suggested by a woman in a black high-necked evening gown in a rocking chair moving to and fro in Samuel Beckett's *Rockaby*. The words fly up, the body remains below always making me aware of the contours of silence on the other side — in this theatre in the void, infinity of the mind, and the desert peopled by the flesh of the world. Maybe, in this space of the now, their words, translated into verbal hallucinations by our technology and mnemotechnics, can materialize in the theatre that cuts through the fidgeting bodies on this side to reveal the delirium of the flesh on that other side:

> close of a long day
> when she said
> to herself
> whom else
> time she stopped
> time she stopped
> going to and fro
> all eyes

> all sides
> high and low
> for another
> another like herself.
> (Beckett, *Rockaby*, 1984, p. 275)

Maybe, in this space of the now, their words, searching for another like herself, can materialize in the theatre that cuts through the limits of what can be thought or said, which 'has the power to arrest the flight of an arrow in a recess of time, in the space proper to it' (Foucault, 1977, pp. 53-4). But, if there is no story to be told, no misfortune to be recorded, no disaster to be averted, there remains only 'the 'invisible reality' that damns the life of the body on earth as a pensum and reveals the meaning of the word: 'defunctus'' (Beckett, *Proust*, 1931, p. 72). The pensum — that which is measured — makes me see, before it reveals in the flesh the meaning of the word 'defunctus' — death that recalls and preserves death, articulates the trace of death:

> close of a long day
> saying to herself
> whom else
> time she stopped
> time she stopped
> going to and fro
> time she went and sat
> at her window
> quiet at her window
> only window
> facing other windows
> other only windows.
> (Beckett, *Rockaby*, 1984, pp. 277-8)

A woman in a black high-necked evening gown in a rocking chair moving to and fro gently and carefully pronounces every word damming the life of the body on earth and reveals the inadequation between the organic exterior and that which materializes in the excess of logos and the fading of the body — in the missing articulation that can only be expressed as the desire to be seen or heard moving like feathers, like leaves, like ashes, like leaves...

A woman in a black high-necked gown in a rocking chair archives the language in which Samuel Beckett bears witness to one's grace (if one ever does) to breathe that void:

so in the end
close of a long day
went down
let down the blind and down
right down
into the old rocker
and rocked
rocked
saying to herself
no
done with that
the rocker
those arms at last
saying to the rocker
rock her off
stop her eyes
fuck life.
(Beckett, *Rockaby*, 1984, pp. 281-2)

But the eye will return to the scene of betrayals — maybe, this is why we are fascinated with Beckett's and our returns, as if every act of repetition allowed us to comprehend the lack of essence and the possibility that 'whatever this new understanding of (death) holds to be irrelevant — shards created by the selection of materials, remainders left aside by an explanation — comes back, despite everything, on the edges of discourse or in its rifts and crannies: "resistances", "survivals", or delays discreetly perturb the pretty order of a line of "progress" or a system of interpretation' (De Certeau, 1988, p. 4).

...A strenuous search for the voice...

Tadeusz Kantor's, Marta Becket's, and Samuel Beckett's theatre abandons the enchantments of reality and is a gesture of space-time-matter that surpasses the visible only to locate itself in the aporia between the living body and Voice or Logos. Faced with a ceaseless renewal of the need to give birth to words that can name the unnameable word, 'defunctus', the living being's speaking and the Logos's becoming living are a eulogy — a eulogy for repetition that suspends life and death in a spectacular play of thought and no relief. The murmurs and the contours of words break the silence of the enchanted reality and create a space where the inaudible lament comes forth to what is audible and sonorous. I am faced with the imperceptible grading of words that both gloss over and are the breath of flight toward and away from that body defined by epistemology as well as material conditions governing everything that has a visible existence in Inigo Jones's anatomy theatre, where Pepys touched the dead body with his bare hand.

The Old People, the 81-year-old Ballerina, and a prematurely old woman with unkempt grey hair, as Samuel Beckett described her, may end up in front of Pepys as cadavers marked by a particular political, social, ideological, and cultural matrices. He may even be able to touch their bodies with his bare hand. Be that as it may. There is always however the fidgety 'liveness' of the flesh, which, on occasions, may disrupt this coding and its critical prose to present the unthinkable, the invisible through the body's being unhoused in being.

The body unhoused in being can no longer be appropriated by the dominant convention. It exists in the space behind the rope, in the desert/the void, and the infinity of the mind. In this space, existing outside the normative categories, the body ceased to be represented by the subject — that is to say, the Old People, the 81-year-old Ballerina, and a prematurely old woman with unkempt grey hair were freed from the bondage of history and utility, dissociated from the assumed or imposed functions and entered into a network of possible relationships with other objects/people in the space of the now.

Tadeusz Kantor, Marta Becket, and Samuel Beckett created a space (literally and metaphorically) in which all categories and concepts were wrestled from the pre-assigned use-value so that they could enter into the closest possible relationships with other categories and objects in order to reinvent and rearticulate themselves. They abandoned visual sovereignty of the eye which produced the representational image in a classic, three-dimensional, pictorial space of the anatomy theatre. Instead, the eye or the hand did not perform a visual or ordering function: rather, it followed the contours of that which organized its field of perception to invoke what Lyotard calls 'the unrepresentable in presentation itself' (Lyotard, 1993, p. 15). This feeling that there is something unrepresentable is invariably accompanied by an enunciation of becoming, rather than being, an enunciation which perturbs the order of things in the space of the now.

The space of the now — the space of self-examination that will always be *in* reality but not *of* it — turns performance into an immense site wherein many poetics proliferate, coalesce, and diverge. This site does not function as an organizing force within a particular system of cultural consumption, but draws attention to a system of the formation and transformation of bodies, objects and thoughts articulating an experience of the aporia that challenges the increasingly mediated surface images; to the theatre reclaiming its right to be an arena for showing that which cannot be grasped or understood, because in the most concrete form it shows nothing. The Old People, the 81-year-old Ballerina, and a prematurely old woman with unkempt grey hair cannot return to their recognizable forms and definitions — delirium of the flesh. Rather, the modalities of being, seeing, and movement proliferate in the unregulated, dynamic (mental and physical) space inhabited by bare life that offers escape from Pepys:

> Estragon: All the dead voices. (...)
> Vladimir: They all speak at once. (...)
> Vladimir: Rather they whisper.
> Estragon: They rustle.
> Vladimir: They murmur. (...)
> Estragon: They talk about their lives. (...)
> Vladimir: They make a noise like feathers.
> Estragon: Like leaves.
> Vladimir: Like ashes.
> Estragon: Like leaves.

Michal Kobialka is Chair and Professor of Theatre at the Department of Theatre Arts & Dance at the University of Minnesota. He is the author of a book on Tadeusz Kantor's theatre, *A Journey Through Other Spaces: Essays and Manifestos, 1944-1990* (1993) and on the early medieval drama and theatre, *This Is My Body: Representational Practices in the Early Middle Ages* (1999); an editor of *Of Borders and Thresholds: Theatre History, Practice, and Theory* (1999); a co-editor (with Barbara Hanawalt) of *Medieval Practices of Space* (2000); as well as author of more than 65 articles, essays and reviews. His new book on Tadeusz Kantor will be published by University of Minnesota Press in 2008.

Notes

1   See Kobialka (1999), chapter 4, for the discussion of the representational practices used after the Fourth Lateran Council in order to secure the visibility of the missing body of Christ.

2   See Calbi (1995) for bibliographic citations.

3   La Mettrie, J. Offray de, *Machine Man and Other Writings*. Cambridge and New York, 1996.

4   Laqueur, T., *Making Sex: Body and Gender*. Cambridge, 1990, chapter 6. Or Laqueur, T., *Solitary Sex: A Cultural History of Masturbation*. New York, 2004, pp. 203-205.

5   Kobialka, M., 'Words and Bodies: A Discourse on Male Sexuality in Late Eighteenth-Century English Representational Practices'. In: *Theatre Research International*, Vol. 28, No. 1, pp. 1-19. 2003.

6   In his *The Production of Space*, Henri Lefebvre proposed a nuanced theoretical model for exploring lived-in space as socially and politically produced. According to Le-

febvre, social space is a particular outcome of the class struggle and actions of self-conscious powers because hegemony makes use of space in establishing and materializing its ideological status. Assigned such a function, 'space may be said to embrace a multitude of intersections, each with its assigned location. As for representations of the relations of production, which subsume power relations, these too occur in space: space contains them in the form of buildings, monuments and works of art. Such frontal (and hence brutal) expressions of these relations do not completely crowd out their more clandestine or underground aspects; all power must have its accomplices — and its police.' This multitude of intersections can be further elaborated on in terms of:

1. *Spatial practice*, which embraces production and reproduction, and the particular locations and spatial sets characteristic of each social formation. Spatial practice ensures continuity and some degree of cohesion. In terms of social space, and of each member of a given society's relationship to that space, this cohesion implies a guaranteed level of *competence* and a specific level of *performance*.

2. *Representations of space*, which are tied to the relations of production and to the 'order' which those relations impose, and hence to knowledge, to signs, to codes, and to 'frontal' relations.

3. *Representational spaces*, embodying complex symbolism, sometimes coded, sometimes not, linked to the clandestine or underground side of social life, as also to art (which may come eventually to be defined less as a code of space than as a code of representational spaces) (See Lefebvre, 1991, p. 31).

7   It should be noted here that there were three versions of *The Dead Class* — version I: 1975-1977; version II: 1977-86 (after 1,500 performances, Kantor made the decision to no longer show *The Dead Class*); and version III recreated by Kantor for a 1989 production filmed by Nat Lilenstein. For a detailed analysis of the literary sources for *The Dead Class* and a performance analysis, see Krzysztof Pleśniarowicz (2004) and Kobialka (1993), chapter 2.

8   This particular waltz, composed by Adam Karasiński with words by Andrzej Własta, is also known in Poland as Waltz François. Kantor used an instrumental version of the waltz in the production.

9   The phrase 'undialectical death' is taken from Barthes (1981).

10   The phrase 'poisonous ingenuity of Time' can be found in Beckett, 1931, p. 4.

References

Agamben, G., *Remnants of Auschwitz: The Witness and the Archive*. (Translated by D. Heller-Roazen.) New York, 1999.

Barthes, R., *Camera Lucida: Reflections on Photography*. (Translated by R. Howard.) New York, 1981.

Beckett, S., *Proust*. London, 1931.

Beckett, S., *Waiting for Godot*. New York, 1954.

Beckett, S., 'Endgame'. In: *Stages of Drama*. (Edited by C. Klaus, M. Gilbert and B. Field Jr.) Glenview, 1981.

Beckett, S., *Ill Seen Ill Said*. London, 1982.

Beckett, S., 'A Piece of Monologue'. In: *The Collected Shorter Plays of Samuel Beckett*. New York, 1984.

Beckett, S., 'Ohio Impromptu'. In: *The Collected Shorter Plays of Samuel Beckett*. New York, 1984.

Beckett, S., 'Rockaby'. In: *The Collected Shorter Plays of Samuel Beckett*. New York, 1984.

Borges, J.L., 'The Analytical Language of John Wilkins'. In: *Other Inquisitions 1937-1952*. (Translated by Ruth Simms.) Texas, 1964.

Calbi, M., *Approximate Bodies: Gender and Power in Early Modern Drama and Anatomy*. London and New York, 1995.

Certeau, M. de, *The Writing of History*. (Translated by T. Conley.) New York, 1988.

Clément, C., *Syncope: The Philosophy of Rapture*. (Translated by S. O'Driscoll and D. Mahoney.) Minneapolis, 1994.

Foucault, M., *The Order of Things: An Archaeology of Human Sciences*. (Translated by A. Sheridan Smith.) New York, 1973.

Foucault, M., *Language, Counter-Memory, Practice: Selected Essays and Interviews*. (Translated by D. Bouchard and S. Simon; edited by D. Bouchard.) Ithaca, 1977.

Fuentes, C., *Terra Nostra*. (Translated by M. Sayers Peden.) New York, 1976.

Goytisolo, J., *State of Siege*. (Translated by H. Lane.) San Francisco, 2002.

Hagens, G. von, *Körperwelten: Fascination Beneath the Surface*. Heidelberg, 2001.

Kantor, T., 'The Infamous Transition from the World of the Dead into the World of the Living', 'Silent Night' and 'The Theatre of Death'. In: *A Journey Through Other Spaces: Essays and Manifestos, 1944-1990*. (Edited and translated with critical commentary by M. Kobialka.) Berkeley, 1993.

Kantor, T., *Umarla klasa — Partytura*. Unpublished manuscript.

Kobialka, M., *A Journey Through Other Spaces: Essays and Manifestos, 1944-1990*. Berkeley, 1993.

Kobialka, M., *This Is My Body: Representational Practices in the Early Middle Ages*. Ann Arbor, 1999.

Lefebvre, H., *The Production of Space*. (Translated by D. Nicholson-Smith.) Oxford, 1991.

Lyotard, J., *The Inhuman: Reflections on Time*. (Translated by G. Bennington and R. Bowlby.) Stanford, 1991.

Lyotard, J., *The Postmodern Explained: Correspondence 1982-1985*. (Translated by D. Barry, B. Maher, J. Pefanis, V. Spate, and M. Thomas.) Minneapolis, 1993.

Merleau-Ponty, M., *The Visible and the Invisible*. (Translated by A. Lingins; edited by C. Lefort.) Evanston, 1968.

Pleśniarowicz, K., *The Dead Memory Machine: Tadeusz Kantor's Theatre of Death*. Wales, 2004.

Sawday, J., *The Body Emblazoned: Dissection and the Human Body in Renaissance Culture*. London and New York, 1995.

Wolska, A., *Dancing in the Desert*. Unpublished manuscript.

Performance Documentation 8:
Körper

The fact that Sasha Waltz decided to inaugurate her position as co-director of the Berlin Schaubühne am Lehniner Platz with a piece called *Körper* is no minor issue. The Schaubühne is considered the 'Holy Grail of dramatic arts' and 'the most fiercely intellectual of German theatres' (Bowen, 2000) and has during the past thirty years promoted some of the greatest names of German text-based theatre. The unprecedented move to not only 'include' but to give a position of such privilege as the artistic direction of the company to a choreographer allows 'the body' to take centre stage.

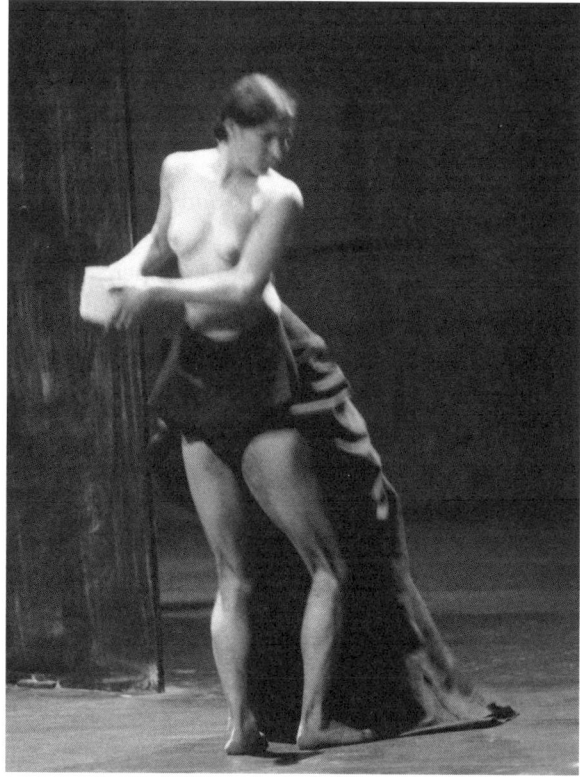

Körper (2000). Choreography by Sasha Waltz. Photo: Bernd Uhlig. Reproduced with permission of Sasha Waltz & Guests.

Sasha Waltz's appointment might be called a sign of the times, now that the body has taken centre stage in much theoretical research as well, and has become an accepted component of discourse for scholars in a variety of subjects. In this cultural context, Sasha Waltz is called upon by the Berlin Schaubühne to take the place of the anatomist in the historical anatomy theatre and *show* us the body. Waltz's works acknowledge that such showing is not without complications.

Visibility promises knowledge about that which previously remained unintelligible, obscure or hidden. This is the promise also presented by the anatomical theatre: namely, that ocular experience corresponds directly to knowledge about the human body and maybe even about the mysteries of the human soul. To see is to know. However, as Joan Scott observes, visibility may actually function to obscure rather than to enlighten. Reflecting on the desire to 'render historical what has hitherto been hidden' by 'document[ing] the lives of those omitted or overlooked in accounts of the past,' Scott warns against the danger implicit in this 'making visible', pointing out that 'it may reproduce rather than contest given ideological systems (...)' (Scott, 1991, p. 775, 778). This, in her view, occurs because when making something or some*body* visible one tends to take for granted that which one is making visible, and thus neglects to enquire upon its constructedness.

With *Körper* Sasha Waltz acknowledges this risk. The show self-consciously presents itself as a survey concerning the 'inner human body and the outer shell', asking itself 'What is the body?' and 'How is it made?' (Sasha Waltz & Guests, 2000). The project has an obvious anatomical ring to it, even more so when we take into account Waltz's choice of the word *Körper*, meaning 'corpse' in German, as opposed to *Leib*, which designates a living body. Interestingly, Waltz initiated her work on this piece in the then-empty building designed by Liebeskind for the Jewish Museum in Berlin, six weeks before it opened to the public. Even though I do not want to speculate about Waltz's intentions, I believe this knowledge provides the show with yet another promise of visibility, the promise of exposing the bare facts and the inescapable truths of history, of destruction, of Holocaust. In the performance, however, Waltz decidedly obscures rather than illuminates the bare body, making ironically evident its constructedness through the constant debunking of the myth of visibility as unmediated experience or access to reality. For what is it that becomes visible in this show, if anything does?

Körper confronts its audience with a myriad of body images, including (in no particular order):

A glass box enclosing semi-nude dancers who slither, curl, twist and step on each other like worms crammed in a jar.

A man and woman placed on opposite sides of a looking glass play with their reflections, producing hybrid images of mixed male and female anatomies.

A body whose legs go backwards; half back to front.

A body with two torsos.

Limbs that pop through holes, thereby appearing as if they were detached from their bodies, and having lives of their own.

A group of dancers manipulating white plates so that the plates look like an exo-skeleton that breaks, comes back together, and then dissolves, becoming separated vertebrals floating in the air.

Naked bodies, stacked on top of each other in various ways.

Bodies from whose sides eggs seem to emerge.

Dancers 'draining' the body of its fluids through what is an obvious optical 'trick' of pouring large amounts of water while turning the body upside down or twisting its joints.

Two dancers slapping price tags onto each others' bodies, representing the market value of certain organs.

Dancers narrating stories and everyday thoughts about their bodies while confidently indicating the wrong anatomical parts as they misname them.

A freak show, or a parade of weird bodily illusions?

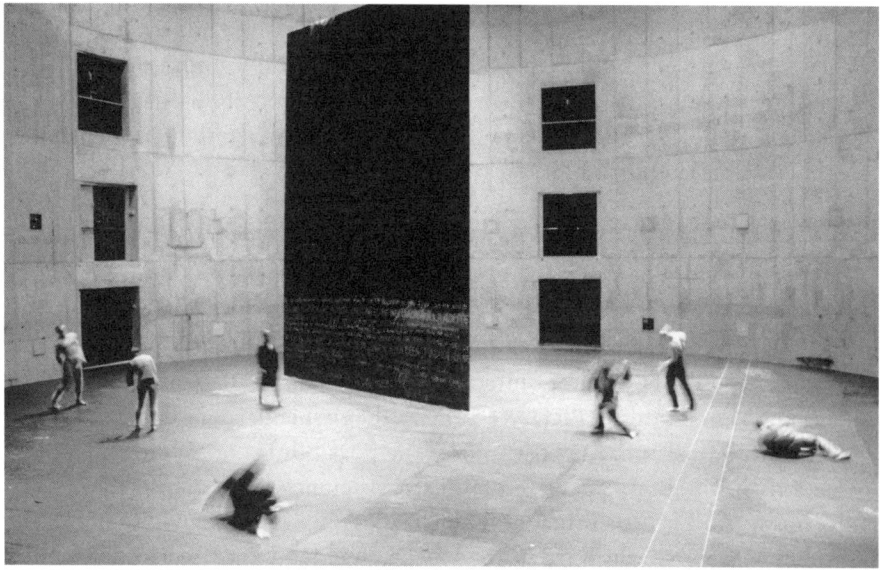

Körper (2000). Choreography by Sasha Waltz. Photo: Bernd Uhlig. Reproduced with persmission of Sasha Waltz & Guests.

Although the stripped-bare aesthetics of this performance promises unrestricted visibility, the dancers show what we think we see to be an optical trick. They do so similarly to how Ian Maxwell describes Da Cortona´s anatomical drawings: 'The images resist a laying-out under the rubric of a democratizing ocular centrism. The cross-hatchings and fecund darknesses remind us of the conditions of their creation as images' (Maxwell, in this volume, p. 59). Similarly, Waltz's piece questions the epistemic hegemony of visibility. These bodies on stage perform images of 'the body', rather than expose or show themselves as bodies. The piece frustrates the desire to see the body in all its 'reality' and prevents the constructedness of the body from being obscured under the conception that visibility works as a transparent reference to the 'real'. The work plays with these expectations (the expectation to see and to know) by frustrating our every desire.

A final, spatial example. A wall standing in the middle of the bare stage divides the space into two halves. One half of the space is exposed to the audience, the other is hidden. During the performance the wall falls violently on the floor exposing its 'back'; still, it does not fall flat. It gains a new, slight, inclination that makes visible what had been invisible, but also hides something new. Maxwell describes a similar frustration in the anatomical theatre as follows: 'This is what is so unsettling about the experience of the anatomical theatre: the epistemological promise made in the name of visibility cannot be delivered upon' (Maxwell, in this volume, p. 62).

The Schaubühne too makes an epistemological promise, by bringing in Sasha Waltz, who herself also makes an epistemological promise by producing *Körper*. Nevertheless, in my view she takes on the responsibility of this promise merely as a rhetorical gesture; one that allows her to make the fall of visibility resound just that much louder.

Text by *Manuela Infante-Guell*

Sasha Waltz founded her company Sasha Waltz & Guests with Jochem Sandig in 1993. In 1999 Waltz was appointed as one of the new artistic directors of the Schaubühne am Lehniner Platz. *Körper* was the first choreography she presented in this new position. *Körper* explores the possibilities of the body, inspired by notions of the body produced by history, science, and architecture. What is the body? And how is it made? The choreographic studies Waltz did in the Judisches Museum in Berlin, designed by Daniel Liebeskind, were of particular influence on the spatial design of the performance.

Manuela Infante-Guell is a theatre maker based in Santiago, Chile. In 2007, she received her MA in Cultural Analysis from the University of Amsterdam.

Performance Data

Direction and choreography: Sasha Waltz
Stage design: Heike Schuppelius, Sasha Waltz, Thomas Schenk
Costumes: Bernd Skodzig
Music: Hans Peter Kuhn
Light: Valentin Gallé, Martin Hauk
Performers: Davide Camplani, Nadia Cusimano, Lisa Densem, Luc Dunberry, Annette Klar, Juan Kruz, Diaz de Garaio Esnaola, Nicola Mascia, Grayson Millwood, Michal Mualem, Joakim NaBi Olsson, Virgis Puodzunias, Claudia de Serpa Soares, Xuan Shi, Takako Suzuki, Laurie Young, Sigal Zouk-Harder

Körper was a production by Schaubühne am Lehniner Platz, presented by Sasha Waltz & Guests. It was co-produced by Théâtre de la Ville.

References

Bowen, C., 'Berlin Waltz Festival'. www.eif.co.uk/pdfs/festmag-aug2000-i.pdf
Maxwell, I., '"Who Were You?": The Visible and the Visceral', pp. 49-66 in this
     volume.
Sasha Waltz & Guests, 'Körper'. Text world premiere January 22, 2000.
     www.sashawaltz.com/a03.php?w=&ID=5&t=1&spr=en.
Scott, J., 'The Evidence of Experience'. In: *Critical Inquiry*, 17, 1991, pp.
     773-797.

Operating Theatres: Body-bits and a Post-apartheid Aesthetics

Rachel Fensham

During the Renaissance, as Jonathan Sawday (1995) argues, the operating theatre provided a frame and lens for examining the society of death, crime, sexual politics, class, and medical knowledge. In this model, an operating theatre could be designed to detach organs from a body in order to perpetuate or produce systems and hierarchies of knowledge. Taking an eye, for instance, a structure of optics dissected from its jelly-like orb will inform the notion of a perspectival view and the lens of the camera, while later systems of power will reassemble the dismembered eyeball in the surveillance camera and the endoscope. It could be argued therefore that the anatomical body had little of absolute value since what became significant was its bit-like propensity for connectivity with other objects, mechanisms and beliefs in an historical situation. Further historicization of the anatomical body, so presciently examined by Sawday as a way of seeing the world, has complex implications for modernity and its history of colonization. One is that the history of modern states and their body politics are already located within a specular regime based on dissection.

In this essay, I want to consider how the bits of bodies that appear in 'operating theatres' connect to political and aesthetic structures, particularly those of a postcolonial situation. I intend to examine 'body-bits' as objects that are tied to a 'landscape-like' reshaping of theatrical form. The restaging of Monteverdi's 1640 opera *Il Ritorno d'Ulisse* by Handspring Puppet Company in association with visual artist William Kentridge has particular resonance for this discussion. Post-apartheid South Africa, like much of the 'postcolony' of Africa, exists in a 'phenomenology of violence', in which human life expectancy is low (Mbembe, 2001, p. 173). Blacks, coloureds and whites still live at stratified distances from one another, and street violence is an everyday reality. In this landscape, different bodies have different life expectancies and thus varied access to medical care or legal rights. On a daily basis postcolonial subjectivity contends with the fragmentation, hybridity and differentiation of time and space left by colonial history, but I want to suggest that contemporary theatre does not merely replicate this fragmentation and hybridity. Through a multilayered revisiting of the operating theatre, as an anatomical space, the postcolonial theatre contests not only its narrative trajectory as subaltern, but also the nihilist aesthetic visions of scientific modernity. This discussion involves therefore both a reflection on contemporary theatre and a political discourse.

In his thesis on postdramatic theatre, Hans-Thies Lehmann (2006) argues that a new paradigm of theatrical representation in the late twentieth century has pushed the multiple logics of language and actors to the limits of signification. When discussing Robert Wilson's work, he identifies the emergence of a *postanthropocentric* theatre, i.e. a theatre which is proposing another kind of post- or passing of an old way of seeing and thinking about human subjectivity. As Lehmann writes: 'Under this heading one could assemble the theatre of objects entirely without human actors, theatre of technology and machines and theatre that integrates the human form mostly as an element in landscape-like spatial structures' (Lehmann, 2006, p. 81). These aesthetic figurations, according to Lehmann, suggest a way of conceiving theatrical performance that veers away from the naturalizing effects that align bodies with characters as well as away from the lingering effects of utopian realism on human representation. Instead, the textual referents of the dramatic world have become subordinated to what he later argues is 'the exposition of intense physicality' (Lehmann, 2006, p. 96). Although I agree with much of his analysis of the restructuring of dramatic form and the popular ambivalence towards the text in contemporary theatre, I want to argue against this idea that 'the body becomes the only subject matter' in this theatrical heightening of corporeal signification (p. 96). The moving body, the excessive body, the animated body, all suggest particular readings of the bodies in a performance, although they all depend on the body imagined as a discrete entity or as a physically potent subjectivity. What I want to suggest is that political theatre in this globalized and postcolonial phase of modernity has to be one of body parts, not seen as intensely physical totalities, but rather as bits that provide evidence of the present time's non-human history.

Bare Life – What Else?

To theorize the body politics of the state, I need to return to two concepts activated in Giorgio Agamben's *Homo Sacer: Sovereign Power and Bare Life* (1998) because they locate the radically dismembered politics of the body in the twentieth century. He writes of the biopolitics which have established the new sovereignty of totalitarian power by producing the juridico-political conditions for the denial of life to individual subjects. In his view, the central political function of modern government has become the connection between governmentality and biological life which can reduce a body to its 'bare life'. Far from the sanctity of the individual integral to earlier political and religious systems, the modern political state no longer uses bodies only as human sacrifice, such as when they serve as soldiers or appear in symbolic form in civic or religious rituals. Instead, the body of *homo sacer* must be disposed of in order to maintain the system since its invisibleness as a discrete human existence becomes in part essential to the operations of the state. In this way, the death of a 'bare life' does not represent loss of life, namely the death of a human being, but is entirely justified in this ideological transformation of a state's power. In apartheid South Africa, for instance, the denial of legal rights to black citizens was justified because they were *homo sacer*, that is bodies with only 'bare life', in relation to the Afrikaans' dominion over the land and its economy.

To maintain this fictional life of the state, according to Agamben, its boundaries can be modified internally in order to regulate the quality of existence for different kinds of subjects. The declaration of a 'state of exception' therefore happens at the level of zoning of geographic space and through ruling on the limits of violence that can be done to particular bodies. These zones organized on the model of the concentration camp, not insignificantly first developed by the British in South Africa against the Afrikaans during the Boer War, function as a 'dislocating localization' in which bodies have little sense of belonging to older forms of social order and geography (Agamben, 1998, p. 20). The abstractness of a 'camp', or 'prison-island', from a knowable reality grants further power to abstract human life from bodily existence. In South Africa, of course, these zones were the townships, from which black workers had to travel to work in the cities, or where the unemployed without a pass could never leave. The realization that the black people who worked daily in the houses and suburbs of white South Africans had a life different from theirs was hidden from consciousness, as Kentridge recalls: 'for a white suburban house the journey through Africa began across the yard in the servants room' (Cameron et al., 1999, p. 109).

A 'state of exception' also establishes a continuity of political configurations that might be called non-human, in their denial of physical life to the subject. Under a 'state of exception' the Nazis could murder 'incurably mentally ill' patients for humanitarian purposes or a modern hospital can decide when a patient is 'brain dead' so that their 'organs may be harvested for science' (Agamben, 1998, pp. 140-141, pp. 163-164). The anatomy theatres of the modern state therefore include laboratories, intensive care units and police morgues in which organs are kept living outside of a body, or reassembled like moving parts, through the 'gift of organs' or their retention as morbid evidence. In the operating theatre, bodies are connected to other machines, that might be sometimes attached to a particular name, or a mode of data collection, but their ongoing existence depends on 'life support'. In a benign form, these medical models of the 'state of exception' may keep bodies alive but more perniciously, they can also determine what minimal sentience is needed for 'bare life' in the modern state (Agamben, 1998, p. 162).

What is significant to my discussion is how this relationship between bare life and the 'state of exception' renders the subject. In the postcolonial state, any citizen can potentially be reduced to bare life since the natural life of the body has already been taken by the act of colonization. The sovereignty of land, law and birth-right have already been possessed by the colonizer, but the more tenuous the state's grip on power, then the more categories of 'exclusion' are required to prevent all bodies from claiming their rights. South Africa's declaration of the First State of Emergency in 1985, for instance, followed years of internal protests against apartheid and violent suppression that led to the state's exclusion from the world political arena. The exercise of sovereign power was therefore to warp the meanings of 'bare life', making white brutality legitimate and black crime illegal. The evidence of this non-human history continues in the daily life of the post-apartheid state: due to an official rate of 18% infection with HIV/AIDS, 43% will not survive past 40 years of age; unemployment among young black South Africans is estimated at as high as 40%; and one in four South African men surveyed by Johannesburg City Council said they had committed rape before they were 18.[1] These facts of 'bare life' accumulate where a historical process, a machinery of dehumanization, turns bodies into virtual corpses. According to Agamben, this new model of political sovereignty can become relocalized in different nations, but it can only persist when this non-human history is erased from consciousness by the state.

Under the Skin: Il Ritorno d'Ulisse (1998) and The History of the Main Complaint (1996)

Theatre, as Lyotard (1997) writes, can be the 'mise-en-scène of the unconscious'. But in a more cognisant way, we also enter its imaginary world through a wilful anaesthesia that begins with blanking out certain features of the real world in order to return to historical memory. Together Kentridge and Handspring have produced several theatre works, such as *Woyczek* and *Faustus in Africa!* (1995) that were embedded in colonial history, or *Ubu and the Truth Commission* (1997), which provided a grotesque response to the official excess of narrative produced by the Final Report of the Truth and Reconciliation Commission in 1998. Contentiously, these hearings that staged the desire for an absolution from guilt wanted by both white and blacks also fed the demand for individual testimony. 'Its repercussions in post-apartheid South Africa continue to spawn a growing discourse on Truth and Reconciliation, both in the civil and political sectors of society,' writes theatre theorist Rustom Bharucha (2002), but the courtroom also made 'only too clear that the teller of factual truth is not a story-teller, or more emphatically, that the story-teller is no teller of facts'.[2] This non-referentiality of narrative form provokes a postdramatic response, and indeed, although the effects of the 'state of exception' produced by the TRC were daily dramatized in the media during the 1998 performance season of *Il Ritorno d'Ulisse*, the restaging of a Baroque opera seemed to be a departure from immediate political concerns. Its more objective question seems to be: How could theatre examine collective responsibility for the 'stranger truths of fiction' in what was left behind? (Cameron et al., 1999, p. 35). Theatrically, the quest to identify individual agency and accountability was 'bypassed' for a more anatomical approach, so that the journey of Ulisse was represented as a kind of postoperative delirium of the modern white subject. As Kentridge explains:

> I was looking at the body as a metaphor for our relationship to memory and the unconscious, acknowledging that there are things happening under the surface, which we hope will be well contained by our skin. We hope that our skin will not erupt, that parts of us will not collapse inside. (Kentridge in Cameron et al., 1999, p. 23)

On one level, the puppet opera *Il Ritorno d'Ulisse* involves a stark retelling of Homer's story of a weary Odysseus returning from the Trojan War. In counterpoint to the many suitors besieging Penelope's good trust, it narrates the steps towards his return, the defeat of the suitors and the marital reunion. The puppets and their manipulators perform in a scale replica of Vesalius's operating theatre complete with mortuary table and raked seating, replicating a mini-chamber opera. But in this reproduction of the anatomical theatre, the half-scale wooden mannequins, the black animators and the singers triangulate and rupture the mechanisms of identification as they watch and wait on the wooden benches for their moment to enter into the formal alternating cadences of the music. Above these spectral figures, Kentridge's animated film, with its grim images of the brutal urban landscapes of contemporary South Africa, scrolls along with the calm efficiency of a modern CAT scan machine. Although the drawings serve a diegetic function, pointing beyond the seventeenth-century libretto and mise en scène, they cannot provide any satisfactory response to the frustrated desire and potent sense of loss explored in the opera. The setting of the operating theatre pertinently returns to and opens up the inner workings of the body in order to investigate whether Ulisse has any surviving function as a sentient being. For Tadeusz Kantor, as Lehmann notes, the figure of Odysseus symbolically returning from the dead sets the stage for a ghostly return from a

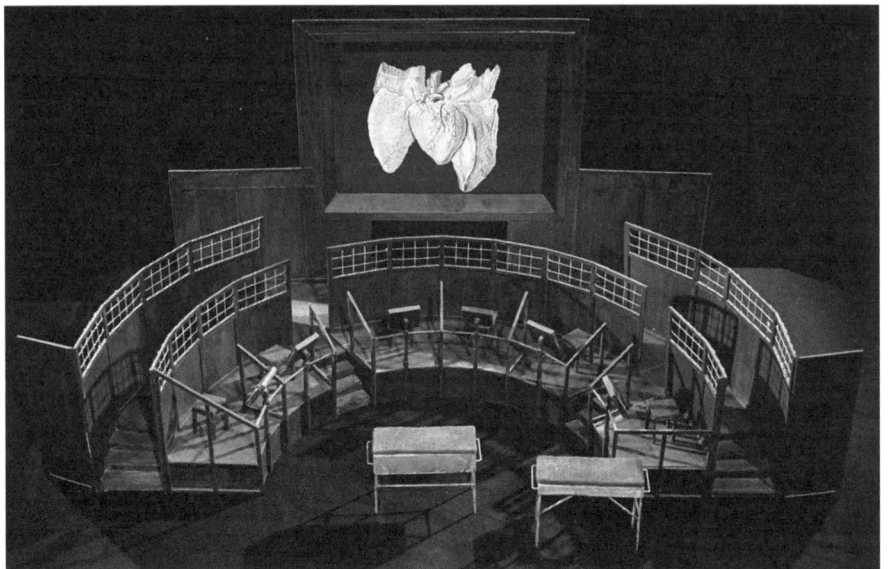

Set of *Il Ritorno d'Ulisse* by Handspring Puppet Company. Photo by Ruphin Coudyzer FPPSA (www.ruphin.com). Reproduced with his permission.

state of terror, and thus does this Ulisse revisit the horrid nightmare memories of post-apartheid South Africa (Lehmann, 2006, p. 71). It is, however, the detailed architecture of the operating theatre that stages the rhetorical architecture of the state of exception in an aesthetics of 'landscape-like' anthropocentrism, as if without human agency. What impresses the watcher is that the metonymy of wooden puppet bodies in juxtaposition with Kentridge's line drawings function only as text fragments or partial objects of the postcolonial condition.

For thirty years, Kentridge has worked between the mediums of drawing, film and theatre, selectively involved in a range of projects including installations, agit-prop theatre, public art and opera. Throughout this body of work, he has been observing the sense of exile, loss and displacement that white South Africans experience in their sense of belonging to an apartheid state. Whether in *Colonial Landscapes* (1995-1996) or *Stereoscope* (1999), his black and white drawings trace the desolate beauty of South Africa, the contradictions of its people and its violent racial politics. Other layers of the charcoal and pastel are semi-autobiographical, and figurative presences accumulate in his film animations from the arduous erasing of gestures and objects as they travel across the screen; he calls his method 'stone-age filmmaking' (Cameron et al., 1999, p. 114). One sequence of drawings shown on the screen suspended above the wooden stage derives from a short film called *The History of the Main Com-*

plaint. It is the sixth in a series of *Drawings for Projection* that 'star' Soho Eckstein and Felix Teitlebaum, although the mine owner Soho is usually attired in a black suit in contrast with the often-naked Felix. In this sequence, however, Soho is in hospital, trapped in a comatose state in which he relives two horrific incidents seen while driving his car: 'a man being beaten in the middle of the road, and a man who suddenly runs in front of his car and is killed' (Cameron et al., 1999, p. 33). Given that driving in post-apartheid South Africa can be considered travelling through combat territory, particularly for whites who fear being robbed or knifed by local gangs, the film asks them to consider how much responsibility or 'indirect guilt' they should feel for their apparent distance and safety from the events and people they see in the street. In what sense is the car as barrier different from earlier barriers between races and classes during apartheid? The film examines both the scenes on the street as well as inner bits of his body, the lungs, nervous system, heart and brain, in order to see where his complaint lies. The doctors crowding around the patient undertake an examination of white guilt but the interior organs do not, as anatomists know, discriminate between perpetrators and victims. This search for a biological basis for evil, like in Edward Bond's play *Lear* in which the monstrous Regan is disembowelled on stage, can provide no direct explanation. The cartoon doctors appear unsure about what they are looking for or seeing as their gaze maps the inner life of the body, and yet Soho finds himself staring blankly at the dead man lying on the road. This Ulisse is waiting either for recovery or death after the operation, but his consciousness stirs above the austerely carved puppet Ulisse for whom male voices sing exquisite laments.

Details from seventeenth-century anatomical drawings are juxtaposed with the scientific imaging of modern medicine including the heart in outline, brain scans in cross-section, and diagrams of the nervous system. These body parts cannot assuage the images of a modern South Africa, also linked in retrospect with an optimistic anatomical theatre where the surgeon Christian Barnard staged the world's first heart transplant operation in 1967. Post-apartheid, there is no hope of a classic return to those failed promises of modernity because the country has been left in ruins, and the film shows burnt-out buildings, a black man being bashed by thugs, and the stumps of trees in a desiccated landscape. As Kentridge writes of this Ulisse-Soho: 'His journey home is a journey through himself' and the cumulative effect of these layered traces of an interior and exterior existence in which bodies have had to undergo 'multiple bypass surgery' (Cameron et al., 1999, p. 130).

The reappearance of anatomical representation in this operating theatre needs a radically different aesthetics of vision. Kentridge deliberately utilizes the medicalized gaze in this work:

> these images – sonar, X-ray, MRI, CAT-scan (...) are by their very nature,
> internal images. Dissect as deep as you like and you will never find the
> mimetic reference of the sonar. They are already a metaphor. They are mes-
> sages from an inside we may apprehend but can never grasp. (Kentridge in
> Cameron et al., 1999, p. 140)

As a way of seeing pain, forgetfulness or damage to vital organs, 'the X-ray al-
ludes to the otherness of our bodies, but also to other less tangible parts of us'
with an uncomfortable history (Cameron et al., 1999, p. 143). In the absence of
other reports or official records, the illuminated CAT and MRI scans circulate,
as he explains, as 'notices from a distant and more dangerous region' (Cameron
et al., 1999, p. 143). From the detached vision of this operating theatre, and its
multiple bodily dissections, I would suggest that Kentridge recuperates a mu-
tability or 'bare life' of bodies. In the state of exception that prevailed in South
Africa in order to profit from the disposability of black bodies, these organs are
suspended messages that ask questions of responsibility for those who witness
this dehumanization of place and peoples. The film ends with Soho looking
through his rearview mirror as he continues to drive on through the darkened
streets of a scorched landscape. And the opera draws to its bittersweet close
with Penelope and Ulisse reunited in old age by a powerful admission of each
other's fallibility.

For the spectator shifting between these different landscapes, there is the
narrative line of the operatic music. It makes associations between the partial objects of violent longing, loss and love through a tissue of song. What
is powerful is the detachment of vision from identification with a particular
landscape and historical condition. The physical landscape, the stage architecture and the filmic presence alert us to the eyes of the man watching himself
being watched in ways that tie subjectivity not to self but to perception. The
spectators are reminded again of their own position as watchers from afar, as
people who observe the unfolding of dehumanizing operations and actions
that differentiate between one type of citizen and another. For Kentridge, the
removal of the body parts in his operating theatre and their animated tracings
make it possible to recognize what bare life becomes when black is not the
same as white.

In the ancient Greek myth of Ulisse returning home to Penelope with his
soul scourged, this production constructs an alternative mythology for the
post-apartheid state. Rather than concluding with a comforting presence in the
hearth, the female puppet suggests the firm authority of a judgment without
penitence for Ulisse at his homecoming. The delusional wanderings of the hero
through the landscape of political nightmare are, it would seem, unable to re-
deem the state of exception, although the endurance of love might assist with

some form of reconciliation. But over and above these terms, the watchful pen and ink drawings of the screenic imagination remain critically prescient about the slow and mournful movement of the puppets in the anatomy theatre. Situated as they, or we, are in the melancholia of postcolonial history, this version of an anthropocentric theatre can only offer an affective, yet ambiguous, response to the journey and compromise politics of modern South Africa.

Body-bits: Metonymy and Non-human History

I have argued that Kentridge transforms Sawday's theatre of dissection by looking at body parts as metonymic of the collective experience. With organs that do not promote individuals, nor depend upon a single racialized or national identity, the body-bits become connective tissues aligned with other textual fragments in psychic or socio-economic structures. Since this postanthropocentric theatre is non-allegorical, it ruthlessly attends to how objects are animated inside and outside of the body. What seems important is that the combination of these elements amplifies a disturbing loss of consciousness, about processes of sovereign power, that would otherwise reduce human beings to 'bare life'. Antonin Artaud's concept of a body without organs, formulated in 1947, was also a plea for freedom from the operating theatres of science, politics, and theatre: 'for tie me down if you want to but there is nothing more useless than an organ; when you make a body without organs you will have delivered man from all his automatisms and returned him to his true freedom' (Artaud, 1988). Having considered this *Il Ritorno d'Ulisse*, however, its concept of a body appears of necessity different to that of Lehmann's 'absolute body' in theatrical representation, since historical amnesia must be resisted even when anatomical bodies have become bits. Earlier, following Mbembe, I suggested that there is a phenomenology of violence in postcolonial society, but in this violence that underpins and surrounds the postdramatic loss of history, the body without organs takes on a new meaning. In South Africa, black bodies were repeatedly and violently exploded, as Kentridge explains:

> The image of a pig's head wearing a Walkman that suddenly explodes [in one of my drawings] is based on South African police photographs of experiments testing a Walkman booby trap on a pig's head which were used as evidence in the Truth and Reconciliation Commission (...). They would take people whom they had killed and blow up the corpses. They would collect the pieces and blow them up again, and again, until no recognizable fragments remained. (Kentridge in Cameron et al., 1999, p. 35)

Beyond the limits of any remainder, freedom or truth, the unintelligibility of these organs without bodies need a theatre that sutures the bits together again. Kentridge refers to Penelope's stitching and restitching of the cloth as she waits for Ulisse, and there are signs of the stitching together of fragments in the delicate drawings and the work of the puppeteers. Slavoj Žižek's theorizing of 'autonomous partial-objects' provides a way to think about how this fragmented historical experience is translated into theatrical representation. The partial-object has a spectral existence because it only figures through a process whereby 'we pass from the wound on the body to the wound as autonomous organ without a body, outside it' (Žižek, 2004, p. 168). In the heart illuminated against a night landscape, or a skull opened for inspection, an infinitely plastic object is transposed from one medium to another by a fine membrane, a thin blue line, or the string of a puppet. The *lamella* between social violence and the vulnerability of the body becomes then a 'way of trying to understand how we operate in the world' (Cameron et al., 1999, p. 35).

When the body-bits trace wilfully repressed memories and events of an historical past, then we are in a different kind of operating theatre. A finely threaded revisiting of connections between body part and burnt-out tree, past and present, differs from the totalizing of the body in postdramatic theatre as well as from a theorizing of postcolonial fragmentation and syncretism. This process of drawing together in the theatre helps to overturn the 'state of exception' which numbs people of affect, and with the singing of different objects can provide a passage for more than 'bare life'. With Ulisse returning through a landscape-like South Africa, an aesthetic paradigm that is somewhere between opera and operating theatre has surfaced.

Rachel Fensham is Professor of Dance and Theatre Studies at the University of Surrey, UK. Her co-authored book *The Dolls' Revolution* (Australian Scholarly Publishing, 2005) established a new paradigm in Australian theatre studies for recognizing women on the national stage. She has published widely on feminist theory, theatre historiography, dance and performance studies and is finalizing a collection of these essays on corporeality, genre and spectatorship (Peter Lang, 2008). With her current focus on postcolonial performance cultures, she is midway through an ARC research grant on transnational and crosscultural choreographies that involves interviewing artists in Malaysia, Australia, New York and the Netherlands.

Notes

1   The United Nations Human Development Index provides reliable data (where available) on economic and social conditions in South Africa. The 'fact' about the crime rate comes from Bharucha (2002).

2   No page number as the quote is taken from an unpublished paper, but the now published essay is given in the bibliography.

References

Agamben, G., *Homo Sacer: Sovereign Power and Bare Life*. (Translated by D. Heller-Roazen.) Stanford, 1998.

Artaud, A., 'To Have Done with the Judgment of God, a radio play (1947)'. In: *Antonin Artaud: Selected Writings*, S. Sontag (ed.), pp. 555-575. Berkeley, 1988.

Bharucha, R., 'Between Truth and Reconciliation: Experiments in Theater and Public Culture'. In: Enwezor, O. and A. Jaar (eds), *Experiments with Truth: Transitional Justice and the Processes of Truth and Reconciliation*: Documenta 11_Platform2. Ostfildern, 2002.

Cameron, D., C. Christov-Bakargiev, J. Coetzee and W. Kentridge, *William Kentridge*. London, 1999.

Lehmann, H., *Postdramatic Theatre*. London and New York, 2006.

Lyotard, J., 'The Unconscious as Mise-en-Scène'. In: T. Murray (ed.), *Mimesis, Masochism, and Mime: The Politics of Theatricality in Contemporary French Thought*. Ann Arbor, 1997.

Mbembe, A., *On the Postcolony*. Berkeley and Los Angeles, 2001.

Sawday, J., *The Body Emblazoned: Dissection and the Human Body in Renaissance Culture*. London and New York, 1995.

Žižek, S., *Organs without Bodies: On Deleuze and Consequences*. London and New York, 2004.

Index